Nail Disorders: Diagnosis and Management

Editor

SHARI R. LIPNER

DERMATOLOGIC CLINICS

www.derm.theclinics.com

Consulting Editor
BRUCE H. THIERS

April 2021 • Volume 39 • Number 2

ELSEVIER

1600 John F. Kennedy Boulevard ● Suite 1800 ● Philadelphia, Pennsylvania, 19103-2899

http://www.theclinics.com

DERMATOLOGIC CLINICS Volume 39, Number 2
April 2021 ISSN 0733-8635, ISBN-13: 978-0-323-70923-1

Editor: Lauren Boyle
Developmental Editor: Karen Justine Solomon

Dermatologic Clinics (ISSN 0733-8635) is published quarterly by Elsevier Inc., 360 Park Avenue South, New York, NY 10010-1710. Months of publication are January, April, July, and October. Business and editorial offices: 1600 John F. Kennedy Blvd., Suite 1800, Philadelphia, PA 19103-2899. Customer service office: 11830 Westline Drive, St. Louis, MO 63146. Periodicals postage paid at New York, NY, and additional mailing offices. Subscription prices are USD 416.00 per year for US individuals, USD 1,000.00 per year for US institutions, USD 456.00 per year for Canadian individuals, USD 1,055.00 per year for Canadian institutions, USD 510.00 per year for international individuals, USD 1,055.00 per year for international institutions, USD 100.00 per year for US students/residents, USD 100.00 per year for Canadian students/residents, and USD 240 per year for international students/residents. International air speed delivery is included in all *Clinics* subscription prices. All prices are subject to change without notice. **POSTMASTER:** Send address changes to *Dermatologic Clinics*, Elsevier Health Sciences Division, Subscription Customer Service, 3251 Riverport Lane, Maryland Heights, MO 63043. **Customer Service: 1-800-654-2452 (U.S. and Canada); 314-447-8871 (outside U.S. and Canada). Fax: 314-447-8029. E-mail: journalscustomerservice-usa@elsevier.com (for print support); journalsonlinesupport-t-usa@elsevier.com (for online support).**

Reprints. For copies of 100 or more, of articles in this publication, please contact the Commercial Reprints Department, Elsevier Inc., 360 Park Avenue South, New York, New York 10010-1710. Tel.: 212-633-3874; Fax: 212-633-3820; Email: reprints@elsevier.com.

The *Dermatologic Clinics* is covered in *MEDLINE/PubMed (Index Medicus)*, *Current Contents/Clinical Medicine*, *Excerpta Medica*, *Chemical Abstracts*, and *ISI/BIOMED*.

Contributors

CONSULTING EDITOR

BRUCE H. THIERS, MD
Professor and Chairman Emeritus, Department
of Dermatology and Dermatologic Surgery,
Medical University of South Carolina,
Charleston, South Carolina, USA

EDITOR

SHARI R. LIPNER, MD, PhD
Associate Professor of Clinical Dermatology,
Director, Nail Division, Department of
Dermatology, Weill Cornell Medicine, New
York, New York, USA

AUTHORS

AURORA ALESSANDRINI, MD
Dermatology, Department of Specialised
Experimental and Diagnostic Medicine,
Dermatology Alma Mater Studiorum -
Università di Bologna, Bologna, Italy

JULIA O. BALTZ, MD
Dermatology Professionals, Inc, East
Greenwich, Rhode Island, USA; Assistant
Clinical Professor, Department of
Dermatology, University of Massachusetts
Medical School, Worcester, Massachusetts,
USA

ROBERT BARAN, MD, PhD
Honorary Professor of Dermatology, Nail
Disease Centre, Cannes, France

JANE SANDERS BELLET, MD
Professor of Pediatrics and Dermatology, Duke
University School of Medicine, Durham, North
Carolina, USA

MARCO ADRIANO CHESSA, MD
Department of Specialised Experimental and
Diagnostic Medicine, Dermatology Alma Mater
Studiorum - Università di Bologna, Bologna,
Italy

FLORENCE DEHAVAY, MD
Saint-Pierre, Brugmann and Queen Fabiola
Children University Hospitals, Université Libre
de Bruxelles, Belgium

EMI DIKA, MD, PhD
Department of Specialised Experimental and
Diagnostic Medicine, Dermatology Alma Mater
Studiorum - Università di Bologna, Bologna,
Italy

ZOE DIANA DRAELOS, MD
Dermatology Consulting Services, PLLC, High
Point, North Carolina, USA

ATHINA FONIA, MBBS, BSc, MRCP
Department of Dermatology, Consultant
Dermatologist, Queen Elizabeth Hospital,
London, United Kingdom

STAMATIOS GREGORIOU, MD, PhD
University Hospital of Venereal and Skin
Diseases "A.Sygros"

MOHIT KUMAR GUPTA, BBA
State University of New York Downstate
College of Medicine, Brooklyn, New York,
USA

ANNA QUINN HARE, MD, MS
Dermatologist, Oregon Dermatology and
Research Center, Portland, Oregon, USA

MATILDE IORIZZO, MD, PhD
Private Dermatology Practice, Bellinzona,
Switzerland

NATHANIEL J. JELLINEK, MD
Dermatology Professionals, Inc, East
Greenwich, Rhode Island, USA; Department of
Dermatology, University of Massachusetts
Medical School, Worcester, Massachusetts,
USA; Department of Dermatology, The Warren
Alpert Medical School at Brown University,
Providence, Rhode Island, USA

SHARI R. LIPNER, MD, PhD
Associate Professor of Clinical Dermatology,
Director, Nail Division, Department of
Dermatology, Weill Cornell Medicine, New
York, New York, USA

CHRISTOPHER J. MILLER, MD
Director, Penn Dermatology Oncology Center,
Associate Professor of Dermatology,
University of Pennsylvania Health System,
Philadelphia, Pennsylvania, USA

MARCEL C. PASCH, MD, PhD
Department of Dermatology, Radboud
University Medical Center, Nijmegen, the
Netherlands

BIANCA MARIA PIRACCINI, MD, PhD
Dermatology, Department of Specialised
Experimental and Diagnostic Medicine,
Dermatology Alma Mater Studiorum -
Università di Bologna, Bologna, Italy

STACY L. McMURRAY, MD
Assistant Professor of Dermatology, University
of Pennsylvania Health System, Philadelphia,
Pennsylvania, USA

JOSE W. RICARDO, MD
Department of Dermatology, Weill Cornell
Medicine, New York, New York, USA

PHOEBE RICH, MD
Adjunct Professor, Dermatology OHSU,
Oregon Dermatology and Research Center,
Portland, Oregon, USA

BERTRAND RICHERT, MD, PhD
Saint-Pierre, Brugmann and Queen Fabiola
Children University Hospitals, Université Libre
de Bruxelles, Belgium

DIMITRIOS RIGOPOULOS, MD, PhD
Professor, University Hospital of Venereal and
Skin Diseases "A.Sygros"

NATALIA ROMPOTI, MD, PhD
University Hospital of Venereal and Skin
Diseases "A.Sygros"

BETH S. RUBEN, MD
Director of Dermatopathology, Palo
Alto Medical Foundation, Medical Group,
Palo Alto, California; Professor, Dermatology
(Dermatopathology), University of California,
San Francisco, San Francisco, California,
USA

MICHELA STARACE, MD, PhD
Dermatology, Department of Specialised
Experimental and Diagnostic Medicine,
Dermatology Alma Mater Studiorum -
Università di Bologna, Bologna, Italy

XIMENA WORTSMAN, MD
Adjunct Professor, Institute for Diagnostic
Imaging and Research of the Skin and Soft
Tissues, Department of Dermatology,
Universidad de Chile and Pontificia
Universidad Católica de Chile, Santiago,
Chile

SOOK JUNG YUN, MD, PhD
Professor, Department of Dermatology,
Chonnam National University Medical School,
Gwangju, Korea (South)

JUNQIAN ZHANG, MD
Department of Dermatology, University of
Pennsylvania Health System, Philadelphia,
Pennsylvania, USA

Contents

Preface: Nail Disorders: Diagnosis and Management   xi

Shari R. Lipner

Nail is Systemic Disorders: Main Signs and Clues   153

Florence Dehavay and Bertrand Richert

> Describing and listing all nail symptoms and signs in systemic disorders has already been widely detailed in dedicated textbooks. To be tutorial, this article described most common nails signs and the systemic disorders one may encounter in routine dermatologic consultation. Capsule summaries are presented for each section.

Cutaneous Paraneoplastic Syndromes with Nail Involvement   175

Athina Fonia and Robert Baran

> The cutaneous paraneoplastic syndromes are rare and intrinsically devoid of any neoplastic nature. The manifestations on the skin and the nails are due to various mechanisms caused by the tumor, either due to production of bioactive substances or in response to it. These disorders evolve in parallel to the malignancy, in that, they regress when the tumor is removed and reappear in the case of tumor recurrence. The aim of this article is to aid with the early recognition of the signs, leading to the early detection of cancer and therefore to better clinical outcomes for the patients.

Nail Psoriasis in Older Adults: Epidemiology, Diagnosis, and Topical Therapy   183

Jose W. Ricardo and Shari R. Lipner

> Nail involvement is common in patients with cutaneous psoriasis, which is prevalent among older adults. Nail psoriasis greatly impacts patients' quality of life and self-esteem. Concomitant psoriatic arthritis is common. Treating nail psoriasis in the geriatric population may be challenging. General nail care measures may prevent exacerbations. Topical therapy is relatively effective, with a low rate of adverse events and little to no risk of systemic toxicity or drug interactions. However, application under occlusion may be cumbersome. There is a need for randomized controlled clinical trials in the elderly population to make more evidence-based treatment guidelines.

Nail Psoriasis in Older Adults: Intralesional, Systemic, and Biological Therapy 195

Jose W. Ricardo and Shari R. Lipner

> Psoriasis may affect the skin, scalp, joints, and nails and is common in older adults. Intramatrical injections with triamcinolone acetonide are safe and effective in older individuals. Conventional systemic medications are relatively effective, but side effects, including laboratory abnormalities and drug interactions, are particularly common among older adults. Biologic medications have shown excellent efficacy in treating nail psoriasis. Their safety profile is favorable, but data assessing long-term safety are lacking. Randomized controlled trials in older adults exclusively are necessary to develop evidence-based treatment guidelines in this population.

Management of Nail Psoriasis   211

Dimitrios Rigopoulos, Natalia Rompoti, and Stamatios Gregoriou

Nail psoriasis is a chronic nail disorder that requires personalized treatment. General prophylactic measures are suggested for all patients. Topical treatment is considered when treating a few-nail disease, with involvement of 3 or fewer nails, without joint involvement and without (or with mild) skin psoriasis. The ideal formulation should be ointment, solution, or foam. When moderate to severe skin psoriasis or psoriatic arthritis coexists, systemic treatment is suggested. This also should be considered when more than 3 nails are affected or significant impairment of quality of life is present. Conventional systemic agents, biologics, and small molecules are highly efficacious.

Review of Nail Lichen Planus: Epidemiology, Pathogenesis, Diagnosis, and Treatment   221

Mohit Kumar Gupta and Shari R. Lipner

Nail lichen planus is an inflammatory disorder of the nails with potential for significant cosmetic disfigurement and functional impairment. Nail manifestations may be isolated or appear concurrently with other forms of lichen planus. Longitudinal ridging is the most common clinical finding, but progressive disease may result in irreversible scarring (dorsal pterygium) or permanent nail loss (anonychia). Data on treatment are limited to retrospective studies and case reports. The mainstays of treatment are intralesional and intramuscular corticosteroid injections and oral retinoids. There is a need for randomized controlled trials on nail lichen planus to more rigorously assess efficacy and outcomes.

Pediatric Nail Disorders   231

Jane Sanders Bellet

Many pediatric nail findings are normal variants and are no cause for alarm. Others represent congenital abnormalities or genetic syndromes for which there is no cure. Still others are inflammatory or infectious entities that require treatment. Pediatric nail disorders are reviewed, along with management.

Bacterial and Viral Infections of the Nail Unit   245

Matilde Iorizzo and Marcel C. Pasch

Bacterial and viral infections of the nail unit are very common as primary infections, especially bacterial paronychia and warts, but they can also be superinfections complicating other nail disorders. In many nail unit infections, the clinical presentation is nonspecific: in these cases, diagnostic tests are mandatory before treatment, to avoid spread of the infection and drug resistance. The most common forms of bacterial and viral infections that may affect the nail unit are herein described in detail, with diagnostic and treatment options provided.

Diagnosis of Melanonychia   255

Aurora Alessandrini, Emi Dika, Michela Starace, Marco Adriano Chessa, and Bianca Maria Piraccini

Melanonychia has many causes and can involve one or several fingernails or toenails, and may occur at any age. Dermoscopy is used routinely in the evaluation of a pigmented nail. If pigmentation is caused by melanin produced by nail matrix, identify whether the pigmentation is caused by an activation or proliferation of nail melanocytes. When melanocytic proliferation is suspected, biopsy with histopathologic examination is the gold standard for diagnosis and is recommended when a longitudinal melanonychia occurs in an adult and is localized in a single digit, in the absence of local or systemic causes that may explain its onset.

Management of Nail Unit Melanoma   269

Junqian Zhang, Sook Jung Yun, Stacy L. McMurray, and Christopher J. Miller

Nail unit melanoma is an uncommon form of melanoma with worse prognosis compared with nonacral cutaneous melanoma. Nail unit melanoma is often diagnosed at a late stage. Clinical and dermoscopic features may suggest a diagnosis of nail unit melanoma, but confirmation requires histologic analysis. Like the clinical diagnosis, histopathologic diagnosis of nail unit melanoma is also difficult. The surgical management of nail unit melanoma has evolved from aggressive amputations to digit-sparing approaches. This article reviews the clinical presentation, diagnosis, and surgical treatment of nail unit melanoma to promote early diagnosis and rational surgery.

Nail Tumors   281

Anna Quinn Hare and Phoebe Rich

This article describes nail tumors and their clinical features, biologic behavior, and treatment. Tumors included are onychopapilloma, onychomatricoma, periungual fibromas/fibrokeratomas, glomus tumors, subungual exostosis, myxoid cysts, and squamous cell carcinoma.

Dermoscopy of the Nail Unit   293

Michela Starace, Aurora Alessandrini, and Bianca Maria Piraccini

Nail dermoscopy (onychoscopy) is being used for a more accurate diagnosis of all nail disorders and has become a routine diagnostic instrument. In daily practice, nail signs can be magnified, and dermoscopy may confirm the clinical diagnosis and guides in management of nail diseases and treatments, permitting a better visualization of symptoms. Onychoscopy is used by the experts in almost all nail diseases. It can be performed dry or with ultrasound gel in order to make the stratum corneum translucent, depending on which part of the nail unit has to be evaluated.

Nail Surgery: Six Essential Techniques   305

Julia O. Baltz and Nathaniel J. Jellinek

Successful nail surgery requires an understanding of specific disease processes, the anatomy of the nail unit, and fluency with only a few key techniques. This article focuses on 6 high-yield procedures, facility with which will allow the clinician to approach most of the clinical scenarios requiring surgical intervention. These encompass surgical approaches to inflammatory nail diseases, melanonychia, erythronychia, and nail melanoma in situ.

Pathology of the Nail Unit   319

Beth S. Ruben

This article discusses the histologic findings in key nail unit diseases, including inflammatory, infectious, and neoplastic conditions. The emphasis is on clinicopathologic correlates, best practices to demonstrate the relevant histopathologic features, and pitfalls in diagnosis. Understanding the pathology of these disorders enhances clinical acumen and may affect the choice of biopsy procedures and treatment measures, with the outcome of better clinical care for patients with nail disease.

Concepts, Role, and Advances on Nail Imaging   337

Ximena Wortsman

This review discusses, from a practical point of view, relevant concepts, the role and advances of the most common imaging techniques that allow studying nail pathologies. There are several imaging techniques for studying the nail, and all of them require proper devices and trained operators. The better axial resolution and a more extensive range of applications are provided by ultrasound, which currently is the first-choice imaging technique for evaluating nail conditions. A discussion on basic concepts, the role of imaging, and the advances on this topic is provided. The correlation of state-of-the-art clinical and imaging figures supports this review well.

Nail Cosmetics and Adornment   351

Zoe Diana Draelos

Nail polish is a nitrocellulose-based film that is modified to create a plastic shiny colored film that can be painted on the nail plate. The desire to develop a long-lasting pigmented film has resulted in the development of nail shellacs based on polymethyl methacrylate (PMMA) designed to polymerize on the nail plate. These films are chip resistant and long wearing, designed to last 3 to 4 weeks. Further polymer use has resulted in the ability to sculpt an elongated nail on the nail plate to create the appearance of long nails.

DERMATOLOGIC CLINICS

FORTHCOMING ISSUES

July 2021
Hair
Neil Sadick, *Editor*

October 2021
COVID-19 and the Dermatologist
Esther Freeman and Devon McMahon *Editors*

January 2022
Pediatric Dermatology Part I
Kelly M. Cordoro, *Editor*

RECENT ISSUES

January 2021
Global Dermatology and Telemedicine
Victoria L. Williams and Carrie L. Kovarik, *Editors*

October 2020
Oral Medicine in Dermatology
Eric T. Stoopler and Thomas P. Sollecito *Editors*

July 2020
Allergic Contact Dermatitis
Christen M. Mowad, *Editor*

SERIES OF RELATED INTEREST

Medical Clinics
https://www.medical.theclinics.com/
Primary Care: Clinics in Office Practice
https://www.primarycare.theclinics.com/

THE CLINICS ARE AVAILABLE ONLINE!
Access your subscription at:
www.theclinics.com

DERMATOLOGIC CLINICS

FORTHCOMING ISSUES

July 2021
Hair
Neil Sadick, Editor

October 2021
COVID-19 and the Dermatologist
Esther Freeman and Devon McMahon, Editors

January 2022
Pediatric Dermatology Part I
Kelly M. Cordoro, Editor

RECENT ISSUES

January 2021
Global Dermatology and Telemedicine
Victoria L. Williams and Carrie L. Kovarik, Editors

October 2020
Oral Medicine in Dermatology
Eric T. Stoopler and Thomas P. Sollecito, Editors

July 2020
Allergic Contact Dermatitis
Christen M. Mowad, Editor

SERIES OF RELATED INTEREST

Medical Clinics
https://www.medical.theclinics.com
Primary Care: Clinics in Office Practice
https://www.primarycare.theclinics.com/

Preface
Nail Disorders: Diagnosis and Management

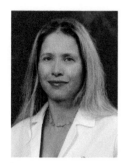

Shari R. Lipner, MD, PhD
Editor

Nail conditions are commonly seen in dermatologic practice with significant impact on quality of life. The purpose of this issue of *Dermatologic Clinics*, authored by international nail experts in the field, is to provide an update on diagnosis and treatment of nail disease. Medical and surgical residency training in nail disease may be quite variable depending on incorporation of nail lectures into didactics, hands-on surgical training sessions, and the presence of a dermatologist that specializes in nail disease on the faculty. Furthermore, dermatology attendings may have little prior training in nail conditions, and there may be a deficiency of lectures on this topic at many conferences and continuing medical education activities.

In this issue, we aim to address these knowledge gaps in nail disease. Nine nail signs of systemic disease are discussed in detail with accompanying images. Key nail findings seen in children are reviewed, including those that are not worrisome as well as those that require prompt diagnosis and treatment. The article on nail infections includes pearls for management of bacterial and viral causes. There are several articles focusing on nail psoriasis, highlighting consensus guidelines on therapies. Two articles focus exclusively on the intricacies of management of nail psoriasis in older adults. While nail lichen planus is relatively uncommon compared with other nail diseases, it is a true nail emergency, requiring prompt diagnosis and treatment. One of the articles reviews this condition along with recent consensus guidelines. Another important topic is cutaneous paraneoplastic syndromes with nail involvement, with key findings shown and accompanying images. A challenging topic for dermatologists at all levels is longitudinal melanonychia, which is included in this series as well as an entire article focused on nail dermoscopy. Common and uncommon nail tumors are reviewed as well as an article devoted to management of nail unit melanoma, including recent data on digit-sparing surgery versus amputation for thin melanomas. Six high-yield procedures are demonstrated in the nail surgery section, and an article on nail unit pathology discusses how understanding nail pathology can enhance clinical acumen and aid in biopsy technique. Nail cosmetics are described in detail, and another article demonstrates how imaging can noninvasively aid in diagnosis of many nail diseases.

We hope that this supplement enhances comfort and knowledge on diagnosis and treatment of nail diseases, ultimately improving patient care and outcomes.

Shari R. Lipner, MD, PhD
Department of Dermatology
Weill Cornell Medicine
1305 York Avenue, 9th floor
New York, NY 10021, USA

E-mail address:
shl9032@med.cornell.edu

Dermatol Clin 39 (2021) xi
https://doi.org/10.1016/j.det.2021.01.002
0733-8635/21/© 2021 Published by Elsevier Inc.

derm.theclinics.com

Nail is Systemic Disorders: Main Signs and Clues

Florence Dehavay, MD[1], Bertrand Richert, MD, PhD*

KEYWORDS

- Nails • Systemic diseases • Clubbing • Yellow nail syndrome • Scleroderma • Lupus
- Connective tissue diseases • Acrokeratosis paraneoplastica

KEY POINTS

- Nail alterations are common in systemic diseases, but most of them are not specific.
- Typical nail signs for systemic disease are rare, but should not be missed.
- Some nail signs should suggest a systemic disease, especially if present on several digits: Beau's lines, onychomadesis, splinter hemorrhages, clubbing, apparent leukonychia, abnormal nail fold capillaries, melanonychia, red lunula and pterygium inversum unguis.

INTRODUCTION

Theoretically, all systemic conditions could result in nail alterations but most of them are reactional and nonspecific but some may be a clue to the diagnosis.

We discuss 9 nail signs that are frequently observed in systemic diseases along with their description and associated diseases. We will then focus on 5 systemic pathologies that could be associated with specific nail changes, hallmarking the condition.

MAIN NAIL SIGNS IN SYSTEMIC DISORDERS
Beau's Lines and Onychomadesis

Beau's lines are transverse superficial grooves of the nail plate. The depression extends across width of the nail and is more visible in the middle part. It is more prominent on the thumb and great toe.[1,2] Beau's lines reflect a transitory damage to the proximal matrix with a decrease in the keratinocyte mitotic activity. The depth of the depression is related to the severity of the matrix injury and the length reflects the duration of the disease. This transverse depression appears 4 to 11 weeks after illness, allowing to date the event.[3] This delay corresponds with the growth of the nail under the proximal nail fold. If it is located on several nails at the same level, a systemic cause is responsible[3] and a thorough history often reveals the culprit (**Box 1**).[1,3]

Onychomadesis corresponds with a complete temporary arrest of the nail production.[2] When the growth restarts, the proximal nail plate will push away the distal part ending with onychoptosis (nail plate shedding) .

Splinter Hemorrhages

Splinter hemorrhages are a frequent but not specific clinical finding.[4,5] Splinter hemorrhages are fine, nonblanchable, red–brown to black longitudinal streaks of 1 to 3 mm visible through the plate, most frequently on its distal third, but they may be seen at any level.[4,6] They are usually asymptomatic and migrate distally with the nail growth.[4,6] Splinter hemorrhages results from bleeding of the nail bed capillaries into the longitudinal ridges of the nail bed.[2] Dermoscopy shows deep red to black lines with typical distal fading of the pigmentation, owing to progressive hemosiderin degradation.[2] Splinter hemorrhages can be idiopathic, traumatic, or associated with a nail tumor or with inflammatory dermatosis.[4,6,7]

Saint-Pierre, Brugmann and Queen Fabiola Children University Hospitals, Université Libre de Bruxelles, Belgium
[1] Present address: boulevard de Waterloo, 129, Bruxelles 1000, Belgium.
* Corresponding author. Place Van Gehuchten, 4, Bruxelles 1020, Belgium.
E-mail address: Bertrand.richert@chu-brugmann.be

Dermatol Clin 39 (2021) 153–173
https://doi.org/10.1016/j.det.2020.12.013
0733-8635/21/© 2020 Elsevier Inc. All rights reserved.

derm.theclinics.com

Box 1
Main systemic causes of Beau's lines
Higher fever
Viral diseases in children
• Hand–foot–mouth disease
Cardiovascular disease
Hepatic, pulmonary, endocrine severe disease
Malnutrition and deficiency
Change in pressure or hypoxia
Drugs (antimitotic drugs, chemotherapeutic agents, ...)
Data from Rubin A, Holzberg M, Baran R. Physical signs. In: Baran R, de Berker DAR, Holzberg M, et al., editors. Baran and Dawber's Diseases of the Nails and their Management, 5th edition. Oxford: Wiley Blackwell; 2019; and Zaiac MN, Walker A. Nail abnormalities associated with systemic pathologies. Clin Dermatol 2013;31(5):627-49.

Box 2
Systemic causes of splinter hemorrhages
Elderly
Cardiovascular diseases
• *Bacterial endocarditis*
• Congenital heart disease
• Arterial/cholesterol emboli
• Mitral stenosis
• Atrial fibrillation
• Raynaud phenomenon
• Aortic dissection
Hematologic diseases
• Anemia
• Thrombocytopenia, thrombotic thrombocytopenic purpura
• Osler–Weber–Rendu syndrome
• Cryoglobulinemia
• Leukemia
• Hypereosinophilic syndrome
Connective tissue diseases and vasculitis
• *Antiphospholipid syndrome*
• Systemic lupus erythematosus
• Dermatomyositis
• Systemic scleroderma
• Rheumatoid arthritis
• Systemic juvenile idiopathic arthritis
• Medium vessels vasculitis
• Thromboangiitis obliterans
• Granulomatosis with polyangiitis
• Behçet disease
Endocrine diseases
• *Diabetes mellitus*
• Hypoparathyroidism
• Thyroid diseases
Gastrointestinal diseases
• Cirrhosis
• Hepatitis
• Hemochromatosis
• Inflammatory bowel disease
Drugs
• *Tyrosine kinase inhibitors* (sunitinib, sorafenib)
• Anti-vascular endothelial growth factor receptor drugs

In systemic diseases, Splinter hemorrhages involve simultaneously several nails, occur mostly on the proximal third and can be painful.[7] Many systemic diseases have been associated with splinter hemorrhages (**Box 2**)[1,4,7] but they rarely are the only manifestation.[4] If splinter hemorrhages are present in more than 1 fingernail, an in-depth medical history and clinical examination are required and will guide the additional diagnostic testing.[4] Treatment is causative

Lichenoid Alterations

Lichenoid alterations are defined as nail changes resembling or mimicking those of matrix nail lichen planus. These alterations can be seen in different systemic disorders . Nail involvement is rare in systemic amyloidosis, but it can be the initial manifestation and sometimes the only cutaneous sign.[8–10] Nail abnormalities can mimic lichen planus with all the nails showing thinned, brittle, longitudinal ridges, distal fissures, and sometimes trachyonychia.[8–11] Splinter hemorrhages are common. Nail involvement can lead to anonychia. Some reports mention chronic paronychia, onycholysis, and severe subungual hyperkeratosis.[12] A histologic examination shows typical amyloid deposits in the dermis and around the vessels in the nail matrix and/or nail bed. The onychodystrophy usually slowly worsens with the disease duration.[10,11] Nail dystrophy resolution has been reported after a successful treatment of multiple myeloma.[13]

In sarcoidosis, nail involvement is also rare, but it indicates a long-lasting systemic disease.[14,15] It is

Others

- *Chronic renal failure* (hemodialysis or peritoneal dialysis)
- Meningococcemia
- Chronic or acute exposure to high altitude
- Systemic amyloidosis
- Scurvy
- Sarcoidosis
- Sweet's syndrome
- Irradiation

Data from Refs.[1,4,7]

mostly associated with bone alteration of the underlying phalanges. Radiology shows osteolysis with a honeycomb trabecular pattern and radiolucent bone cysts and could help in the diagnosis of nail sarcoidosis. However, nail sarcoidosis without bone involvement and in the absence of any systemic manifestation has been described.[16] Nail manifestations are diverse and related to the presence of noncaseating granulomas in the dermis.[17] A case of isolated hyponychium sarcoidosis[18] and a case with longitudinal erythronychia[19] have been reported. Skin sarcoidosis as lupus pernio and dactylitis can be associated with nail abnormalities, which are a sign of severe disease.[14] Finger clubbing and osteoarthropathy are rarely associated to pulmonary sarcoidosis.[20] Nail disease can be treated with high-potency topical steroids, intralesional steroid injection, or systemic treatment (oral corticosteroids and/or hydroxychloroquine), but with poor effect on the bony alteration.[14–16]

In cutaneous graft-versus-host disease (GVHD), nails are involved in one-third to one-half of the patients.[21–23] In children, nail involvement is related to severe cutaneous GVHD and pterygium is associated with severe lung disease.[22] In adults, nail dystrophy seems to be more related to the duration of the disease[21] (**Fig. 1**). Nail changes are often associated with scleroderma-like or lichenoid cutaneous lesions, but it may be the first manifestation of chronic cutaneous GVHD.[24] Treatment is the same as that for chronic cutaneous GVHD and should involve hematologists. Systemic corticosteroids are of some help.

D congenita is an exceptional heterogenous inherited syndrome related to a defective telomere maintenance, associated with bone marrow failure, premature aging, and cancer predisposition.[25,26] This genetic disorder is characterized by the triad associating nail dystrophy, oral leukoplakia, and reticular pigmentation of the neck or the body.[25,26] Nail alterations are present in 90% of patients, usually before the age of 10 years and affects the fingernails first. Allogenic hematopoietic stem cell transplantation is the only curative treatment for bone marrow failure.[25,26]

Clubbing

Digital clubbing, also known as Hippocratic fingers, is defined by morphologic changes[1]:

- Soft tissue hypertrophy with bulbous enlargement of the distal digit.
- Increased transverse and longitudinal curvature of the nail.

Clubbing can be obvious on clinical examination, but subtle presentations can be missed.[27] Different signs may help to differentiate clubbing from pseudoclubbing[27,28]:

- Lovibond's angle measures the angle between the proximal nail fold and the nail plate on a lateral view. Physiologically the angle is lower than 165° but exceeds 180° in clubbing (**Fig. 2**).[29]
- A positive Schamroth's sign shows an obliteration of the normal rhomboidal space created by placing the dorsal aspects of opposite symmetric terminal phalanxes together in clubbed fingers (**Fig. 3**).[30]
- The ratio of Rice and Rowland is the ratio between the thickness of the middle finger on a lateral view, at the level of the proximal nail fold and the distal interphalangeal joint. If it exceeds 1, clubbing is confirmed (see **Fig. 2**).[31]

Clubbing can be congenital (associated or not with various genetic syndromes) or acquired and unilateral or bilateral.[27,28] It can be isolated or occur as part of the hypertrophic osteoarthropathy syndrome, characterized by periostosis of long bones, arthralgia, and clubbing.[27,28] This syndrome can be primary (also known as pachydermoperiostosis, an autosomal-dominant disorder) or secondary. Clubbing is more frequent in the hands, but can also be seen in the feet. The evolution is slow without pain, but stiffness and discomfort can occur. Interestingly, many patients do not notice the clubbing.[27] Secondary hypertrophic osteoarthropathy syndrome and clubbing can be associated with many different diseases, particularly neoplastic, pulmonary, digestive, or cardiac pathologies (**Boxes 3** and **4**).[1,27,28] Secondary hypertrophic osteoarthropathy syndrome is more often paraneoplastic, with 90% of adults who have or will develop neoplasia (especially

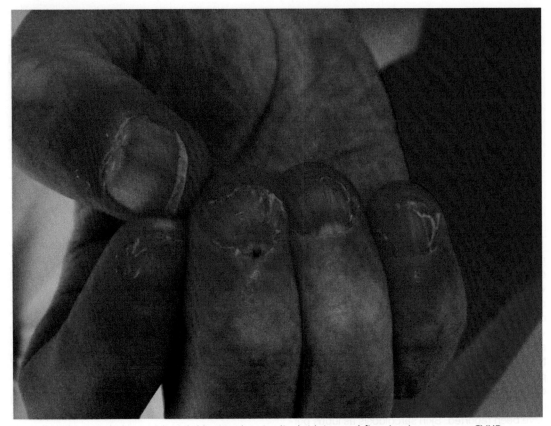

Fig. 1. Lichenoid alterations with nail thinning, longitudinal ridging and fissuring in cutaneous GVHD.

pulmonary malignancy with non-small cell lung carcinoma).[32] Pathogenesis remains unclear although several hypotheses have been proposed.[27,28] Currently, the most accepted hypothesis is an abnormal expression of fibroblast growth factors.[33] This overexpression is induced by different pathogenetic mechanisms, according to the underlying disease, leading to a common final pathway: the production of vascular endothelial growth factor and platelet-derived growth factor.[27,28,33] Vascular endothelial growth factor and platelet-derived growth factor promote synergistically edema, vascular hyperplasia, fibroblast proliferation, collagen synthesis, and new bone formation, all symptoms observed in clubbing or hypertrophic osteoarthropathy syndrome.[33]

Acquired clubbing requires a complete work-up looking for the cause.[27,28]

- In acquired unilateral clubbing
  ○ Complete history and clinical examination
  ○ Angiography
- In acquired bilateral clubbing
  ○ Complete history and clinical examination
  ○ If no relevant symptoms or signs: chest radiography

  ○ Work-up and specialist referral according to symptoms/signs[27,28]
- In acquired bilateral hypertrophic osteoarthropathy syndrome or clubbing with joint pain: more aggressive screening for malignancy need to be done considering the higher association with malignancy

Finally, clubbing can be idiopathic, but this is an exclusion diagnosis.[27,28,34] Patient reassurance is mandatory after a complete negative work-up, but ensure that the patient has the regular cancer screenings.[27,28,34]

The treatment of secondary clubbing or hypertrophic osteoarthropathy syndrome is the treatment of the underlying cause.[27,28,35] In case of painful hypertrophic osteoarthropathy syndrome, selective cyclo-oxygenase-2 inhibitors, bisphosphonates, or octreotide can alleviate symptoms.[35]

Leukonychia

The term leukonychia (LK) describes white nails. It can be divided into 3 subtypes[1]:

1. True LK, with nail plate alteration, originating from altered keratinization in the distal matrix;

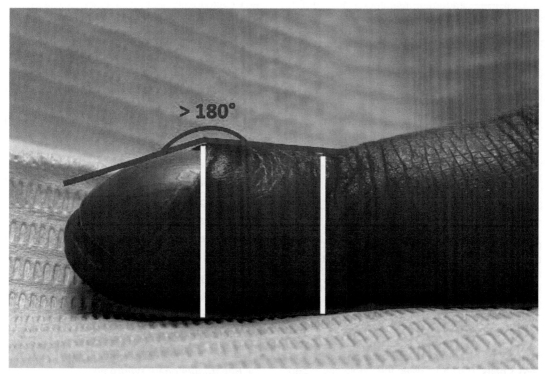

Fig. 2. Lovibond's angle (*red*) and the ratio of Rice and Rowland (*white*) in clubbing.

2. Apparent LK, with involvement of the subungual tissue, through a normal nail plate; and
3. Pseudo-LK, with nail plate alteration, not related to the matrix but external factors.

True LK can be totalis, partialis, striata, or punctate. In this rare condition, the nail seems to be opaque milky to bulky white. The LK does not fade with pressure and moves distally with the nail growth.[1,3]

LK can be traumatic, inherited (related or not to genetic syndrome), or associated to a systemic condition. The historical Mee's lines are due to arsenic intoxication and present as 2 transverse bands of 1 to 2 mm wide, parallel to the lunula, located on the same level of several nails.[1] Other intoxications like thallium, selenium and fluorine as well as other conditions like trauma and drugs (chemotherapy) may also induce transverse white lines. They should not however be called Mee's line, which refers only to arsenic intoxication.[36] Many drugs and chemical are accumulated and stored in nails, reflecting an exposure period of several months. Toenails are used as exposure biomarkers in environmental and forensic medicine.[37]

Apparent LK is the main type observed in systemic diseases. It presents as a white

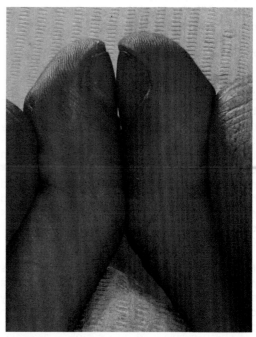

Fig. 3. A positive Schamroth's sign in clubbing, showing an obliteration of the normal rhomboidal space.

<table>
<tr><td>

Box 3
Diseases associated with unilateral clubbing

Neurologic
- Hemiplegia

Vascular
- Aneurysm
- Dialysis fistula
- Infected arterial graft
- Takayasu's arteritis

Data from Refs.[1,27,28]

</td><td>

Box 4
Systemic diseases associated with bilateral clubbing

Malignancy
- *Non-small cell lung carcinoma*
- *Bronchogenic carcinoma*
- Mesothelioma
- Lymphoma
- Nasopharyngeal carcinoma
- Pulmonary metastases
- Esophageal carcinoma
- Gastric adenocarcinoma
- Renal cell carcinoma
- Thyroid cancer

Pulmonary diseases
- *Bronchiectasis*
- *Chronic obstructive pulmonary disease*
- *Idiopathic fibrosis*
- *Pulmonary arteriovenous malformations*
- *Hepatopulmonary syndrome*
- Asbestosis
- Cystic fibrosis
- Sarcoidosis
- Extrinsic allergic alveolitis
- Emphysema
- Tuberculosis
- Pleural empyema
- Pulmonary abscess

Cardiovascular diseases
- *Cyanotic heart disease*
- Congestive heart failure
- Endocarditis
- Aortic aneurysm
- Atrial myxoma

Gastrointestinal diseases
- *Crohn's disease*
- *Cirrhosis (biliary and alcoholic)*
- *Chronic hepatitis*
- Ulcerative colitis
- Chronic parasitic infections
- Malabsorption syndromes

Endocrine diseases
- Grave's disease
- Secondary hyperparathyroidism

</td></tr>
</table>

discoloration of the plate related to bed alterations, mainly abnormal vascularization, through a normal translucent nail plate. Typically, it fades with pressure and does not migrate with nail growth.[1,3] Apparent LK can be seen in healthy individuals, but it might be the sign of an underlying systemic disease.

Four types of apparent leukonychia

Terry's nails The LK involves the whole nail except the last distal 0.5 to 3.0 mm forming a pink to brownish distal band on the free edge. The lunula may or may not be visible. Usually, all the fingernails are involved but this condition is more pronounced on the first and second fingers.[38] Different associations have been reported (**Box 5**)[1,3,38–41] but liver cirrhosis is the most common (in up to 82%).[38,39,42]

Half and half nails, also called Lindsay's nails The LK involves the proximal part of the nail bed and a distal pink, red to brownish area involving 20% to 60% of the total length. The 2 parts are separated transversely by a well-defined line.[43,44] Half and half nails were first described in chronic kidney disease and are present in approximatively one-third of patients on hemodialysis.[43] The relation between half and half nails and hemodialysis remains controversial. For some authors, half and half nails is related to the long-term uremia and not to the dialysis itself.[45,46] This apparent LK could disappear after kidney transplantation.[45] Other associations are cited in **Box 6**.[3,20,41]

Muehrcke's lines These transverse white bands parallel to the lunula, are most prominent on the second, third, and fourth fingernails, and rarely observed on the thumbs.[47] The first association described and one of the main causes of Muehrcke's lines is hypoalbuminemia (albumin <2.2 g/dL). Typically, Muehrcke's lines disappear when the albumin levels return to normal and

Systemic diseases

- Systemic lupus erythematous

Others

- Human immunodeficiency virus
- Syphilis
- Polyneuropathy, organomegaly, endocrinopathy, monoclonal protein, skin changes (POEMS) syndrome

Data from Refs.[1,27,28]

comes back if they decrease again.[47,48] However, we can see Muehrcke's lines in patients with normal albuminemia[48] (**Box 7**).[3,20,41,48]

Neapolitan nails Neapolitan nails are characterized by a loss of the lunula and 3 transverse bands: the proximal one with apparent leukonychia, a normal pink band, and a distal opaque band at the free edge of the nail.[20,49] It is present in 20% of patients older than 70 years and should not be misinterpreted as Terry or Lindsay's nails. Neapolitan nails are also described in patients with hemiplegia[50]

Nail Fold Capillaries

The microvasculature is easily seen in the proximal nailfold because the dermal capillary loops are horizontal and run parallel to the skin surface, visible throughout their length. The nailfold capillary network can be evaluated by microscopy (called nailfold capillaroscopy), nailfold videocapillaroscopy, and dermoscopy.[51]

The dermoscope is helpful for the identification of major qualitative abnormalities, such as giant capillaries.[52] However, nailfold capillaroscopy and nailfold videocapillaroscopy offer a more detailed imaging with a semiquantitative approach and cannot be replaced by dermoscopy.[53] To have a complete interpretation of images, nailfold capillaroscopy is performed on all fingers, except the thumb.[53,54]

Through (semi)-quantitative and qualitative assessment, a normal capillaroscopy can be distinguished from an abnormal one.[55,56] A normal capillary looks like a thin, regular hairpin, with an afferent, transitional, and efferent limb.[51,53] Normal capillaries are homogeneously sized and regularly arranged in a parallel fashion. Nevertheless, there can be subtle morphologic variations or even nonspecific abnormalities of capillaroscopic characteristics[51,55] (**Fig. 4**).

In systemic sclerosis (SSc) and diseases of the scleroderma spectrum (mixed connective tissue disease, dermatomyositis, undifferentiated connective tissue disorders), specific (pathognomonic) abnormalities or a pathognomonic combination of specific anomalies occur: giant capillaries, hemorrhages, loss of capillaries and abnormal shapes (ie, "neoangiogenesis"). These pathognomonic abnormalities form the scleroderma pattern. This scleroderma pattern is found in 86% to 100% of patients with SSc, but also in 30% to 75% of patients with dermatomyositis, in 50% to 65% of patients with mixed connective tissue disease, and in 14% of patients with undifferentiated connective tissue disorders.[53]

Recently, a fast track algorithm has been proposed and validated multicentrally which allows capillaroscopists with any level of experience to correctly classify images as nonscleroderma pattern or scleroderma pattern.[57] This algorithm relies on 3 rules[57]:

1. The presence of 7 or more capillaries AND the absence of giant capillaries allows to call the capillaroscopic image a nonscleroderma pattern. This comprises perfectly normal

---

Box 5
Diseases associated with Terry's nails

Age

Liver cirrhosis

Congestive heart failure

Diabetes mellitus

Infectious

- Human immunodeficiency virus/AIDS
- Leprosy
- Tuberculosis

Hematological disorders

Chronic renal failure

Neoplastic (pancreatic carcinoma, plasmacytoma)

Rheumatologic

- Reactive arthritis
- Rheumatoid arthritis
- Systemic sclerosis

Malnutrition

Drugs (cyclophosphamide, itraconazole, vincristine)

Data from Refs.[1,3,38,39,40,41]

images but also images with nonspecific abnormalities.
2. The presence of giant capillaries or the presence of an extremely lowered capillary density (≤3 capillaries) in combination with abnormal shapes (a late scleroderma pattern) allows the capillaroscopist to call the capillaroscopic image a scleroderma pattern.
3. If the image does not meet rule number 1 or 2, then the image is automatically classified as a nonscleroderma pattern.

There is a dynamic evolution of the microvascular alterations in SSc and 3 progressive patterns have been described to evaluate the level of microangiopathy: early, active, and late scleroderma patterns.[51,58] Giant capillaries are the hallmark of the early and active scleroderma patterns, and a severe loss of capillaries with abnormal shapes characterize the late pattern.[51,57,58]

Nailfold capillaroscopy is mainly indicated in diagnosing connective tissue diseases associated

with a prominent microangiopathy.[51] It can differentiate primary from secondary Raynaud phenomenon. Also, it is useful in diagnosing early SSc and scleroderma spectrum diseases.[51,53] Beside its diagnostic purposes, nailfold capillaroscopy also has a prognostic value.[51,53]

- The Raynaud phenomenon can be the first sign of scleroderma spectrum disease. Nailfold capillaroscopy and antinuclear antibodies, together with a complete medical history and physical examination, are part of the initial mandatory work-up to differentiate primary from secondary Raynaud phenomenon. Giant capillaries are the most striking feature of Raynaud phenomenon secondary to scleroderma spectrum diseases.[51] The risk of developing SSc in patients with Raynaud phenomenon, is up to 65% in 5 years if patients have both specific positive antinuclear antibodies and a scleroderma pattern on nailfold capillaroscopy.[53,59] A regular follow-up is mandatory.
- In SSc, nailfold capillaroscopy allows an early diagnosis and is now considered as a major diagnostic criterium[60] and moreover has a prognostic interest. It evaluates the severity of SSc and helps to identify patients at risk of visceral involvement. The evolution of nailfold capillaroscopy images to a late pattern is associated with a higher modified Rodnan skin score, with an increased risk of pulmonary arterial hypertension, interstitial lung disease, cardiac and vascular pathology, and an increased mortality.[51,53] Patients with SSc with a nonscleroderma pattern have less severe skin and pulmonary involvement.[61] Some studies have described an improvement in nailfold capillaroscopy abnormalities under systemic treatment.[62,63]
- In dermatomyositis, the scleroderma-like pattern is observed with usually a more anarchic picture with a higher capillary density (no capillary dropout), more neo-formed capillaries (ramified capillaries) and capillary disorganisation.[64] Some authors report a normalization of the nailfold capillaries under immunosuppressive treatment, especially rituximab.[65]
- In the others autoimmune disease, nailfold capillaroscopy is less specific and is not paramount in the diagnosis.[51] For systemic lupus erythematosus, there is no specific capillaroscopic pattern but tortuous capillaries, hemorrhages and abnormal morphology are more prevalent than in the normal

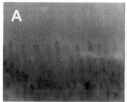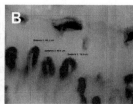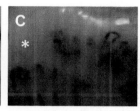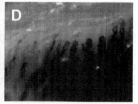

Fig. 4. Normal capillaroscopy image with thin regular hairpin loops with a homogeneous distribution (*A*), an active scleroderma pattern with giant capillaries and hemorrhages (*B*), a late scleroderma pattern with avascular areas (*asterisk*), abnormal capillary shapes (*C*), and tortuous capillaries in systemic lupus erythematosus (*D*).

population.[56] There is also no specific pattern on nailfold capillaroscopy for rheumatoid arthritis[66]

Melanonychia

Longitudinal melanonychia describes a longitudinal gray to brown–black band extending from the proximal nail fold to the free edge. It corresponds to the presence of melanin within the nail plate resulting from activation or proliferation of matrix melanocytes.[67] Causes of melanonychia are multiple and here will be cited only those related to systemic disorders. Melanonychia can be longitudinal or diffuse. Muehrcke's lines may be associated with endocrinopathies (acromegaly, Addison disease, Cushing syndrome, hyperthyroidism), nutritional deficiencies, infections (eg, human immunodeficiency virus), and connective tissue diseases.[3,68] Many drugs can lead to melanonychia, the main being chemotherapeutic agents (hydroxyurea, doxorubicin, fluorouracil, taxanes, cyclophosphamide); tetracyclines; antiretroviral drugs like nucleotide reverse transcriptase inhibitors and antimalarial agents.[40,41]

Peutz-Jeghers syndrome, a rare genetic autosomal-dominant disease, is characterized by mucocutaneous pigmentation and multiple intestinal polyps associated with an increased risk for

---

Box 8
Diseases associated with red lunula

Connective tissue diseases

- **Rheumatoid arthritis**
- **Systemic lupus erythematosus**
- Dermatomyositis/polymyositis
- Sjögren syndrome
- Polymyalgia rheumatica

Cardiac diseases

- Congestive heart failure
- Myocardial infarction
- Rheumatic heart disease
- Hypertension
- Conduction abnormalities
- Atherosclerotic disease

Hematologic malignancies

Pulmonary diseases

- Chronic obstructive pulmonary
- Chronic bronchitis
- Emphysema

Gastrointestinal diseases

- Hepatic cirrhosis

Renal: proteinuria

Toxicity: alcohol or tobacco use, carbon monoxide poisoning

Drugs: corticosteroids, procainamide

Data from Refs.[1,3,20,72,73,74]

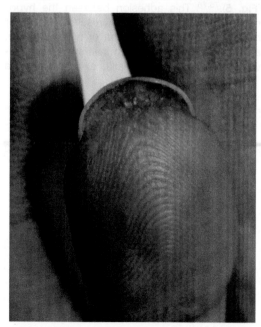

Fig. 5. Pterygium inversum unguis showing an obliteration of the distal nail groove.

malignancies.[69] Brown–blue macules are localized on acral sites particularly the lips, oral mucosa, palms, and soles. Longitudinal melanonychia have been exceptionally described.[69] The main differential diagnosis is the Laugier–Hunzinker–Baran syndrome.[70,71] This syndrome associates lenticular hyperpigmentation of the oral and anogenital mucosal with frequent longitudinal melanonychia without any systemic involvement.[69] Longitudinal melanonychia are present in 60% of the cases, more frequently on the fingernails and pseudo-Hutchinson has been described[69]

Red Lunula

Red lunula is defined by red–pink to dusky redness of the lunula. It can be complete or partial, with persistence of a narrow white band at the distal portion of the lunula. It fades under pressure on the nail plate.[72] All the nails can be affected but red lunula is more frequent on fingernails, especially the thumb where the distal matrix is more visible.[20] Red lunula can be associated with systemic disorders (**Box 8**)[1,3,20,72–74] and be the first sign of the underlying disease.[73] Red lunula can also be seen with medications as amoxicillin/clavulanic acid (fixed drug eruption), corticosteroid and procainamide.[20] The physiopathology of red lunula remains unclear.[72]

Pterygium Inversum Unguis

Pterygium inversum unguis, or ventral pterygium, is the obliteration of the distal groove (**Fig. 5**).[75,76] This adhesion between the hyponychium and the nail plate results in pain or bleeding with minimal trauma or when the nails are trimmed.[75–77] Pterygium inversum unguis involves mainly the fingernails, exceptionally the toenails.[76,77] Pterygium inversum unguis can be congenital, but the majority are acquired (idiopathic or secondary).[76,77] Secondary pterygium inversum unguis most commonly occurs in auto-immune diseases, especially SSc or systemic lupus erythematosus. Caputo and colleagues[77] evaluated that pterygium inversum unguis occurs in 16% of these patients. For this reason, women are more prone to develop a pterygium inversum unguis.[76,77] Other associations are reported in **Box 9**.[1,20,76–79] The physiopathology is not fully understood and could be different according to the etiology.[76] Microvascular ischemic lesions with subsequent scarring are suspected in connective tissue diseases and leprosy.[77–79] There is not treatment for pterygium inversum unguis as it results from scarring. Surgery is not an option in systemic disorders

SELECTED SYSTEMIC DISORDERS WITH NAIL INVOLVEMENT
Gout

Tophi are more frequent in chronic stage but they can also be the first clinical sign of gout.[80] Gouty tophi, pink to whitish firm nodules or swelling, could be periungual with perionychium deformation and Beau's lines or longitudinal groove owing

---

Box 9
Systemic diseases associated to pterygium inversum unguis

Connective tissue diseases
- **Systemic sclerosis**
- **Systemic lupus erythematosus**
- **Dermatomyositis**

Diabetes mellitus

Leprosy

Cerebral vascular accident with hemiparesis (unilateral pterygium inversum unguis)

Drugs: beta-blockers

Data from Refs.[1,20,76,77,78,79]

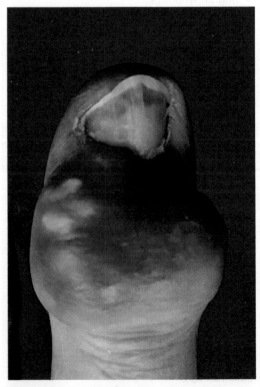

Fig. 6. Voluminous tophi.

to matrix compression[20] (**Fig. 6**). When tophi are located at the tip of a toe, friction may lead to a chronic, crusted, nonhealing wound.[81] Besides the classical tophi, gout may manifest as abrupt and acute isolated painful hallux in the early morning. Less frequently, gout tophi could involve finger pad with a sometimes challenging clinical presentation as periungual hyperkeratotic lesion mimicking squamous cell carcinoma.[82] Radiology, although frequently normal, may be useful in chronic stage showing asymmetrical swelling and subcortical cysts without erosion.[83] It is not specific in early or acute gout.[83] Diagnosis is based on a combination of clinical findings, laboratory tests and imaging.[80,83] A demonstration of monosodium urate crystals deposition permits a definitive diagnosis of gout.[83] Interestingly, urate crystals may be found in the nail plate and could be, according some authors, a new noninvasive diagnostic method for gout.[84] Once installed, tophi may last years before resolving or remain forever, even with appropriate medical treatment.[85] Thus, early urea-lowering treatment is mandatory.[86]

Surgery may be an option in selected cases, but delayed healing is the rule.[87]

Yellow Nail Syndrome

The yellow nail syndrome is an acquired rare entity affecting middle-age adults of unknown etiology characterized by the triad: yellow nails, chronic respiratory diseases, and lymphedema.[88,89] The 3 symptoms are not always present, but the typical nail alterations are sufficient.[90,91] Nails are the only manifestation in one-third of patients with yellow nail syndrome. Hereditary cases are anecdotal.[92–94] Nail changes are pathognomonic: the nail growth is much decreased or stopped; the nail plate is thick with an opaque yellow–green to brownish discoloration; there is a lack of cuticle with paronychia and a transverse and longitudinal overcurvature leading to onycholysis and sometimes nail shedding[90,92] (**Fig. 7**). This nail was described by Moffitt and de Berker[95] as the nail that grows one-half as fast but twice as thick. Both fingernails and toenails are affected, and usually all the nails involved. The diagnosis of yellow nail syndrome is clinical and anamnesis often

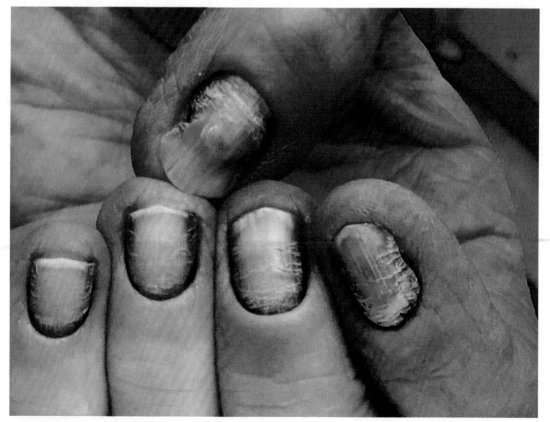

Fig. 7. Pathognomonic nail changes in yellow nail syndrome: thick opaque yellow nail plate with missing cuticle and multiple transversal lines.

unveil some chronic symptoms such as respiratory manifestations (56%–71%) like chronic cough, pleural effusion, chronic obstructive lung disease, chronic bronchitis, recurrent pneumonia, bronchiectasis, and sinusitis.[92,93]

Lymphedema is observed in 29% to 80% of patients with yellow nail syndrome.[92,93] It is a nonpitting edema usually involving symmetrically the lower limbs, but the hands or the face can be involved.[93] Yellow nail syndrome has also been described in association with various diseases, but most of them are anecdotal[92,93] (**Box 10**).[20,90,92,93] Amazingly, nail changes similar to yellow nail syndrome have been exceptionally reported with nail lichen planus.[96] Recently, several reports suggest titanium as a potential cause of yellow nail

syndrome.[97] Titanium may be encountered in implants, foods, personal care products, or medications.[97,98] Eviction of titanium sources may allow partial or complete healing, but it remains controversial.[97,98] Spontaneous improvement of the nails has been reported in 10% to 30% of cases.[90,94] Improvement or even resolution of the nail disease has been described with the treatment of the respiratory or lymphedema manifestations of the yellow nail syndrome.[90,92] There is no therapeutic consensus for yellow nail syndrome. High-dose vitamin E (1000–1200 IU/d) has been effective in some case studies.[90,92] Its association with systemic antifungals (itraconazole [400 mg/d a wk/mo] or fluconazole [300 mg/wk]) for at least 6 months, can be beneficial for their stimulating nail growth effect[92,99]

Connective Tissue Diseases

Many nonspecific nail alterations can be observed in autoimmune diseases and only few of them are suggestive for a specific disease (**Table 1**). Nevertheless, nail abnormalities are frequent and can be the initial sign of these diseases.[100] The most affected part is the proximal nail fold, especially on fingernails.[100] Periungual erythema, telangiectasia, and hemorrhages are observed commonly.[100,101] These nail signs should alert the clinicians and nailfold capillaroscopy is mandatory for differential diagnosis (see below nail fold capillary).

In SSc, fingernails changes are present in up to 80% and seem to be associated with more severe diseases.[101] Raynaud phenomenon is one of the earlier symptoms of SSc. Proximal nailfold erythema, telangiectasias and hemorrhages are frequent.[20,101,102] Chronic paronychia and a

---

Box 10
Systemic diseases associated with yellow nail syndrome

Neoplasia

- Lung cancer
- Larynx carcinoma
- Breast carcinoma
- Hodgkin lymphoma
- Multiple myeloma
- Melanoma
- Mycosis fongoides
- Renal cell carcinoma
- Endometrial adenocarcinoma
- Gallbladder adenocarcinoma

Immunodeficiency states

Infectious disease

- Tuberculosis
- Syphilis

Autoimmune disease

- Rheumatoid arthritis
- Systemic lupus erythematosus
- Guillain-Barré syndrome
- Raynaud phenomenon

Endocrine disorders

- Diabetes mellitus
- Thyroid disease

Myocardial infarction

Nephrotic syndrome

Data from Refs.[20,90,92,93]

Table 1
Suggestive nail abnormalities in connective tissue diseases

	Suggestive Nail Abnormalities
SSc	Parrot beak nails Pterygium inversum unguis
SLE	Onycholysis Pterygium inversum unguis
DE	Hypertrophic cuticles (Manicure's sign) and cuticular hemorrhages Gottron's papules
AR	Bywaters lesions

Data from Refs.[20,100,101,114]

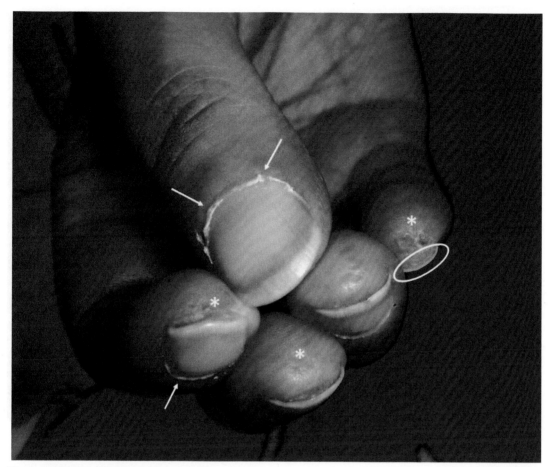

Fig. 8. Digital ulcerations (*white asterisk*), pterygium inversum unguis (*white ring*), and thickened cuticules (*white arrows*) in patient with systemic sclerosis.

thickening and enlarged cuticle can be seen[20,101,102] (**Fig. 8**). Other features reported are absent or red lunula, a white dull color of the plate, splinter hemorrhages, nail plate thinning and ridging, trachyonychia, and transverse overcurvature of the nail plate.[20,100–102] The latter is associated with disease activity.[100] In the most severe cases, destruction of the terminal phalanges leads to brachyonychia or even anonychia.[20] Two specific nail changes can be observed in SSc, namely, parrot beak nail and pterygium inversum unguis[20] (see **Fig. 8**). Parrot beak nails is the bending of the nail plate around the fingertip resulting from soft tissue atrophy in severe acrosclerosis[20] (discussed elsewhere in this article). Sclerodactyly—a localized skin thickening of the extremities in advanced cases—is observed in up to 90% of these patients.[20] Ischemic changes of the fingertip with ulcerations are common (see **Fig. 8**) and digital gangrene can occur.[20,101]

In systemic lupus erythematosus (SLE), a wide range of nail abnormalities may be observed in 25% to 55% of patients.[103,104] None of them are sufficiently distinctive to allow a definitive diagnosis.[103,105,106] Erythema and telangiectasia of the proximal nailfold (**Fig. 9**), splinter hemorrhages, thinning of the plate, longitudinal ridging, melanonychia, ventral pterygium, and red lunula are frequently described.[100,106] Many other nail changes have been reported in systemic lupus erythematosus, including Beau's lines, onychomadesis, pitting, chronic paronychia, subungual hyperkeratosis, leukonychia, increased transverse or longitudinal nail curvature, pincer nails, and clubbing.[20,105,107] Onycholysis seems to be the most common finding (25%–40%).[103,104] Red lunula can be the presenting sign of systemic lupus erythematosus[73] and has been found in up to 20% of patients with lupus.[74] Longitudinal melanonychia or diffuse blue–black chromonychia can occur in systemic lupus erythematosus, especially in patients with darker skin.[20,108] These pigmentations could result from the direct involvement of the nail matrix by lupus or be drugs related (antimalarial agents).[108] Different studies reported an

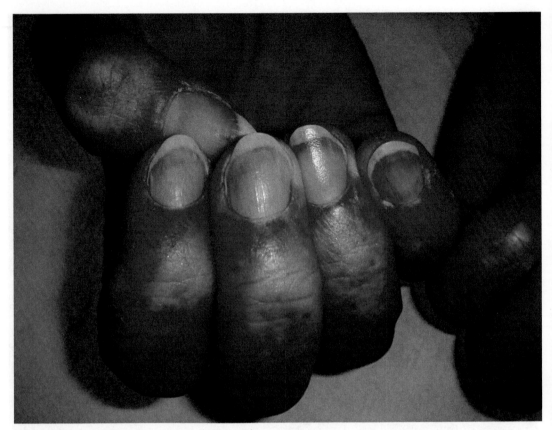

Fig. 9. Periungual erythema in systemic lupus erythematosus.

association between splinter hemorrhages[100] or nailfold erythema and onycholysis[106] with disease activity. Overall, patients with systemic lupus erythematosus with nail abnormalities have a higher damage organ index, disease activity, and nailfold capillaroscopy abnormalities, suggesting that nail involvement might be related to chronic microvascular damages.[104,105] In discoid lupus erythematosus, nail involvement is unusual and never restricted to the nail unit.[103] Severe subungual hyperkeratosis, longitudinal ridging, and nail atrophy can occur with sometimes the typical discoid lupus erythematosus lesions on the perionychium (**Fig. 10**).[103] Patients with discoid lupus erythematosus with nail changes are at a higher risk to develop systemic lupus erythematosus.[109]

In dermatomyositis (DM), hyperkeratotic and thickened cuticles are common with frequent nailfold erythema and telangiectasia associated (**Fig. 11**). This condition may be painful and is called the manicure's sign. It is not pathognomonic and can be observed in SSc and systemic lupus erythematosus. The parallelism between cuticular changes and dermatomyositis activity are controversial.[110] Gottron's papules—

violaceous flattened papules on the dorsum of the metacarpophalangeal and interphalangeal joints—can be observed[20] (see **Fig. 11**). Other findings are splinter hemorrhages, red lunula, trachyonychia, pitting, Terry's nail, and pterygium inversum unguis (less frequent than in SSc and systemic lupus erythematosus).[20] Periungual ischemic lesions can occur and might be a predictive sign of malignancy in adult dermatomyositis.[111] Mechanic's hands are nonpruritic hyperkeratotic scaly eruption of the lateral surfaces of the digits with sometimes a fissuring pulpitis, mimicking the hands of a manual labourer.[112,113] It is observed in antisynthetase syndrome, which is associated with diffuse interstitial lung disease, inflammatory myopathy, polyarthritis, and cutaneous signs.[112] Mechanic's hands are also described in patients with dermatomyositis, systemic lupus erythematosus, and SSc.[113]

In patients with rheumatoid arthritis, small punctiform painless hemorrhagic lesions on the nailfold and pulp, named the Bywaters lesions, are specific.[114] These lesions are small infarcts from necrotizing vasculitis.[20,114] Splinter hemorrhages,

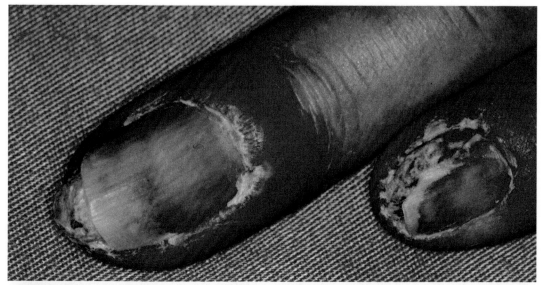

Fig. 10. Erythema and scaling of the perionychium with severe subungual hyperkeratosis in discoid lupus erythematosus.

red lunula (mottled red lunula), longitudinal ridging, onycholysis, and a white dull color of the nail plate are frequent.[20,100] Muehrcke's lines were also reported.[115] Gangrene is rare and observed in severe form of rheumatoid vasculitis.[20] Rheumatoid nodules can be localized in the perionychium.[20] In rheumatoid arthritis, yellow nail syndrome can occur spontaneously or after treatment initiation (D-penicillamine or bucillamine)[116]

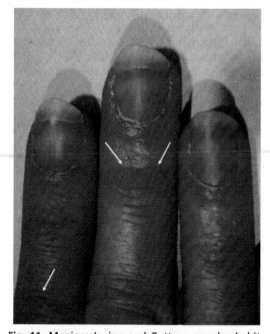

Fig. 11. Manicure's sign and Gottron papules (*white arrows*) in dermatomyositis.

Tuberous Sclerosis Complex

Tuberous sclerosis complex (TSC) is a multisystemic autosomal dominant genetic disorder related to mutation of tumor suppressor genes: TSC1 or TSC2, coding respectively for hamartin and tuberin protein, important regulators of the mechanistic target of rapamycin complex 1 pathway, which controls cell growth and proliferation.[117,118] This syndrome predisposes to hamartoma formation in many organs, especially in central the nervous system, kidneys, lungs, heart, and skin.[117,118] Ungual fibromas are the last skin manifestations of TSC, occurring at puberty and increasing in number with age.[117] Ungual fibromas are usually not present at the time of the initial diagnosis, but multiple ungual fibromas (Koenen tumors) must alert the clinician (**Fig. 12**). They are a major diagnostic criterion of TSC and involve 20% to 80% of patients.[117,119]

Ungual fibromas are pedunculated, flesh-colored benign tumors, with a pointed hyperkeratotic extremity. When located beneath the proximal nail fold, ungual fibromas can rest on a longitudinal groove, which are sometimes the only sign of ungual fibromas.[119]

The majority of ungual fibromas are periungual and located on toenails (especially the fifth), but subungual and fingernails lesions are also seen.[119] Others nail abnormalities have been reported in TSC; longitudinal leukonychia, splinter hemorrhages, onychogryphosis, and cuticular hyperkeratosis.[119] Red comets are a recently described sign that could be specific of TSC. Red comets are partially blanchable reddish

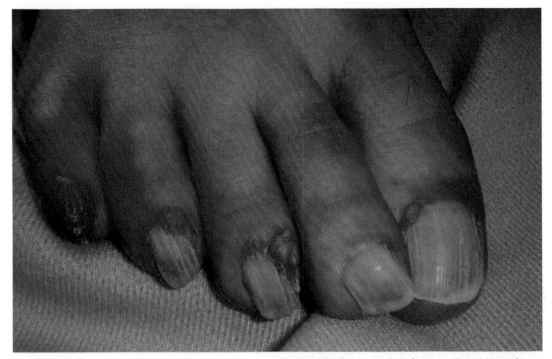

Fig. 12. Multiples ungual fibromas (Koenen tumors) and longitudinal grooves in tuberous sclerosis complex.

longitudinal streaks with a narrow proximal tail and a dilated distal head with sometimes a surrounding whitish halo. They affect fingernails most frequently and could be multiple[119,120]

Acrokeratosis Paraneoplastica of Bazex and Dupré

Acrokeratosis paraneoplastica (AP), also called Bazex syndrome, is a rare but distinctive paraneoplastic dermatosis. It is mostly associated with squamous cell carcinomas of the upper respiratory or digestive tracts but other malignancies have been described.[121–124] It is always associated with malignancy, and in the majority of the cases (63%) cutaneous lesions precede the symptoms with a mean time of 11 months.[124] The pathogenesis remains unclear.[122,124] Acrokeratosis paraneoplastica is typically seen in Caucasian males more than 40 years old.[122,124] Initially, the lesions are ill-defined erythematosquamous plaques symmetrically located on the acral sites: ears, nose, feet, and hands. Parallel to cancer progression, skin lesions evolve to the palms, soles, and cheeks and finally to the arms, legs, scalp, and trunk. Typically, plantar and palmar keratoderma spares the central part of the soles, which can be a clue to the diagnosis.[122–124] Violaceous erythema, erosions, and crusts might be present, and the distribution could be asymmetrical.[122,124] In dark-skinned patients,

hyperpigmentation predominates.[123,124] Some cases of vesicular to bullous lesions are reported, particularly on the digits, mimicking autoimmune bullous disorders. Most of the lesions are asymptomatic, but intensive itch and pain are mentioned.[122,124] The nails are almost always involved (75%)[124] and one of the earliest manifestations.[125] The toenails are more severely affected than the fingernails.[125] First, nail plates are thin, brittle, and cracked. Then they become thick with subungual hyperkeratosis, onycholysis and white to yellowish color, mimicking nail psoriasis.[124,125] Longitudinal and transversal lines are seen.[124,125] Onychomadesis, paronychia, and pigmentation may occur.[123,124] Nail changes could be quite variable, ranging from simple thickening to complete nail atrophy.[125] The perionychium Is typically covered with erythematosquamous papules.[124,125] Histopathology is often nonspecific.[122,124] Upon suspicion, a complete physical examination and an exhaustive work-up (otolaryngologic examination, chest radiographs, blood tests with complete blood cell count, erythrocyte sedimentation rate, biochemistry profile, tumor markers, and a test for occult blood in stool) should be performed.[122,123] If this first work-up is unrevealing, gastrointestinal endoscopy and colonoscopy and further medical imaging should be done.[122,123] For highly suspicious acrokeratosis paraneoplastica with no malignancy detected, a close follow-up every 3 months seems appropriate.[123] The classical therapies for inflammatory skin diseases (steroids, retinoids, and phototherapy) are not efficient in these paraneoplastic lesions, except sometimes to control the symptoms.[122] The only effective therapeutic option is the treatment of the underlying neoplasia, leading to a rapid regression of the cutaneous lesions in 90% of patients.[122,124] Unlike the skin, nail changes often remain or show a really slow regression.[122,124] In case of malignancy recurrence, the skin lesions often relapse[122,124]

CLINICS CARE POINTS

- Beau's lines are frequent.
- If multiples Beau's lines, check history for the culprit.
- Splinter hemorrhages are frequent but not specific.
- If occurring in more than one fingernail, a systemic disease has to be ruled out.
- When facing lichenoid alterations perform a biopsy to rule out:
    Amyloidosis
    Sarcoidosis
    Graft-versus-host disease
    Dyskeratosis congenita
- Clubbing should be differentiated from pseudoclubbing.
- It may arise from many severe systemic diseases especially neoplastic, pulmonary, cardiac and digestive.
- Complete history and physical examination are mandatory. Additional exams will be performed according to symptoms and signs.
- Hypertrophic osteoarthropathy syndrome is often paraneoplastic and need an aggressive screening.
- Terry's nails first exclude hepatic diseases.
- Half and half nails first exclude renal diseases.
- Muehrcke's nails first check albuminemia.
- Nailfold capillaroscopy is a standard noninvasive and reproductive diagnostic tool, assessing microcirculation.
- The main indications for nailfold capillaroscopy are:
- Differentiate primary to secondary Raynaud phenomenon
- Work-up of all connective tissue disorders
- Systemic sclerosis diagnosis and prognosis
- In systemic disorders, longitudinal melanonychia are multiples.
- In case of multiples acquired pterygium inversum unguis, rule out autoimmune disease, especially systemic sclerosis and systemic lupus erythematosus.
- Slowed or no nail growth.

- Yellow to green to brown discoloration.
- Chronic or subacute proximal nail fold inflammation and disappearance of cuticle.
- Thick, hard and opaque nail plate.
- Patients with yellow nail syndrome:
    Ask about sinusal/pulmonary symptoms.
    Perform chest imaging.
    Involve ENT and pneumologist.
    Treat underlying disease aggressively.
    Vitamin E and fluconazole are first line treatment.
    Keep titanium in mind.
- In connective tissue diseases, nail changes are frequent and mainly non specific but can be the presenting sign.
- Fingernails and proximal nailfold are mostly affected.
- Some nail abnormalities are associated with disease activity.
- Nails should always be evaluated in autoimmune diseases.
- If more than one periungual fibrokeratoma rule out tuberous sclerosis complex.
- Acrokeratosis paraneoplastica is always paraneoplastic and mostly associated with squamous cell carcinomas of the upper respiratory or digestive tracts.
- Nails are almost always involved and one of the earliest manifestations.
- If acrokeratosis paraneoplastica is suspected, a detailed patient history, a complete physical examination and an exhaustive diagnostic work-up needs to be performed.

ACKNOWLEDGMENTS

The authors wish to thank Yora Mostmans, MD from the department of immunology and allergology and the department of dermatology in Brugmann hospital Belgium, for her contribution in the nailfold capillaroscopy section.

DISCLOSURE

The authors have no conflict of interest for this publication. No founding sources were received for this work.

REFERENCES

1. Rubin A, Holzberg M, Baran R. Physical signs. In: Baran R, de Berker D, Holzberg M, et al, editors. Baran & Dawber's diseases of the nails and their management. 5th edition. Oxford (United Kingdom): Wiley Blackwell; 2019. p. 59–104.
2. Piraccini BM. Nails signs. In: Nail disorders: a practical guide to diagnosis and management. Milan (Italy): Springer; 2014. p. 2–22.

3. Zaiac MN, Walker A. Nail abnormalities associated with systemic pathologies. Clin Dermatol 2013;31:627–49.

4. Haber R, Khoury R, Kechichian E, et al. Splinter hemorrhages of the nails: a systematic review of clinical features and associated conditions. Int J Dermatol 2016;55:1304–10.

5. Monk BE. The prevalence of splinter haemorrhages. Br J Dermatol 1980;103:183–5.

6. Miller A, Vaziri ND. Recurrent atraumatic subungual splinter hemorrhages in healthy individuals. South Med J 1979;72:1418–20.

7. Saladi RN, Persaud AN, Rudikoff D, et al. Idiopathic splinter hemorrhages. J Am Acad Dermatol 2004;50:289–92.

8. Fanti PA, Tosti A, Morelli R, et al. Nail changes as the first sign of systemic amyloidosis. Dermatologica 1991;183:44–6.

9. Mancuso G, Fanti PA, Berdondini RM. Nail changes as the only skin abnormality in myeloma-associated systemic amyloidosis. Br J Dermatol 1997;137:471–2.

10. Renker T, Haneke E, Röcken C, et al. Systemic light-chain amyloidosis revealed by progressive nail involvement, diffuse alopecia and sicca syndrome: report of an unusual case with a review of the literature. Dermatology 2014;228:97–102.

11. Fujita Y, Tsuji-Abe Y, Sato-Matsumura KC, et al. Nail dystrophy and blisters as sole manifestations in myeloma-associated amyloidosis. J Am Acad Dermatol 2006;54:712–4.

12. Tausend W, Neill M, Kelly B. Primary amyloidosis-induced nail dystrophy. Dermatol Online J 2014;20:21247.

13. Oberlin KE, Wei EX, Cho-Vega JH, et al. Nail changes of systemic amyloidosis after bone-marrow transplantation in a patient with multiple myeloma. JAMA Dermatol 2016;152:1395–6.

14. Momen SE, Al-Niaimi F. Sarcoid and the nail: review of the literature. Clin Exp Dermatol 2013;38:119–24.

15. Santoro F, Sloan SB. Nail dystrophy and bony involvement in chronic sarcoidosis. J Am Acad Dermatol 2009;60:1050–2.

16. Moulonguet I, Abimelec P. An unusual case of dactylitis with nail unit involvement: answer. Am J Dermatopathol 2018;40:701.

17. Losada-Campa A, De la Torre-Fraga C, Gomez de Liaño A, et al. Histopathology of nail sarcoidosis. Acta Derm Venereol 1995;75:404–5.

18. Rajan S, Melegh Z, de Berker D. Subungual sarcoidosis: a rare entity. Clin Exp Dermatol 2014;39:720–2.

19. van Lümig PPM, Pasch MC. Nail sarcoidosis presenting with longitudinal erythronychia. Skin Appendage Disord 2018;4:156–9.

20. Holzberg A, Piraccini BM. The nail in systemic disease. In: Baran R, de Berker D, Holzberg M, et al, editors. Baran & Dawber's diseases of the nails and their management. 5th edition. Oxford (United Kingdom): Wiley Blackwell; 2019. p. 481–573.

21. Sanli H, Arat M, Oskay T, et al. Evaluation of nail involvement in patients with chronic cutaneous graft versus host disease: a single-center study from Turkey. Int J Dermatol 2004;43:176–80.

22. Huang JT, Duncan CN, Boyer D, et al. Nail dystrophy, edema, and eosinophilia: harbingers of severe chronic GVHD of the skin in children. Bone Marrow Transplant 2014;49:1521–7.

23. Nanda A, Husain MAA, Al-Herz W, et al. Chronic cutaneous graft-versus-host disease in children: a report of 14 patients from a tertiary care pediatric dermatology clinic. Pediatr Dermatol 2018;35:343–53.

24. Palencia SI, Rodríguez-Peralto JL, Castaño E, et al. Lichenoid nail changes as sole external manifestation of graft vs. host disease. Int J Dermatol 2002;41:44–5.

25. Fernández García MS, Teruya-Feldstein J. The diagnosis and treatment of dyskeratosis congenita: a review. J Blood Med 2014;5:157–67.

26. Sharma RK, Gupta M, Sood S, et al. Dyskeratosis congenita: presentation of cutaneous triad in a sporadic case. BMJ Case Rep 2018;11(1).

27. Callemeyn J, Van Haecke P, Peetermans WE, et al. Clubbing and hypertrophic osteoarthropathy: insights in diagnosis, pathophysiology, and clinical significance. Acta Clin Belg 2016;71:123–30.

28. Spicknall KE, Zirwas MJ, English JC 3rd. Clubbing: an update on diagnosis, differential diagnosis, pathophysiology, and clinical relevance. J Am Acad Dermatol 2005;52:1020–8.

29. Lovibond JL. Diagnosis of clubbed fingers. Lancet 1938;1:363–4.

30. Schamroth L. Personal experience. S Afr Med J 1976;50:297–300.

31. Rice RE, Rowland PW. A quantitative method for the estimation of clubbing. Scientific Session of the Senior Class of Tulane University Medical School 1961;11:302–15.

32. Kurzrock R, Cohen PR. Cutaneous paraneoplastic syndromes in solid tumors. Am J Med 1995;99:662–71.

33. Martinez-Lavin M. Exploring the cause of the most ancient clinical sign of medicine: finger clubbing. Semin Arthritis Rheum 2007;36(6):380–5.

34. Piraccini BM. Nails signs of systemic diseases and drug-induced nail changes. In: Nail disorders: a practical guide to diagnosis and management. Milan (Italy): Springer; 2014. p. 117–24.

35. Nguyen S, Hojjati M. Review of current therapies for secondary hypertrophic pulmonary osteoarthropathy. Clin Rheumatol 2011;30:7–13.

36. Baran R. Mees' lines. Br J Dermatol 1999;141:1152.

37. Daniel CR 3rd, Piraccini BM, Tosti A. The nail and hair in forensic science. J Am Acad Dermatol 2004;50:258–61.

38. Terry R. White nails in hepatic cirrhosis. Lancet 1954;266:757–9.

39. Holzberg M, Walker HK. Terry's nails: revised definition and new correlations. Lancet 1984;1:896–9.

40. Piraccini BM. Drug-induced nail disorders. In: Baran R, de Berker D, Holzberg M, et al, editors. Baran & Dawber's diseases of the nails and their management. 5th edition. Oxford (United Kingdom): Wiley Blackwell; 2019. p. 574–603.

41. Sibaud V, Baran R, Piraccini BM, et al. Anticancer therapies. In: Baran R, de Berker D, Holzberg M, et al, editors. Baran & Dawber's diseases of the nails and their management. 5th edition. Oxford (United Kingdom): Wiley Blackwell; 2019. p. 604–16.

42. Nelson N, Hayfron K, Diaz A, et al. Terry's nails: clinical correlations in adult outpatients. J Gen Intern Med 2018;33:1018–9.

43. Lindsay PG. The half-and-half nail. Arch Intern Med 1967;119:583–7.

44. Baran R, Gioanni T. Half and half nail (equisegmented azotemic fingernail). Bull Soc Fr Dermatol Syphiligr 1968;75:399–400.

45. Saray Y, Seçkin D, Güleç AT, et al. Nail disorders in hemodialysis patients and renal transplant recipients: a case-control study. J Am Acad Dermatol 2004;50:197–202.

46. Salem A, Al Mokadem S, Attwa E, et al. Nail changes in chronic renal failure patients under haemodialysis. J Eur Acad Dermatol Venereol 2008;22:1326–31.

47. Muehrcke RC. The finger-nails in chronic hypoalbuminaemia; a new physical sign. Br Med J 1956;1:1327–8.

48. Short N, Shah C. Muehrcke's lines. Am J Med 2010;123:991–2.

49. Horan MA, Puxty JA, Fox RA. The white nails of old age (Neapolitan nails). J Am Geriatr Soc 1982;30:734–7.

50. Siragusa M, Schepis C, Cosentino FI, et al. Nail pathology in patients with hemiplegia. Br J Dermatol 2001;144:557–60.

51. Cutolo M, Sulli A, Smith V. How to perform and interpret capillaroscopy. Best Pract Res Clin Rheumatol 2013;27:237–48.

52. Bergman R, Sharony L, Schapira D, et al. The handheld dermatoscope as a nail-fold capillaroscopic instrument. Arch Dermatol 2003;139:1027–30.

53. Senet P, Fichel F, Baudot N, et al. Nail-fold capillaroscopy in dermatology. Ann Dermatol Venereol 2014;141:429–37.

54. Dinsdale G, Roberts C, Moore T, et al. Nailfold capillaroscopy-how many fingers should be examined to detect abnormality? Rheumatology (Oxford) 2019;58:284–8.

55. Smith V, Beeckman S, Herrick AL, et al. EULAR study group on microcirculation. An EULAR study group pilot study on reliability of simple capillaroscopic definitions to describe capillary morphology in rheumatic diseases. Rheumatology (Oxford) 2016;55:883–90.

56. Cutolo M, Melsens K, Wijnant S, et al. Nailfold capillaroscopy in systemic lupus erythematosus: a systematic review and critical appraisal. Autoimmun Rev 2018;17:344–52.

57. Smith V, Vanhaecke A, Herrick AL, et al. EULAR study group on microcirculation in rheumatic diseases. fast track algorithm: how to differentiate a "scleroderma pattern" from a "non-scleroderma pattern". Autoimmun Rev 2019;18:102394.

58. Cutolo M, Sulli A, Pizzorni C, et al. Nailfold videocapillaroscopy assessment of microvascular damage in systemic sclerosis. J Rheumatol 2000;27:155–60.

59. Koenig M, Joyal F, Fritzler MJ, et al. Autoantibodies and microvascular damage are independent predictive factors for the progression of Raynaud's phenomenon to systemic sclerosis: a twenty-year prospective study of 586 patients, with validation of proposed criteria for early systemic sclerosis. Arthritis Rheum 2008;58:3902–12.

60. Van den Hoogen F, Khanna D, Fransen J, et al. 2013 classification criteria for systemic sclerosis: an American College of Rheumatology/European League against Rheumatism collaborative initiative. Arthritis Rheum 2013;65:2737–47.

61. Fichel F, Baudot N, Gaitz JP, et al. Systemic sclerosis with normal or nonspecific nailfold capillaroscopy. Dermatology 2014;228:360–7.

62. Vilela VS, da Silva BRA, da Costa CH, et al. Effects of treatment with rituximab on microcirculation in patients with long-term systemic sclerosis. BMC Res Notes 2018;11:874.

63. Trombetta AC, Pizzorni C, Ruaro B, et al. Effects of longterm treatment with bosentan and iloprost on nailfold absolute capillary number, fingertip blood perfusion, and clinical status in systemic sclerosis. J Rheumatol 2016;43:2033–41.

64. Pizzorni C, Cutolo M, Sulli A, et al. Long-term follow-up of nailfold videocapillaroscopic changes in dermatomyositis versus systemic sclerosis patients. Clin Rheumatol 2018;37:2723–9.

65. Argobi Y, Smith GP. Tracking changes in nailfold capillaries during dermatomyositis treatment. J Am Acad Dermatol 2019;81:275–6.

66. Sag S, Sag MS, Tekeoglu I, et al. Nailfold videocapillaroscopy results in patients with rheumatoid arthritis. Clin Rheumatol 2017;36:1969–74.

67. Moulonguet I, Goettmann-Bonvallot S. Longitudinal melanonychia. Ann Dermatol Venereol 2016;143(1):53–60.

68. Braun RP, Baran R, Le Gal FA, et al. Diagnosis and management of nail pigmentations. J Am Acad Dermatol 2007;56:835–47.

69. Lampe AK, Hampton PJ, Woodford-Richens K, et al. Laugier-Hunziker syndrome: an important differential diagnosis for Peutz-Jeghers syndrome. J Med Genet 2003;40:e77.

70. Laugier P, Hunziker N. Essential lenticular melanic pigmentation of the lip and cheek mucosa. Arch Belg Dermatol Syphiligr 1970;26:391–9.

71. Baran R. Longitudinal melanotic streaks as a clue to Laugier-Hunziker syndrome. Arch Dermatol 1979;115(12):1448–9.

72. Morrissey KA, Rubin AI. Histopathology of the red lunula: new histologic features and clinical correlations of a rare type of erythronychia. J Cutan Pathol 2013;40:972–5.

73. García-Patos V, Bartralot R, Ordi J, et al. Systemic lupus erythematosus presenting with red lunulae. J Am Acad Dermatol 1997;36:834–6.

74. Wollina U, Barta U, Uhlemann C, et al. Lupus erythematosus-associated red lunula. J Am Acad Dermatol 1999;41:419–21.

75. Caputo R, Prandi G. Pterygium inversum unguis. Arch Dermatol 1973;108:817–8.

76. Richert BJ, Patki A, Baran RL. Pterygium of the nail. Cutis 2000;66:343–6.

77. Caputo R, Cappio F, Rigoni C, et al. Pterygium inversum unguis. Report of 19 cases and review of the literature. Arch Dermatol 1993;129:1307–9.

78. Vadmal M, Reyter I, Oshtory S, et al. Pterygium inversum unguis associated with stroke. J Am Acad Dermatol 2005;53:501–3.

79. Patki AH. Pterygium inversum unguis in a patient with leprosy. Arch Dermatol 1990;126:1110.

80. Thissen CA, Frank J, Lucker GP. Tophi as first clinical sign of gout. Int J Dermatol 2008;47(Suppl 1):49–51.

81. Simman R, Kirkland B, Jackson S. Posttraumatic tophaceous gout: a case report and literature review. J Am Col Certif Wound Spec 2009;1:114–6.

82. Dacko A, Hardick K, McCormack P, et al. Gouty tophi: a squamous cell carcinoma mimicker? Dermatol Surg 2002;28:636–8.

83. Zhang W, Doherty M, Pascual E, et al. EULAR standing committee for international clinical studies including therapeutics. EULAR evidence based recommendations for gout. Part I: diagnosis. Report of a task force of the standing committee for international clinical studies including therapeutics (ESCISIT). Ann Rheum Dis 2006;65:1301–11.

84. Tirado-González M, González-Serva A. The nail plate biopsy may pick up gout crystals and other crystals. Am J Dermatopathol 2011;33:351–3.

85. Perez-Ruiz F, Calabozo M, Pijoan JI, et al. Effect of urate-lowering therapy on the velocity of size reduction of tophi in chronic gout. Arthritis Rheum 2002;47:356–60.

86. Zhang W, Doherty M, Bardin T, et al. EULAR standing committee for international clinical studies including therapeutics. EULAR evidence based recommendations for gout. Part II: management. Report of a task force of the EULAR standing committee for international clinical studies including therapeutics (ESCISIT). Ann Rheum Dis 2006;65:1312–24.

87. Kasper IR, Juriga MD, Giurini JM, et al. Treatment of tophaceous gout: when medication is not enough. Semin Arthritis Rheum 2016;45:669–74.

88. Samman PD, White WF. The "yellow nail" syndrome. Br J Dermatol 1964;76:153–7.

89. Hiller E, Rosenow EC 3rd, Olsen AM. Pulmonary manifestations of the yellow nail syndrome. Chest 1972;61:452–8.

90. Piraccini BM, Urciuoli B, Starace M, et al. Yellow nail syndrome: clinical experience in a series of 21 patients. J Dtsch Dermatol Ges 2014;12:131–7.

91. Baran LR. Yellow nail syndrome and nail lichen planus may be induced by a common culprit. focus on dental restorative substances. Front Med (Lausanne) 2014;1:46.

92. Vignes S, Baran R. Yellow nail syndrome: a review. Orphanet J Rare Dis 2017;12:42.

93. Maldonado F, Ryu JH. Yellow nail syndrome. Curr Opin Pulm Med 2009;15:371–5.

94. Hoque SR, Mansour S, Mortimer PS. Yellow nail syndrome: not a genetic disorder? Eleven new cases and a review of the literature. Br J Dermatol 2007;156:1230–4.

95. Moffitt DL, de Berker DA. Yellow nail syndrome: the nail that grows half as fast grows twice as thick. Clin Exp Dermatol 2000;25:21–3.

96. Tosti A, Piraccini BM, Cameli N. Nail changes in lichen planus may resemble those of yellow nail syndrome. Br J Dermatol 2000;14:848–9.

97. Decker A, Daly D, Scher RK. Role of titanium in the development of yellow nail syndrome. Skin Appendage Disord 2015;1:28–30.

98. Ataya A, Kline KP, Cope J, et al. Titanium exposure and yellow nail syndrome. Respir Med Case Rep 2015;16:146–7.

99. Luyten C, André J, Walraevens C, et al. Yellow nail syndrome and onychomycosis. Experience with itraconazole pulse therapy combined with vitamin E. Dermatology 1996;192:406–8.

100. Tunc SE, Ertam I, Pirildar T, et al. Nail changes in connective tissue diseases: do nail changes provide clues for the diagnosis? J Eur Acad Dermatol Venereol 2007;21:497–503.

101. Sherber NS, Wigley FM, Scher RK. Autoimmune disorders: nail signs and therapeutic approaches. Dermatol Ther 2007;20:17–30.

102. Marie I, Gremain V, Nassermadji K, et al. Nail involvement in systemic sclerosis. J Am Acad Dermatol 2017;76:1115–23.

103. Richert B, André J, Bourguignon R, et al. Hyperkeratotic nail discoid lupus erythematosus evolving towards systemic lupus erythematosus: therapeutic difficulties. J Eur Acad Dermatol Venereol 2004; 18:728–30.

104. Higuera V, Amezcua-Guerra LM, Montoya H, et al. Association of nail dystrophy with accrued damage and capillaroscopic abnormalities in systemic lupus erythematosus. J Clin Rheumatol 2016;22:13–8.

105. Trüeb RM. Involvement of scalp and nails in lupus erythematosus. Lupus 2010;19:1078–86.

106. Wagner C, Chasset F, Fabacher T, et al. Ungual lesions in lupus erythematosus: a literature review. Ann Dermatol Venereol 2020;147:18–28.

107. Azevedo THV, Neiva CLS, Consoli RV, et al. Pincer nail in a lupus patient. Lupus 2017;26:1562–3.

108. Skowron F, Combemale P, Faisant M, et al. Functional melanonychia due to involvement of the nail matrix in systemic lupus erythematosus. J Am Acad Dermatol 2002;47:S187–8.

109. Chong BF, Song J, Olsen NJ. Determining risk factors for developing systemic lupus erythematosus in patients with discoid lupus erythematosus. Br J Dermatol 2012;166:29–35.

110. Ekmekci TR, Ucak S, Aslan K, et al. Exaggerated cuticular changes in a patient with dermatomyositis. J Eur Acad Dermatol Venereol 2005;19:135–6.

111. Lu X, Yang H, Shu X, et al. Factors predicting malignancy in patients with polymyositis and dermatomyostis: a systematic review and meta-analysis. PLoS One 2014;9(4):e94128.

112. Gusdorf L, Morruzzi C, Goetz J, et al. Mechanics hands in patients with antisynthetase syndrome: 25 cases. Ann Dermatol Venereol 2019;146:19–25.

113. Concha JSS, Merola JF, Fiorentino D, et al. Reexamining mechanic's hands as a characteristic skin finding in dermatomyositis. J Am Acad Dermatol 2018;78:769–75.e2.

114. Bywaters EG. Peripheral vascular obstruction in rheumatoid arthritis and its relationships to other vascular lesions. Ann Rheum Dis 1957;16:84–103.

115. Chávez-López MA, Arce-Martínez FJ, Tello-Esparza A. Muehrcke lines associated to active rheumatoid arthritis. J Clin Rheumatol 2013;19: 30–1.

116. Mishra AK, George AA, George L. Yellow nail syndrome in rheumatoid arthritis: an aetiology beyond thiol drugs. Oxf Med Case Reports 2016;2016: 37–40.

117. Northrup H, Krueger DA, International Tuberous Sclerosis Complex Consensus Group. Tuberous sclerosis complex diagnostic criteria update: recommendations of the 2012 International Tuberous Sclerosis Complex Consensus Conference. Pediatr Neurol 2013;49:243–54.

118. Curatolo P, Bombardieri R, Jozwiak S. Tuberous sclerosis. Lancet 2008;372:657–68.

119. Aldrich CS, Hong CH, Groves L, et al. Acral lesions in tuberous sclerosis complex: insights into pathogenesis. J Am Acad Dermatol 2010;63:244–51.

120. Sechi A, Savoia F, Patrizi A, et al. Dermoscopy of subungual red comets associated with tuberous sclerosis complex. Pediatr Dermatol 2019;36: 408–10.

121. Bazex A, Griffiths A. Acrokeratosis paraneoplastica–a new cutaneous marker of malignancy. Br J Dermatol 1980;103:301–6.

122. Räßler F, Goetze S, Elsner P. Acrokeratosis paraneoplastica (Bazex syndrome) - a systematic review on risk factors, diagnosis, prognosis and management. J Eur Acad Dermatol Venereol 2017;31:1119–36.

123. Valdivielso M, Longo I, Suárez R, et al. Acrokeratosis paraneoplastica: Bazex syndrome. J Eur Acad Dermatol Venereol 2005;19:340–4.

124. Bolognia JL, Brewer YP, Cooper DL. Bazex syndrome (acrokeratosis paraneoplastica). An analytic review. Medicine (Baltimore) 1991;70:269–80.

125. Baran R. Paraneoplastic acrokeratosis of Bazex. Arch Dermatol 1977;113:1613.

Cutaneous Paraneoplastic Syndromes with Nail Involvement

Athina Fonia, MBBS, BSc, MRCP[a],*, Robert Baran, MD, PhD[b]

KEYWORDS

- Cutaneous paraneoplastic syndromes • Nail involvement
- Acrokeratosis paraneoplastica of Bazex and Dupré • Necrolytic migratory erythema
- Malignant acanthosis nigricans • Tripe palms • Clubbing • Acquired hypertrophic osteoarthropathy

KEY POINTS

- The cutaneous paraneoplastic syndromes are rare and intrinsically devoid of any neoplastic nature.
- The cutaneous paraneoplastic syndromes most commonly disappear after treatment of the malignancy and reappear in the case of tumor recurrence.
- Acrokeratosis paraneoplastica of Bazex and Dupré: the commonest malignancy seen is squamous cell carcinoma of the aerodigestive tract.
- Malignant acanthosis nigricans: the nails may appear with leukonychia, a pathognomonic sign.

INTRODUCTION

The cutaneous paraneoplastic syndromes are rare and intrinsically devoid of any neoplastic nature and do not originate in the skin as a direct consequence of compression or by metastasis. They are, however, due to various mechanisms caused by the tumor, either due to production of bioactive substances or in response to the tumor. They have a statistically significant association with the presence of malignancy in internal organs, which triggers several cutaneous manifestations.[1]

The time relation between the cutaneous manifestations and the responsible malignancy varies: the dermatosis may arise when the malignancy has already clearly developed and is evident, or it may be the revealing sign of small-sized tumor that has not yet manifested or may precede the onset.

These disorders evolve in parallel to the malignancy, in that, they regress when the tumor is removed and reappear in the case of tumor recurrence.

The recognition of the signs is of paramount importance, and in this article the authors present the cutaneous and nail signs of the paraneoplastic dermatoses (**Table 1**), which will lead to the early detection of cancer and therefore a better prognosis for the patient.

Dermatoses Where the Search for a Malignancy is Mandatory (The Percent with Cancer Reaches Nearly 100%)

Acrokeratosis paraneoplastica of Bazex and Dupré

Acrokeratosis paraneoplastica or acrokeratosis paraneoplastica of Bazex and Dupré is a paraneoplastic dermatosis that usually affects middle-aged men, smokers, and those with a previous alcohol dependency (**Table 2**). It may precede, accompany, and even follow the tumor.

Malignancies: it is almost always seen in squamous cell carcinomas of the upper aerodigestive tract and cervical lymphadenopathy from metastatic disease. Other malignancy associations

[a] Department of Dermatology, Queen Elizabeth Hospital, London SE18 4QH, UK; [b] Nail Disease Centre, Rue des Serbes 42, Cannes 06400, France
* Corresponding author.
E-mail address: afonia@doctors.org.uk

Dermatol Clin 39 (2021) 175–182
https://doi.org/10.1016/j.det.2020.12.003

Table 1
Cutaneous paraneoplastic syndromes, their associated malignancies, and the nail signs they present with

Paraneoplastic Syndrome	Malignancy Association	Nail Signs
Acrokeratosis paraneoplastica of Bazex and Dupré	Squamous cell carcinoma of the upper aerodigestive tract, lymphoma, multiple myeloma, lung cancer, cutaneous squamous cell carcinoma, gastric/esophageal, hepatocellular, genitourinary cancers	Dystrophic nails with subungual debris with horizontal/vertical ridging. Periungual erythematous discolouration with overlying psoriatic-like scales
Necrolytic migratory erythema (glucagonoma)	Pancreatic tumors (alpha-cell secreting)	Onychoschizia (more pronounced on the thumb and index fingers), longitudinal ridging, recurrent brittle nails *Attention*: paronychia in *benign* glucagonoma
Malignant acanthosis nigricans	Gastric adenocarcinoma mainly but less associations with ovarian, endometrial, cervical, thyroid, breast, lung, pharyngeal, renal, pancreatic, prostate cancers	Brittle nails with leukonychia. Symmetric hyperpigmented, hyperkeratotic, verrucous plaques that bestow a velvety appearance on the periungual skin
Clubbing	Lung cancer, thyroid, Hodgkin, POEMS	Clubbing
Acquired Hypertrophic Osteoarthropathy	Lung cancer (non–small cell), melanoma	Clubbing
Yellow nail syndrome	Bronchial carcinoma, non-Hodgkin lymphoma, gallbladder, melanoma, multiple myeloma	Thickened, yellow overcurved nails with smooth surface, invisible lunula, nail fold inflammation, and slow growth
Multicentric reticulohistiocytosis	Acute myeloid leukemia, liver, breast, colon, lung, thymic, melanoma, endometrial, peritoneal	"Coral beads" of papules/nodules on the periungual skin
Raynaud phenomenon	Adenocarcinoma of the lung	Acrocyanosis (painful)
Acute digital ischemia	Adenocarcinoma and squamous cell carcinoma, lymphoid neoplasia	Acrocyanosis (painful), ulceration, necrosis
Pincer nails (and alopecia)	Gastrointestinal tract cancer	Pincer nails

include small cell lung cancer, adenocarcinoma of the lung, thymus cancer, gastric/esophageal cancers cutaneous squamous cell carcinoma, multiple myeloma, lymphoma, hepatocellular carcinoma, and genitourinary cancers.[2]

Cutaneous manifestations: the lesions are usually erythematous/violaceous with overlying psoriatic-like scales not well defined, affecting the distal portion of the last phalanges of hands and feet. The acral sites are affected (**Fig. 1**A) in a symmetric fashion (helices and nose bridge) with extension to the cheeks as butterfly wings,

occasionally. This diagnosis should be considered for any acral site eruption or in patients with psoriasiform eruption that does not respond to psoriasis treatment.

Nail signs: dystrophic nails with subungual debris (**Fig. 1**B) especially on thumbs and big toes. In addition, usually only the last phalanges are involved. There may be horizontal or vertical ridging. Nail fold disease (paronychia) (**Fig. 1**C) is a prominent feature, often the first sign of nail involvement and the nonspecific pathology rules out psoriasis.

Table 2
The three main types of paraneoplastic dermatosis involving the nail

1 Dermatoses where the search for a malignancy is *mandatory.*
   - Acrokeratosis paraneoplastica of Bazex and Dupré
   - Necrolytic migratory erythema (glucagonoma)

2 Dermatoses where the search for a malignancy is *suggested*
   - Malignant acanthosis nigricans
   - Tripe palms
   - Clubbing
   - Acquired hypertrophic osteoarthropathy

3 Dermatoses where the search for a malignancy is *rare*
   - Yellow nail syndrome
   - Multicentric reticulohistiocytosis
   - Raynaud phenomenon
   - Acute digital ischemia
   - Pincer nail

Treatment: the most effective treatment is treatment of the underlying malignancy. Conservative treatment for the skin pain and pruritus.

Necrolytic migratory erythema (in glucagonoma)

Glucagonoma is a rare disorder caused by alpha-cell secreting pancreatic tumors that most commonly presents with necrolytic migratory erythema, which has a very characteristic eruption. Fever, abdominal pain, diarrhea, and weight loss may be the presenting symptoms.[3] Glucagonoma is commoner in patients with diabetes and is highly suggests a pancreatic malignancy. Half of tumors are metastatic at the time of diagnosis, with most of the cases occurring in the fifth decade; it is exceptional in children. Zinc deficiency presents with very similar intertriginous lesions, and therefore serum zinc levels should be checked in order to rule it out.

Malignancies: pancreatic alpha-cell tumors.

Cutaneous manifestations: the necrolytic migratory erythema is a distinctive pruritic, painful, bullous dermatosis that evolves over a 2-week period. It has a migrating "wood-grain" pattern, erythematous, annular, scaly rash that presents with papules, patches, and plaques with superficial necrosis leading to erosions and bullae classically located in intertriginous areas. After the vesicles and bullae rupture, they spread outward with crusting and postinflammatory hyperpigmentation. The lesions wax and wane. The distribution involves the perioral region, intergluteal region, genital area, trunk, lower extremities, and fingers. When necrolytic migratory erythema presents in patients with normal glucagon levels and the absence of glucagonoma, then inflammatory bowel disease, nonpancreatic cancers, chronic liver disease, and malabsorption disorders should be considered.

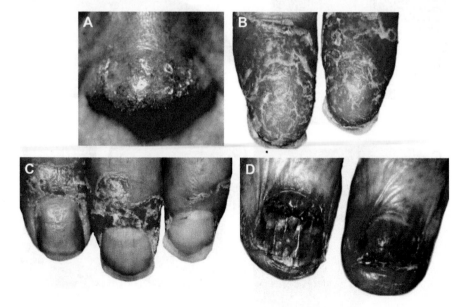

Fig. 1. Acrokeratosis paraneoplastica of Bazex and Dupré. (*A*) Involvement of the tip of the nose (acral site). (*B, C*) Psoriasiform presentation on the tips of fingers and periungual skin. (*D*) Necrolytic migratory erythema: dystrophic nails with onychoschizia and longitudinal ridging.

Nail signs: onychoschizia with lamellar splitting and irregularity of distal nail plate with longitudinal ridging of the nail surface (**Fig. 1**D) and recurrent nail fragility. The signs are more marked on the thumb and index fingers.

Attention: there is a benign variety of glucagonoma when alpha-cell pancreatic tumor is absent with normal glucagon levels and the nails present with paronychia.

Treatment: surgical debulking or excision of the pancreatic cancer may induce improvement or resolution of the clinical picture.

Dermatoses Where the Search for a Malignancy Is Suggested

Malignant acanthosis nigricans

Acanthosis nigricans is a skin condition classified into the following (see **Table 2**):

- Benign
- Malignant: usually of sudden onset with rapid progression and extensive skin involvement

It is characterized by symmetric, hyperpigmented, hyperkeratotic, verrucous plaques that bestow a velvety structure that tends to affect intertriginous areas, although any part of the body can be affected. Malignant acanthosis nigricans is the most common of paraneoplastic dermatosis in older individuals. It tends to be more pruritic and can involve the mucous membranes and lips. The mechanism postulated is that tumor-derived growth factor (especially transforming growth factor-α [TGF-α]) acts as the key cytokine to mediate epidermal cell proliferation and therefore the clinical presentation of acanthosis nigricans.

Malignancies: adenocarcinoma of the gastrointestinal tract mainly, although other tumors have been implicated (ovarian, endometrial, cervical, breast, testicular, pulmonary, renal, pancreatic, liver, esophageal, prostatic, thyroid, pharyngeal)[4] and even mucosal surfaces. Malignancy-associated acanthosis nigricans might be explained by elevated levels of growth factors such as TGF-α, which can stimulate epidermal growth factor receptor EGFR.[5]

Cutaneous manifestations: hyperpigmentation with verrucous thickening of the skin in the flexures (axillary and anogenital) with a special affinity for the umbilicus, areola of the breast, surrounding the nares and the lips as greyish and papillomatous lesions. The face, neck, hands, and feet may also be affected.

Nail signs: brittle nails with leukonychia, a pathognomonic sign (**Fig. 2**A).

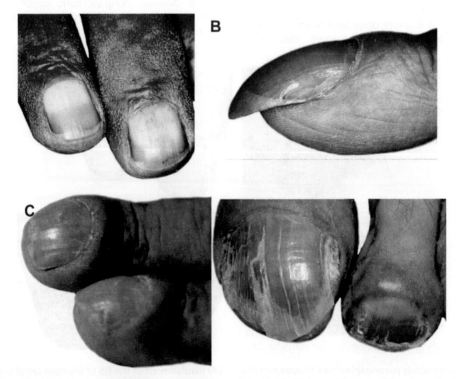

Fig. 2. Acanthosis nigricans. (*A*) Malignancy can be associated with leukonychia, a pathognomonic sign. (*B–D*) Clubbing: clubbing with transverse overcurvature with the "snake head" sign (*C*).

Treatment: treatment of the tumor improves the clinical picture.

Tripe palms

Tripe palms are a rare paraneoplastic presentation coexisting with malignant acanthosis nigricans in 75% of cases.[6] Tripe palms may precede the malignancy by many months. The cause is not clearly understood, but as acanthosis nigricans, it is thought to be due to tumor-derived substances (epidermal growth factor) to stimulate the proliferation of palmar skin cells. Only 1 in 4 cases of tripe palms is not associated with acanthosis nigricans.

Malignancies: in patients with both tripe palms and acanthosis nigricans, gastric carcinoma is the most common with lung cancer but gynecologic and urogenital malignancy can be observed. In contrast to nonmalignant acanthosis nigricans, mucous membranes (oral in particular) can be affected in more than 50%.

Cutaneous manifestations: it is characterized by thickening of the palms, with enhanced ridges and velvety brownish-yellow hyperkeratosis mimicking the mucosa of the stomach of a ruminant, and the dermatoglyphic ridges and sulci become accentuated.

Nail signs: same signs found in acanthosis nigricans, as the 2 co-exist.

Treatment: treatment of the tumor improves the clinical picture.

Clubbing (Hippocratic fingers)

Hippocrates first described digital clubbing in patients with empyema; however, it is associated with many diseases. It is classified as follows:

- Primary: idiopathic, hereditary or
- Secondary: pulmonary, cardiovascular, mediastinal, gastrointestinal, hepatobiliary, endocrine, infectious, neoplastic diseases.
- Symmetric bilaterally or unilateral or one-digit involvement only.

Clubbing is a clinical description referring to increased soft tissue between the nail bed and the bone and the subsequent loss of the angle between the nail plate and the proximal nail fold.[7] It is postulated that cytokines, especially vascular endothelial growth factor and platelet-derived growth factor from aggregated platelets and megakaryocytes, are behind the mechanism of the soft tissue swelling. Clubbing is typically painless, although it may rarely present with pain in the fingertips.

Malignancies: lung cancer[8] is the commonest, although other cancers have been implicated, such as thyroid cancer, thymus cancer, Hodgkin disease,[9] and disseminated chronic myeloid leukemia (POEMS syndrome: polyneuropathy, organomegaly, endocrinopathy, monoclonal gammopathy, and skin changes). POEMS is a rare paraneoplastic syndrome secondary to a plasma cell dyscrasia in which clubbing and white nails may be seen.[10]

Cutaneous manifestations: possible local cyanosis.

Nail signs: bird beak longitudinal exaggerated curvature (**Fig. 2**B). The following are observed:

- Transverse curvature « snake head » (**Fig. 2**C, D)
- Curth angle, normal greater than 180°, clubbing less than 160°
- Lovibond's angle, normal less than 160°, clubbing greater than 180°
- Schamroth sign: prominent angle between the distal part of the nails (with obliteration of the diamond-shaped window produced proximally when the dorsum of the fingers of each hand are opposed) (**Fig. 3**A, B)

Treatment: treatment of the underlying pathologic condition may decrease the clubbing or, potentially, reverse it, if performed early enough. Once substantial chronic tissue changes, including increased collagen deposition, have occurred, reversal is unlikely. Prognosis of the underlying disease should be determined on an individual basis.

Acquired hypertrophic osteoarthropathy (pachydermoperiostosis)

Hypertrophic osteoarthropathy presents as a primary hereditary disease (pachydermoperiostosis) or, more commonly, as secondary to several pathologies, although lung cancer is the commonest (up to 90%).[11]

Hypertrophic osteoarthropathy is a triad of the following:

- Clubbing
- Periosteal new bone formation (of the long bones)
- Arthritis (in the setting of bronchogenic carcinoma)

A complete form of hypertrophic osteoarthropathy is diagnosed when all 3 signs are present, but it can present with clubbing being absent.

Its diagnosis tends to be difficult, as it can mimic rheumatic diseases, especially rheumatoid arthritis.[12]

The radiographs show a characteristic picture, the "sunburst" or "hair-on-end" periosteal reaction, described by Ragsdale in 1981.[13]

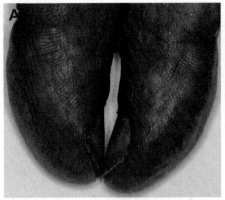
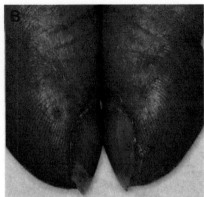
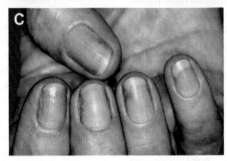

Fig. 3. (*A*): Normal nails with a diamond-shaped window. (*B*) Schamroth sign with obliteration of the diamond-shaped window. (*C*) Yellow nail syndrome.

Bone malignancies are usually located close to the knee and far from the elbow. In contrast to the primary type, epiphyses are spared in the acquired pachydermoperiostosis. Inflammation of the long bones and pain are common symptoms and may be more severe and debilitating.

Malignancies: it is most commonly associated with non–small cell lung cancer, although it may occur with metastatic melanoma and other cancers.[11]

Cutaneous manifestations: acrocyanosis.

Nail signs: clubbing stops abruptly at the distal interphalangeal joint.

Asymmetrical distribution is frequent.

Treatment: nonsteroidal antiinflammatories may help relieve symptomatic pain. The condition typically resolves on treatment of the tumor.

Dermatoses Where the Search for a Malignancy Is Rare

Yellow nail syndrome

Yellow nail syndrome is a rare disorder characterized by the triad of the following (see **Table 2**):

- Yellow nails
- Lymphedema involving mainly lower limb
- Respiratory disorders

Yellow nail syndrome (YNS) can be found by the following: systemic causes (autoimmune hypothyroidism, drugs, common variable immunodeficiency, familial) and rarely malignancy, as a paraneoplastic presentation, still controversial. The cause is unknown, but so far the following have been proposed: primarily lymphatic drainage abnormalities leading to subungual tissue sclerosis and lymphatic obstruction and secondarily microvasculopathy with the occasional dilated, tortuous capillary loops seen in nailfold capillaroscopy.[14] Recently it has been suggested[15] that titanium dioxide may be responsible for some of the cases of the formation of YNS by the release of its ions through the galvanic interaction of amalgam, gold, and oxidative stress of fluorides. Titanium dioxide is commonly found in tooth inlays/crown, joint implants, medications, cosmetics, sunscreens, and confectionaries.

Malignancies: bronchial carcinoma[16] is the commonest association with yellow nail syndrome but various others types of cancers have also been associated: breast,[17] non-Hodgkin lymphoma,[18] gallbladder,[19] melanoma,[20] multiple myeloma after hematopoietic stem-cell transplantation,[21] or precancerous mycosis fungoides.[22]

Cutaneous manifestations: symmetric and nonpitting lymphedema of mainly the lower limbs.

Nail signs: thickened nails with increased curvature on both axis, often with onycholysis and missing cuticle with nailfold inflammation being a frequent sign. The surface of the nail plate may be smooth or there may be occasional transverse ridging due to periods of growth and arrest, as the nails grow very slowly. The nails have a prominent yellow color (**Fig. 3**C) or they may have a green hue secondary to *Pseudomonas* contamination. As a result of the hyperkeratosis and yellow color the lunula becomes invisible.

Treatment: there is attenuation/resolution of the nail signs after chemotherapy; however, long-standing YNS is difficult to reverse.

Multicentric reticulohistiocytosis

Multicentric reticulohistiocytosis (MRH) is a rare disorder that affects the joints, the skin, and the mucous membranes and typically appears in the fourth decade of life. It is of unknown cause, and patients often have anemia, elevated ESR, and dyslipidemia, and there is a rare association with hypergammaglobulinemia and cryoglobulinemia. In more than half of the cases the articular disease is preceded even 3 years before the presentation on the skin.

Malignancies: malignancy is observed in 25% of MRH cases: acute myeloid leukemia, colon cancer,[23] thymic carcinoma,[24] melanoma, lung cancer, endometrial, liver, breast, peritoneal cancer[25] have been reported.

Cutaneous manifestations: the cutaneous signs are symmetric with the appearance of multiple firm, translucent, papules/nodules of erythematous/brown color that appear in a widespread fashion or are grouped and are found on the acral skin sites (head, hands) and over the joints with underlying arthropathy. The same presentation of multiple papules/nodules appears in the perioral and the perinasal areas as well as the mucosa of the nasopharynx.

Nail signs: the nails show the characteristic "coral beads," which is the array of papules/nodules on the periungual skin.

Treatment: the course of the disease does not consistently parallel the activity of the underlying malignancy.

Raynaud phenomenon

Raynaud phenomenon is a reversible episodic vasospastic disorder, is common, and has 2 clinical subtypes: the primary and the secondary. Primary Raynaud (idiopathic) is when there is no associated illness or any other cause of Raynaud phenomenon. Secondary Raynaud phenomenon occurs when the patient suffers from rheumatic diseases (ie, systemic lupus erythematosus, systemic sclerosis, mixed connective tissue disease primary Sjögren syndrome), occlusive vasculopathies, hematologic disorders, use of vibrating tools, use of some medications, and rarely a result of neoplasia (adenocarcinoma of the lung).[26,27]

Malignancies: adenocarcinoma of the lung.

Cutaneous manifestations: acrocyanosis.

Nail signs: the signs are paroxysms of painful acrocyanosis involving a few digits. There is improvement after initiation of chemotherapy.

Treatment: treatment of the cancer.

Acute digital ischemia

Acute digital ischemia is an uncommon pathology (incidence 2/100,000 people per year).[28] Inadequate blood flow to a living tissue is painful and results in disfigurement and loss of function. Arterial blood supply can be compromised by thrombosis, vasculopathy, vasculitis, trauma (hypothenar hammer syndrome), drugs (chemotherapy, cannabis) extrinsic vascular compression, or be a paraneoplastic phenomenon. Acute occurrence of digital ischemia and gangrene without pathologic laboratory findings and negative past medical history should suggest this paraneoplastic syndrome, as it could be the first presentation of an occult neoplasia.

Malignancies: digital ischemia associated with cancer is rare and is observed with adenocarcinomas[29] or other malignancies (squamous cell carcinoma and lymphoid neoplasia).[30]

Cutaneous manifestations/Nail signs: the patient presents with acrocyanosis, Raynaud phenomenon, pain, ulceration, or even necrosis.

Proposed mechanisms for the digital ischemia are hyperviscosity, hypercoagulability, tumor invasion of the sympathetic nerves, tumor-secreted substances, and immunologic mechanisms.[31]

Treatment: treatment of the tumor usually resolves the vascular involvement.

Pincer nails

A case of metastatic adenocarcinoma of the sigmoid colon manifested with pronounced pincer nails and alopecia universalis.[32]

Malignancies: gastrointestinal tract.

Cutaneous manifestations: alopecia.

Nail signs: pincer nails.

Treatment: treatment of the tumor improves the cutaneous signs.

SUMMARY

Recognizing the cutaneous paraneoplastic syndromes and their nail changes can prove vital for the patients' well-being. The manifestation of the cutaneous and nail signs before the neoplasia, as well as the early and quick diagnosis and treatment can give the patient a better prognosis and therefore good quality of life.

DISCLOSURE

The authors have nothing to disclose.

REFERENCES

1. Silva JA, Mesuita Kde C, Igreja AC, et al. Paraneoplastic cutaneous manifestations: concepts and updates. An Bras Dermatol 2013;88(1):9–22.

2. Räßler F, Goetze S, Elsner P. Acrokeratosis paraneoplastica (Bazex syndrome) - a systematic review on risk factors, diagnosis, prognosis and management. J Eur Acad Dermatol Venereol 2017;31(7):1119–36.

3. Toberer F, Hartschuh W, Wiedemeyer K. Glucagonoma-associated necrolytic migratory erythema: the broad spectrum of the clinical and histopathological findings and clues to the diagnosis. Am J Dermatopathol 2019;41(3):e29–32.

4. Rigel DS, Jacobs MI. Malignant acantosis nigricans: a review. J Dermatol Surg Oncol 1980;6:923–7.

5. Wollina U, Hansel G, Lotti T, et al. Acanthosis nigricans. A two-sided coin: consider metabolic syndrome and malignancies. Maced J Med Sci 2019. https://doi.org/10.3889/oamjms.2019.258.

6. Cohen PR, Grossman ME, Almeida L, et al. Tripe palms and malignancy. J Clin Oncol 1989;7:669–78.

7. Spicknall KE, Zirwas MJ, English JC 3rd. Clubbing: an update on diagnosis, differential diagnosis, pathophysiology and clinical relevance. J Am Acad Dermatol 2005;52(6):1020–8.

8. Sridhar KS, Lobo CF, Altman RD. Digital clubbing and lung cancer. Chest 1998;114(6):1535–7.

9. Mullins GM, Lenhard RE Jr. Digital clubbing in Hodgkin's disease. Johns Hopkins Med J 1971; 128(3):153–7.

10. Miest RY, Comfere NI, Dispenzieri A, et al. Cutaneous manifestations in patients with POEMS syndrome. Int J Dermatol 2013;52(11):1349–56.

11. Yap FY, Skalski MR, Patel DB, et al. Hypertrophic Osteoarthropathy: clinical and imaging features. Radiographics 2017;37(1):157–95.

12. Farhey Y, Luggen M. Seropositive, symmetric polyarthritis in a patient with poorly differentiated lung carcinoma: carcinomatous polyarthritis, hypertrophic osteoarthropathy, or rheumatoid arthritis? Arthritis Care Res 1998;11(2):146–9.

13. Ragsdale BD, Madewell JE, Sweet DE. Radiologic and pathologic analysis of solitary bone lesions. Part II: periosteal reactions. Radiol Clin North Am 1981;19(4):749–83.

14. Vignes S, Baran R. Yellow nail syndrome: a review. Orphanet J Rare Dis 2017;12(1):42.

15. Berglund F, Carlmark B. Titanium, sinusitis, and the yellow nail syndrome. Biol Trace Elem Res 2011;143:1–7.

16. Carnassale G, Margaritora S, Vita ML, et al. Granone PM Lung cancer in association with yellow nail syndrome. J Clin Oncol 2011;29(7):e156–8.

17. Iqbal M, Rossoff LJ, Marzouk KA, et al. Yellow nail syndrome: resolution of yellow nails after successful treatment of breast cancer. Chest 2000;117:1516–8.

18. Sève P, Thieblemont C, Dumontet C, et al. Skin lesions in malignancy. Case 3. Yellow nail syndrome in non-Hodgkin's lymphoma. J Clin Oncol 2001;19: 2100–1.

19. Burrows NP, Jones RR. Yellow nail syndrome in association with carcinoma of the gall bladder. Clin Exp Dermatol 1991;16:471–3.

20. Emerson PA. Yellow nails, lymphoedema, and pleural effusions. Thorax 1966;21:247–53.

21. Grégoire C, Guiot J, Vertenoeil G, et al. Yellow nail syndrome after allogeneic hematopoietic stem cell transplantation in two patients with multiple myeloma. Acta Clin Belg 2016;6:1–3.

22. Stosiek N, Peters KP, Hiller D, et al. Yellow nail syndrome in a patient with mycosis fungoides. J Am Acad Dermatol 1993;28:792–4.

23. Montesu MA, Onnis G, Lissia A, et al. Multicentric reticulohistiocytosis and metastatic colon carcinoma: an uncommon neoplasm recurrence manifestation. G Ital Dermatol Venereol 2018;153(3):447–9.

24. Rudha Y, Starobinska E, Abdulqader Y, et al. Multicentric reticulohistiocytosis associated with thymic carcinoma. Rheumatology (Oxford) 2017;56(10): 1706.

25. Sanchez-Alvarez C, Sandhu AS, Crowson CS, et al. Multicentric reticulohistiocytosis: the Mayo Clinic experience (1980-2017. Rheumatology (Oxford) 2019. https://doi.org/10.1093/rheumatology/kez555 [pii: kez555].

26. Sutić A, Gračanin G, Morović-Vergles J. Raynaud's phenomenon - first sign of malignancy: case report. Acta Med Croatica 2014;68(3):295–8.

27. Madabhavi I, Revannasiddaiah S, Rastogi M, et al. Paraneoplastic Raynaud's phenomenon manifesting before the diagnosis of lung cancer. BMJ Case Rep 2012;2012 [pii:bcr0320125985].

28. Poszepczynska-Guigné E, Viguier M, Chosidow O, et al. Paraneoplastic acral vascular syndrome: epidemiologic features, clinical manifestations, and disease sequelae. J Am Acad Dermatol 2002; 47(1):47–52.

29. Mahler V, Neureiter D, Kirchner T, et al. Digital ischemia as paraneoplastic marker of metastatic endometrial carcinoma. Hautarzt 1999;50(10): 748–52.

30. Le Besnerais M, Miranda S, Cailleux N, et al. Digital ischemia associated with cancer: results from a cohort study. Medicine (Baltimore) 2014;93(10): e47.

31. Gambichler T, Strutzmann S, Tannapfel A, et al. Paraneoplastic acral vascular syndrome in a patient with metastatic melanoma under immune checkpoint blockade. BMC Cancer 2017;17(1):327.

32. Jemec GB, Thomsen K. Pincer nails and alopecia as markers of gastrointestinal malignancy. J Dermatol 1997;24(7):479–81.

Nail Psoriasis in Older Adults
Epidemiology, Diagnosis, and Topical Therapy

Jose W. Ricardo, MD[a], Shari R. Lipner, MD, PhD[b],*

KEYWORDS

- Nails • Nail psoriasis • Psoriatic arthritis • Quality of life • Onycholysis • Subungual hyperkeratosis
- Elderly • Older adults

KEY POINTS

- Psoriasis is a prevalent in older adults, and nail involvement is common in patients with skin disease, especially when psoriatic arthritis is present.
- Diagnosing nail psoriasis in elderly individuals may be challenging because physiologic age-related nail changes are common.
- Because nail psoriasis may have less impact on quality of life in the elderly population compared with the general population, a more conservative treatment approach may be considered.
- General nail care measures and precautions are of utmost importance in nail psoriasis treatment; Koebner's phenomenon may exacerbate signs and symptoms.
- Topical therapy for nail psoriasis avoids systemic toxicity, but efficacy is limited, and compliance may be decreased in elderly individuals secondary to mental and/or physical disabilities.

INTRODUCTION

Psoriasis is a common chronic inflammatory condition that causes significant morbidity with a substantial negative effect on quality of life (QOL).[1] The worldwide prevalence is 0.09% to 5.10%, with a higher prevalence in geographic regions more distant from the equator.[2] There is a bimodal incidence distribution, with peaks at 30 to 39 years of age, and secondary peaks at 50 to 59 or 60 to 69 years of age.[3] Therefore, psoriasis is an important condition in older adults.

Psoriasis often presents with well-demarcated, erythematous plaques with silvery scales primarily located on extensor surfaces; some patients may have scalp, joint, and nail involvement, even in the absence of skin lesions. About 40.9% of patients with cutaneous psoriasis also present with nail involvement, and men are 11.2% more frequently affected than women.[4] There is a positive association between nail involvement and a longer disease duration, greater disease severity, and a greater frequency of psoriatic arthritis, as well as scalp and palmoplantar psoriasis, and greater impairment in QOL.[4,5] It is estimated that 80% to 90% of patients with psoriasis will present with nail involvement at some point during their lifetime, 5% of patients present with isolated nail involvement, and up to 85.7% of patients with psoriatic arthritis present concomitant nail disease.[4,6,7]

[a] Department of Dermatology, Weill Cornell Medicine, New York, NY, USA; [b] Department of Dermatology, Weill Cornell Medicine, 1305 York Avenue, New York, NY 10021, USA
* Corresponding author.
E-mail address: shl9032@med.cornell.edu

Dermatol Clin 39 (2021) 183–193
https://doi.org/10.1016/j.det.2020.12.011

EPIDEMIOLOGY OF NAIL PSORIASIS IN THE ELDERLY

Most studies have not demonstrated a correlation between advanced age or age of psoriasis onset and the presence of nail psoriasis. Nail involvement was assessed in a retrospective study of 4049 psoriatic patients, 129 of whom had disease onset after 60 years of age, and nail involvement was present in 27.9% of these patients.[8] Notably, nail involvement was less common in the group with age of onset after 60 years compared with the group with age of onset before 60 years, but the difference was not statistically significant ($P>.005$).[8] Similarly, in a cross-sectional study on 228 psoriatic patients, no significant correlation was observed between age of psoriasis onset and number of affected nails.[9] Furthermore, in a survey-based study of 1728 psoriatic patients, there was no correlation between age and the presence of nail psoriasis.[10] In a retrospective review of 3615 patients with psoriasis, nail involvement was more frequent in those 35 to 64 years (55.5%; $P\leq.001$) compared with groups aged 18 to 34 years and those 65 years or older.[11] Patients aged 35 to 64 years also had more nails involved (6.9 ± 3.3) compared with the remaining groups, but this difference was not statistically significant.[11]

In 1 study, there was a correlation between advancing age and the presence of nail psoriasis. In a cross-sectional study of 410 patients with psoriasis, nail changes were more common in those with psoriasis for 5 years or more compared with patients who had psoriasis for less than 5 years, and in patients 50 years or older compared with those aged less than 50 years. However, the subset of patients 65 and older was not analyzed specifically.[12]

CLINICAL AND HISTOLOGIC PRESENTATION OF PSORIATIC NAILS IN THE ELDERLY

A diagnosis of nail psoriasis in older adults is challenging because there are many physiologic nail changes in this population that may resemble or confound the diagnosis. Nail plate color often changes from a pale pink to a yellow, white, or gray; and a "Napolitan" nail plate pattern, with an absence of the lunula, a white appearance of the proximal one-half of the nail, a pink band, and an opaque free edge of the nail, has been described.[13,14] Older patients may also develop multiple transverse white bands or longitudinal dark bands.[15,16] Additional changes include a slower nail growth rate, thickening of toenails and thinning of fingernails, increased transverse

curvature of the toenails, flattening of fingernails in the transverse and longitudinal directions, longitudinal ridging, horizontal peeling of layers, and an increased incidence of brittle nails and overall fragility of the nail plate.[17–22] In a prospective study conducted on 400 healthy patients, one-half of whom were 60 years and older, nail changes including pale, dull, opaque, and lusterless nails; brittle nails; decreased lunula visibility; and onychorrhexis were significantly more prevalent in the older age group compared with those less than 60 years of age.[23]

The clinical presentation of nail psoriasis in older adults seems to be similar to that of younger populations; however, the available data are limited. For all ages, fingernails are more frequently affected than toenails, and nail changes may be more common in individuals who have had psoriasis for longer duration, from 5.0 to 11.5 years.[12,24–26] Nail matrix psoriasis presents with nail pitting, leukonychia, and red spots in lunula, whereas nail bed psoriasis shows onycholysis, oil drops, splinter hemorrhages, and nail bed hyperkeratosis.[24,27,28] Additional findings include transverse grooves, paronychia, and crumbling of the nail plate.[17] In 1 study of 410 patients with psoriasis, the most common nail changes were pitting (67.5%) and onycholysis (67.2%), followed by nail dystrophy (35.0%), subungual hyperkeratosis (24.7%), discoloration (18.4%), nail loss (2.8%), and pustulation (1.3%) (**Fig. 1**).[12] In a retrospective study on 400 healthy patients, the most common nail changes in patients aged 60 and older were nail pitting (2.5%), followed by onychauxis, onychomadesis, onycholysis, and transverse ridging.[23]

Histopathologically, age-related nail changes include larger nail plate keratinocytes, an increase in the number of pertinax bodies, increased carbon and decreased nitrogen content, thickening of the blood vessels, and degeneration of the

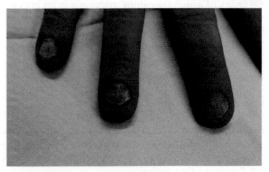

Fig. 1. Sixty-seven-year-old male patient with nail pitting, leukonychia and onycholysis of his right third, fourth, and fifth fingernails.

elastic tissue.[21,29,30] Nonetheless, there are no data regarding specific histopathologic features of nail psoriasis in the elderly. In a prospective study of 60 patients ages 18 to 70 years (mean, 39.7 ± 14.63 years), with clinical examination consistent with nail psoriasis, the most common histologic features were hyperkeratosis and parakeratosis (78.3%), neutrophils (63.3%), hypergranulosis (58.3%), psoriasiform hyperplasia (53.3%), dilated capillaries (46.6%), and serum exudates (43.3%).[31]

IMPACT ON QUALITY OF LIFE IN THE ELDERLY

Nail psoriasis has been shown to greatly impact patients' QOL, including physical symptoms, psychological burden, and restricting of daily activities and employment.[10] It may present in highly visible locations, particularly the fingernails, which has a detrimental cosmetic effect and exacerbates its psychological burden. In a survey-based study of 2449 psoriatic patients using the Dermatology Life Quality Index, those with nail involvement had a higher impairment of QOL compared with those without nail involvement (7.2 vs 5.3; $P \leq .001$).[32] Similarly, in another survey-based study on 5400 patients with psoriasis, nail psoriasis more significantly impacted QOL ($P \leq .001$) and correlated with more severe cutaneous disease compared with patients with psoriasis without nail involvement ($P \leq .001$).[33] In addition, the coexistence of nail bed and matrix disease more greatly affected QOL compared with patients with involvement of 1 of the 2 exclusively ($P = .003$), and patients with nail bed features alone presented with greater QOL impairment when compared with patients with nail matrix features alone.[33] Nail psoriasis impairs functionality most in putting on shoes or socks (21.2% and 25.1%, respectively) and household activities.[33] Nail psoriasis may also cause pain in up to 35.8% of patients, which may further compromise QOL.[33]

Nonetheless, the impact of nail psoriasis on QOL may be less significant with advancing age.[34] In a survey-based study (n = 1111) using the Dermatology Life Quality Index, there was a negative correlation between age and QOL impairment in patients with nail psoriasis.[34] The Dermatology Life Quality Index scores were significantly higher for those 39 years or younger (9.4), followed by individuals 40 to 54 years (9.2), 55 to 64 years (7.8), and those 65 years and older (6.7) ($P<.0001$).[34] Although further research is needed, existing data suggest that more conservative treatment may be indicated in elderly patients with nail psoriasis with a minimal impact on QOL.

TREATMENT OF NAIL PSORIASIS IN THE ELDERLY

Inarguably, treatment should be individualized according to individual patient needs. The extent of skin, nail, and joint involvement must be considered, as well as the patient's concerns, functionality, and support network. The elderly may pose greater challenges in this regard than younger populations, because advanced age often correlates with physical disabilities, including poor sight, coordination, flexibility, and dexterity. For instance, a patient with nail psoriasis ideally limited to a few digits would benefit from topical treatment as first-line management; however, elderly patients with a physical disability may have difficulty applying topicals to fingernails, and even more difficulty with toenails, limiting compliance. In addition, some older individuals may feel that their nail disease does not greatly impact their QOL. For these patients, the pros and cons of treatment must be balanced, and expectant management may be appropriate in the absence of joint involvement.[27]

The presence of onychomycosis should be ruled out when nail psoriasis is suspected, because an overlapping presentation may occur and fungal infection may exacerbate psoriatic nail changes.[35] Furthermore, the prevalence of onychomycosis increases with age, and psoriatic patients may be 50% more likely to develop onychomycosis.[36,37]

Regardless of the treatment modality, it is important to educate patients on general nail care measures and precautions to prevent further damage to their nails. As with cutaneous psoriasis, nail changes have strongly been linked to Koebner's phenomenon.[38] Therefore, patients are counseled to avoid manicures, nail biting, nail picking, and wearing tight-fitting shoewear.[27] Additionally, special precautions such as wearing protective gloves are recommended with intensive manual labor or prolonged exposure to chemical solvents and wet work.[27] In general, applying emollients to nails and trimming them regularly is advised to prevent further damage, and a nail lacquer may improve the cosmetic appearance by partially concealing discoloration and superficial irregularities.[27]

There are a variety of therapeutic options for nail psoriasis. Modalities can be broadly classified into topical therapy, intralesional therapy, and systemic therapy, including immunotherapy with biologic agents.[27] Combined therapy targeting different disease pathways is often required for efficacy.[24]

TOPICAL THERAPY

Success in treating nail psoriasis with topical agents depends on the penetrability of the agent to the site of inflammation. Therefore, special consideration should be given to distinguishing nail matrix and nail bed features.[39] A recent expert panel consensus provided recommendations for the treatment of nail psoriasis with limited or no skin involvement and 3 or fewer nails affected, classifying according to the presence of nail matrix or bed features, or both.[40] Among the recommendations, the combination of topical superpotent steroids and vitamin D analogues (ie, clobetasol propionate and calcipotriene) should be considered as a first-line treatment for patients with nail matrix features exclusively, as an alternative to intralesional steroids injections.[40] For these patients, second-line treatment includes topical steroids, topical vitamin D analogues, combinations of topical D analogues with topical steroids, topical retinoids, topical keratolytic agents (ie, urea nail lacquer, salicylic acid), or topical 0.1% tacrolimus ointment.[40] When signs of nail matrix psoriasis are present, the topical agent is applied directly to the proximal nail fold.[39,41] For patients with 3 or fewer nails affected and nail bed features alone, the panel favored the use of topical alternatives as mentioned (except keratolytic agents), as first-line treatment (**Fig. 2**). In cases where both the nail matrix and the nail bed are involved, the combination of superpotent steroids and calcipotriene may or may not be added to intralesional steroid injections as a first-line treatment.[40] Topicals may also be considered based on patients' preferences or when other treatment alternatives are contraindicated.[42] Clipping the onycholytic nail plate enhances penetrability for nail bed disease.[39,40]

The existing evidence regarding efficacy of topical therapeutic agents used in nail psoriasis is summarized in **Table 1**. It is important to mention that the studies included in this analysis only provide mean ages and age ranges, or one of them exclusively, in the vast majority of studies.

Therefore, larger randomized controlled studies on topical therapy for nail psoriasis in older individuals are needed to make strong evidence-based recommendations.

TOPICAL CORTICOSTEROIDS

Topical corticosteroids are the most frequently used topical medications for the treatment of nail psoriasis. A variety of formulations are available including ointments, creams, emulsions, lotions and nail lacquers, and they are usually applied once or twice daily. Topical steroids are often prescribed as combination therapy with other topical or systemic medications; thus, studies assessing their efficacy as monotherapy are sparse. A study of patients with nail psoriasis (mean age, 48.4 years; range, 25.0–81.0 years) who were treated with 8% clobetasol in a lacquer vehicle applied once daily for 21 days and then twice weekly for 9 months, showed improvement in onycholysis, pitting, and salmon patches in 9 of the 10 patients as early as 4 weeks after the initiation of treatment, with a more marked improvement at the end of the study.[43] Pain disappeared after 4 weeks of treatment in the 3 patients who reported this symptom at baseline.[43] Similarly, a randomized controlled trial (RCT) on 15 patients with nail psoriasis (mean age, 48.7 years; range, 26–76 years) assessing the efficacy of 0.05%, 1.00%, and 8.00% clobetasol nail lacquer applied twice weekly for 16 weeks showed a 51.5% decrease in the Nail Psoriasis Severity Index (NAPSI) score for all 3 groups combined ($P = .0001$).[44] The group receiving 8% clobetasol had the greatest improvement, which was not statistically significant. An RCT (n = 30) comparing tazarotene 0.10% cream with clobetasol propionate 0.05% cream under occlusion once daily for 12 weeks for the treatment of nail psoriasis showed significant improvement in pitting,

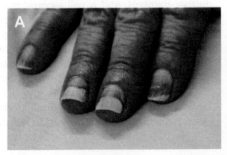
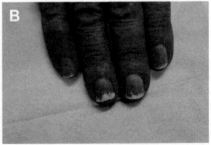

Fig. 2. A 74-year-old female patient showing mainly nail bed psoriasis features, including onycholysis, salmon spots and subungual hyperkeratosis on her right second, third, and fourth fingernails. (*A*) Before treatment (June 2018). (*B*) After treatment (August 2018) with betamethasone ointment applied nightly to the nail bed after clipping off the onycholytic part of the nail plate, under occlusion.

Table 1
Studies on topical therapies for the treatment of nail psoriasis

Author, Year	Number of Patients	Age Range (y)	Mean Age (y)	Medication	Dosage Regimen	Outcome Measure	Clinical Result
Scher et al,[51] 2001	31 (21 tazarotene, 10 vehicle)	Unknown	43	Tazarotene 0.1% gel	Nightly for up to 24 weeks; 1 target nail occluded, 1 nonoccluded	Visual Assessment Score	Treatment with tazarotene showed a favorable response over placebo in reducing onycholysis in occluded and unoccluded nails. In occluded nails, tazarotene was also more effective than placebo in reducing pitting.
Bianchi et al,[52] 2003	35 (25 completed)	22–66	Unknown	Tazarotene 0.1% gel	Nightly for 12 wk		19/25 showed good clinical response at week 12.
Rigopoulos et al,[45] 2007	46 (23 tazarotene, 16 completed, 23 clobetasol, 14 completed)	Unknown	Unknown	Tazarotene 0.1% cream or clobetasol propionate 0.05% cream	Nightly under occlusion for 12 wk	NAPSI	Significant time-effect improvement in all NAPSI parameters (pitting, onycholysis, hyperkeratosis and salmon patches) for both treatments. There were no significant differences between the 2 treatments.
Sanchez Regana et al,[43] 2005	10	25–81	48.4	8% clobetasol-17-propionate lacquer	Daily for 21 d, then twice a week for 9 mo		9/10 patients showed good clinical response. Among clinical signs, onycholysis, pitting and salmon patches showed best improvement. Complete resolution of pain after 4 wk.
Nakamura et al,[44] 2012	15	26–76	48.7	0.05%, 1.00%, or 8.00% clobetasol nail lacquer	Twice a week for 16 wk	Modified NAPSI	Improvement of 51.5% in all groups. Improvement was not significant at the 5% level for the individual groups.

(continued on next page)

Table 1
(continued)

Author, Year	Number of Patients	Age Range (y)	Mean Age (y)	Medication	Dosage Regimen	Outcome Measure	Clinical Result
Rigopoulos et al,[49] 2002	62 (60 completed; 48 fingernails, 53 toenails)	Unknown	48.4	Clobetasol propionate cream, calcipotriol cream	Clobetasol propionate twice a week (on weekends) for 6 mo, then twice a week for a further 6 mo; calcipotriol nightly 5 times/wk (during weekdays) for 6 mo		Reduction in mean thickness of hyperkeratosis: at 2 mo, 35.2% of fingernails, 32.6% of toenails; at 6 mo, 72.3% of fingernails, 69.9% of toenails; at 12 mo, 81.2% of fingernails, 72.5% of toenails.
Tosti et al,[47] 1998	58 (total); 29 calcipotriol (23 completed), 29 betamethasone + salicylic acid (21 completed)	Unknown	51.8	Either calcipotriol ointment (50 μg/g) or betamethasone dipropionate (64 mg/g) + salicylic acid (0.03 g/g) ointment	Twice daily for 3 mo (5 mo for responders)		Eight of 23 patients given calcipotriol and 10/21 patients in the betamethasone + salicylic acid showed a >50% improvement in fingernail subungual hyperkeratosis. Subungual hyperkeratosis showed 40.7% and 51.9% improvements in toenails in the calcipotriol and betamethasone + salicylic acid, respectively, by the end of the fifth month.
Tzung et al,[50] 2008	40 (32 completed)	Unknown	53.2	Group A: 0.005% calcipotriol + 0.05% betamethasone	Group A: daily for 12 wk Group B:	Investigator's global assessment, NAPSI	Of patients treated with either group, 53% showed at least moderate improvement using the investigator's

Study	No. of patients	Age	Mean age	Treatment	Dosing	Assessment	Results
				dipropionate ointment; group B: 0.005% calcipotriol ointment	twice daily for 12 wk		global assessment. Reduction in NAPSI was noted for both groups. Differences between groups were not significant.
Cannavò et al,[54] 2003	16 (8 in the treatment group and 8 in the placebo group)	46–80	61.1	70 mg/mL maize-oil-dissolved oral cyclosporine solution	Twice daily for 12 wk	Clinical Assessment of Nail Involvement and Efficacy	A 70% improvement was seen in the treatment group, and 12% improvement in the placebo group. Best results were obtained in onycholysis and hyperkeratosis.
De Simone et al,[55] 2013	21 (20 patients completed)	Unknown	44.3	Tacrolimus 0.1% ointment	Nightly without occlusion for 12 wk	NAPSI, target NAPSI	Improvement of 57% and 67% in the NAPSI, and target NAPSI scores. Similar improvement between nail bed and matrix features was noted.

Abbreviations: NAPSI, Nail Psoriasis Severity Index; target NAPSI, Nail Psoriasis Severity Index of one target nail.
Data from Refs.[43–45,47,49–52,54,55]

onycholysis, hyperkeratosis, and salmon patches in both groups.[45] Only mild side effects (desquamation, erythema, and irritation of surrounding skin) were reported by 18.8% of patients.[45] The combination of topical steroids and keratolytic agents for the treatment of psoriatic nails has also been used with relatively good success. Steroids may be helpful in decreasing the inflammation caused by keratolytic agents, while at the same time enhancing the therapeutic response by targeting different disease pathways.[46] In 1 study involving 44 patients with nail psoriasis (mean age, 51.8 years) with nail bed findings, the application of betamethasone dipropionate (64 mg/g) and salicylic acid (0.03 g/g) ointment was compared with calcipotriol ointment (50 μg/g) applied twice daily for 3 to 5 months.[47] Subungual hyperkeratosis of the fingernails and toenails showed improvement (20%–30% after 3 months) with both treatments, with a slightly more marked improvement in the group receiving clobetasol dipropionate and salicylic acid, although the difference was not statistically significant.[47] The overall safety profile of superpotent topical steroids for nail psoriasis is favorable, with only mild side effects reported.

COMBINATION THERAPY WITH VITAMIN D₃ ANALOGS

Combination therapy with topical steroids and vitamin D_3 analogs is often used to treat nail psoriasis. Vitamin D_3 analogs regulate epidermal cell proliferation and differentiation, and are also anti-inflammatory.[48] Sixty patients with psoriasis (mean age, 48.4 years) with nail findings were treated using calcipotriol cream 5 times per week at night (on weekdays), and clobetasol propionate was applied twice weekly (on weekends) for 6 months; patients then applied clobetasol propionate cream for another 6 months.[49] At 12 months, there was an 81.2% and 72.5% mean decrease in hyperkeratosis of the fingernails and toenails, respectively.[49] In another nail psoriasis study (mean age, 53.2 years), calcipotriol (0.005%) plus betamethasone dipropionate (0.050%) ointment applied once daily was compared with calcipotriol (0.005%) ointment as monotherapy applied twice daily for 12 weeks.[50] Of the patients in both groups, 53% showed at least moderate improvement in the investigator's global assessment, and overall improvement in the NAPSI score ($P \leq .045$).[50] Combining topical steroids and vitamin D_3 analogs is an effective and safe alternative for the treatment of nail psoriasis, with only 2 patients reporting mild side effects (a burning sensation).[49]

TAZAROTENE

Tazarotene under occlusion has good efficacy as a topical treatment for psoriatic nails. Tazarotene 0.1% gel was applied to 2 nails, 1 under occlusion and 1 unoccluded, nightly for 24 weeks for the treatment of nail psoriasis in an RCT (n = 21 patients; mean age, 43 years).[51] Unoccluded nails showed improvement in onycholysis, whereas occluded nails showed improvement in onycholysis and pitting ($P \leq .05$).[51] Five patients reported mild side effects, including irritation, erythema, or peeling of the surrounding skin.[51] One open, prospective study involving 25 psoriatic patients (age range, 22–66 years) with nail findings assessed the efficacy of tazarotene 0.1% applied nightly (unoccluded) to fingernails and toenails for 12 weeks.[52] Nineteen patients showed a good clinical response with better and more rapid improvement in hyperkeratosis and oil spots, whereas nail pitting was more persistent.[52] Mild erythema, peeling, and burning were reported as side effects of therapy.[52] Tazarotene is tolerable, with only mild side effects reported (peeling, erythema, and burning of the surrounding skin); nonetheless, tazarotene seems to lack efficacy in treating nail matrix psoriasis, limiting its clinical usefulness.

TOPICAL CALCINEURIN INHIBITORS

The inhibition of the serine–threonine protein phosphatase calcineurin suppresses the activity of the genes that code for IL-2, causing suppression of T-cell activation.[53] Topical cyclosporine and tacrolimus are the most frequently used calcineurin inhibitors for the treatment of nail psoriasis; however, there are few data. One RCT involving 16 patients with nail psoriasis (mean age, 61.1 years; range, 46.0–80.0 years) showed improvement in nail findings after 12 weeks of treatment with a 70 mg/mL maize-oil–dissolved oral cyclosporine solution applied twice daily.[54] The treatment group showed 77% improvement, whereas patients in the placebo group (maize oil alone) showed 12% improvement.[54] Onycholysis and hyperkeratosis improved most dramatically, although improvement was also noted in pitting, oil drops, and nail crumbling.[54] Tacrolimus was used without occlusion nightly in a 12-week RCT involving 21 patients with nail psoriasis (mean age, 44.3 years).[55] At the end of the study, there was a mean decrease of 57% and 67% in the NAPSI and target NAPSI scores, respectively.[55] A similar improvement in nail matrix and bed signs was noted.[55] Acute paronychia was the only adverse effect reported by 1 patient.[55]

The treatment of nail psoriasis with calcineurin inhibitors is highly tolerable, and only mild side effects have been reported. These medications may be considered when there are concerns about skin atrophy secondary to steroid use or irritation caused by keratolytic agents. However, compared with topical corticosteroids, topical calcineurin inhibitors have a lower skin penetrance because of their lipophilic nature; thus, their efficacy in treating nail psoriasis is likely compromised.[56]

SUMMARY

Even with reliable application, success with topical treatment is low. Compliance is difficult to achieve with topical nail psoriasis regimens, and it may be further compromised in the elderly owing to physical and/or mental limitations. Additionally, physiologic nail changes inherent to advanced age may also influence efficacy of topicals in this population. Older adults are likely under-represented in nail psoriasis studies to date. More extensive RCT are needed in this population to make more evidence-based treatment guidelines.

CLINICS CARE POINTS

- Diagnosis of nail psoriasis in older adults is challenging due to physiologic nail changes that are common in this population.
- Impact on quality of life is an important consideration in deciding on optimal treatment for nail psoriasis.
- Assessment of functionality, support network and disease severity is necessary before prescribing topical treatment for nail psoriasis.

DISCLOSURE

Dr J.W. Ricardo and Dr S.R. Lipner have no conflicts of interest relevant to the content of the submission. Funding sources: none. No reprints requested. This work has not been previously published or presented.

REFERENCES

1. Stern RS, Nijsten T, Feldman SR, et al. Psoriasis is common, carries a substantial burden even when not extensive, and is associated with widespread treatment dissatisfaction. J Investig Dermatol Symp Proc 2004;9(2):136–9.
2. Michalek IM, Loring B, John SM. A systematic review of worldwide epidemiology of psoriasis. J Eur Acad Dermatol Venereol 2017;31(2):205–12.
3. Parisi R, Symmons DP, Griffiths CE, et al. Identification, Management of P, et al. Global epidemiology of psoriasis: a systematic review of incidence and prevalence. J Invest Dermatol 2013;133(2):377–85.
4. Augustin M, Reich K, Blome C, et al. Nail psoriasis in Germany: epidemiology and burden of disease. Br J Dermatol 2010;163(3):580–5.
5. Callis Duffin K, Mason MA, Gordon K, et al. Characterization of patients with psoriasis in challenging-to-treat body areas in the corrona psoriasis registry. Dermatology 2020;1–10. https://doi.org/10.1159/000504841.
6. Brazzelli V, Carugno A, Alborghetti A, et al. Prevalence, severity and clinical features of psoriasis in fingernails and toenails in adult patients: Italian experience. J Eur Acad Dermatol Venereol 2012; 26(11):1354–9.
7. Salomon J, Szepietowski JC, Proniewicz A. Psoriatic nails: a prospective clinical study. J Cutan Med Surg 2003;7(4):317–21.
8. Kwon HH, Kwon IH, Youn JI. Clinical study of psoriasis occurring over the age of 60 years: is elderly-onset psoriasis a distinct subtype? Int J Dermatol 2012;51(1):53–8.
9. Kyriakou A, Patsatsi A, Sotiriadis D. Detailed analysis of specific nail psoriasis features and their correlations with clinical parameters: a cross-sectional study. Dermatology 2011;223(3):222–9.
10. de Jong EM, Seegers BA, Gulinck MK, et al. Psoriasis of the nails associated with disability in a large number of patients: results of a recent interview with 1,728 patients. Dermatology 1996;193(4): 300–3.
11. Trettel A, Spehr C, Korber A, et al. The impact of age on psoriasis health care in Germany. J Eur Acad Dermatol Venereol 2017;31(5):870–5.
12. Tham SN, Lim JJ, Tay SH, et al. Clinical observations on nail changes in psoriasis. Ann Acad Med Singap 1988;17(4):482–5.
13. Murdan S. Nail disorders in older people, and aspects of their pharmaceutical treatment. Int J Pharm 2016;512(2):405–11.
14. Horan MA, Puxty JA, Fox RA. The white nails of old age (Neapolitan nails). J Am Geriatr Soc 1982; 30(12):734–7.
15. Baran R. Frictional longitudinal melanonychia: a new entity. Dermatologica 1987;174(6):280–4.
16. Baran R, Perrin C. Transverse leukonychia of toenails due to repeated microtrauma. Br J Dermatol 1995;133(2):267–9.
17. Rich PA, Scher RK. An Atlas of Diseases of the Nail2003.
18. Hamilton JB, Terada H, Mestler GE. Studies of growth throughout the lifespan in Japanese: growth and size of nails and their relationship to age, sex, heredity, and other factors. J Gerontol 1955;10(4): 401–15.
19. Baran R. Nail care in the "golden years' of life. Curr Med Res Opin 1982;7(Suppl 2):95–7.

20. Cohen PR, Scher RK. Geriatric nail disorders: diagnosis and treatment. J Am Acad Dermatol 1992; 26(4):521–31.

21. Lewis BL, Montgomery H. The senile nail. J Invest Dermatol 1955;24(1):11–8.

22. Chessa MA, Iorizzo M, Richert B, et al. Pathogenesis, clinical signs and treatment recommendations in brittle nails: a review. Dermatol Ther (Heidelb) 2020;10(1):15–27.

23. El-Domyati M, Abdel-Wahab H, Abdel-Azim E. Nail changes and disorders in elderly Egyptians. J Cosmet Dermatol 2014;13(4):269–76.

24. Jiaravuthisan MM, Sasseville D, Vender RB, et al. Psoriasis of the nail: anatomy, pathology, clinical presentation, and a review of the literature on therapy. J Am Acad Dermatol 2007;57(1):1–27.

25. van der Velden HM, Klaassen KM, van de Kerkhof PC, et al. Fingernail psoriasis reconsidered: a case-control study. J Am Acad Dermatol 2013; 69(2):245–52.

26. Klaassen KM, van de Kerkhof PC, Pasch MC. Nail psoriasis: a questionnaire-based survey. Br J Dermatol 2013;169(2):314–9.

27. Tan ES, Chong WS, Tey HL. Nail psoriasis: a review. Am J Clin Dermatol 2012;13(6):375–88.

28. Rich P, Scher RK. Nail Psoriasis Severity Index: a useful tool for evaluation of nail psoriasis. J Am Acad Dermatol 2003;49(2):206–12.

29. Germann H, Barran W, Plewig G. Morphology of corneocytes from human nail plates. J Invest Dermatol 1980;74(3):115–8.

30. Dittmar M, Dindorf W, Banerjee A. Organic elemental composition in fingernail plates varies between sexes and changes with increasing age in healthy humans. Gerontology 2008;54(2):100–5.

31. Kaul S, Singal A, Grover C, et al. Clinical and histological spectrum of nail psoriasis: a cross-sectional study. J Cutan Pathol 2018;45(11):824–30.

32. Radtke MA, Langenbruch AK, Schafer I, et al. Nail psoriasis as a severity indicator: results from the PsoReal study. Patient Relat Outcome Meas 2011;2:1–6.

33. Klaassen KM, van de Kerkhof PC, Pasch MC. Nail Psoriasis, the unknown burden of disease. J Eur Acad Dermatol Venereol 2014;28(12):1690–5.

34. Taieb C, Corvest M, Voisard J, et al. PSN16 Nail psoriasis: impact on quality of life. Poster session presented at: ISPOR Eighth Annual European Congress; Florence, Italy: Value in Health; 2005; 8(6):A147.

35. Crowley JJ, Weinberg JM, Wu JJ, et al. Treatment of nail psoriasis: best practice recommendations from the Medical Board of the National Psoriasis Foundation. JAMA Dermatol 2015;151(1):87–94.

36. Polat M, Ilhan MN. Dermatological complaints of the elderly attending a dermatology outpatient clinic in turkey: a prospective study over a one-year period. Acta Dermatovenerol Croat 2015;23(4):277–81.

37. Lipner SR, Scher RK. Onychomycosis: clinical overview and diagnosis. J Am Acad Dermatol 2019; 80(4):835–51.

38. Ghosal A, Gangopadhyay DN, Chanda M, et al. Study of nail changes in psoriasis. Indian Journal of Dermatology; 2004;49(1):18.

39. Pasch MC. Nail psoriasis: a review of treatment options. Drugs 2016;76(6):675–705.

40. Rigopoulos D, Baran R, Chiheb S, et al. Recommendations for the definition, evaluation, and treatment of nail psoriasis in adult patients with no or mild skin psoriasis: a dermatologist and nail expert group consensus. J Am Acad Dermatol 2019;81(1):228–40.

41. Piraccini BM, Starace M. Optimal management of nail disease in patients with psoriasis. Psoriasis (Auckl) 2015;5:25–33.

42. Bardazzi F, Starace M, Bruni F, et al. Nail psoriasis: an updated review and expert opinion on available treatments, including biologics. Acta Derm Venereol 2019;99(6):516–23.

43. Sanchez Regana M, Martin Ezquerra G, Umbert Millet P, et al. Treatment of nail psoriasis with 8% clobetasol nail lacquer: positive experience in 10 patients. J Eur Acad Dermatol Venereol 2005;19(5):573–7.

44. Nakamura RC, Abreu L, Duque-Estrada B, et al. Comparison of nail lacquer clobetasol efficacy at 0.05%, 1% and 8% in nail psoriasis treatment: prospective, controlled and randomized pilot study. An Bras Dermatol 2012;87(2):203–11.

45. Rigopoulos D, Gregoriou S, Katsambas A. Treatment of psoriatic nails with tazarotene cream 0.1% vs. clobetasol propionate 0.05% cream: a double-blind study. Acta Derm Venereol 2007;87(2):167–8.

46. Dehesa L, Tosti A. Treatment of inflammatory nail disorders. Dermatol Ther 2012;25(6):525–34.

47. Tosti A, Piraccini BM, Cameli N, et al. Calcipotriol ointment in nail psoriasis: a controlled double-blind comparison with betamethasone dipropionate and salicylic acid. Br J Dermatol 1998;139(4):655–9.

48. Kim GK. The rationale behind topical vitamin d analogs in the treatment of psoriasis: where does topical calcitriol fit in? J Clin Aesthet Dermatol 2010;3(8):46–53.

49. Rigopoulos D, Ioannides D, Prastitis N, et al. Nail psoriasis: a combined treatment using calcipotriol cream and clobetasol propionate cream. Acta Derm Venereol 2002;82(2):140.

50. Tzung TY, Chen CY, Yang CY, et al. Calcipotriol used as monotherapy or combination therapy with betamethasone dipropionate in the treatment of nail psoriasis. Acta Derm Venereol 2008;88(3):279–80.

51. Scher RK, Stiller M, Zhu YI. Tazarotene 0.1% gel in the treatment of fingernail psoriasis: a double-blind, randomized, vehicle-controlled study. Cutis 2001;68(5):355–8.

52. Bianchi L, Soda R, Diluvio L, et al. Tazarotene 0.1% gel for psoriasis of the fingernails and toenails: an open, prospective study. Br J Dermatol 2003;149(1):207–9.

53. Malecic N, Young H. Tacrolimus for the management of psoriasis: clinical utility and place in therapy. Psoriasis (Auckl) 2016;6:153–63.

54. Cannavo SP, Guarneri F, Vaccaro M, et al. Treatment of psoriatic nails with topical cyclosporin: a prospective, randomized placebo-controlled study. Dermatology 2003;206(2):153–6.

55. De Simone C, Maiorino A, Tassone F, et al. Tacrolimus 0.1% ointment in nail psoriasis: a randomized controlled open-label study. J Eur Acad Dermatol Venereol 2013;27(8):1003–6.

56. Hermann RC, Taylor RS, Ellis CN, et al. Topical ciclosporin for psoriasis: in vitro skin penetration and clinical study. Skin Pharmacol 1988;1(4):246–9.

Nail Psoriasis in Older Adults
Intralesional, Systemic, and Biological Therapy

Jose W. Ricardo, MD, Shari R. Lipner, MD, PhD*

KEYWORDS

- Nails • Psoriasis • Nail psoriasis • Psoriatic arthritis • Older adults • Methotrexate • Cyclosporine
- Acitretin

KEY POINTS

- Intralesional therapy is a safe, efficacious, cost-effective treatment for nail psoriasis in older adults.
- With oral and biologics medications, there are risks of systemic toxicity, limiting widespread use, particularly in older individuals.
- Polypharmacy is common among older adults; therefore, drug interactions must be assessed before prescribing systemics.
- Biologic medications are very effective for nail psoriasis. Although further studies are needed, current data support its use in older adults.

INTRODUCTION

Psoriasis is a common chronic inflammatory condition causing significant morbidity with a negative effect on quality of life (QOL).[1] It may affect the skin, scalp, joints, and nails and is common in older individuals.[2]

Although the pathogenesis of psoriasis has not completely been elucidated, genetic predisposition, altered function of keratinocytes, and alteration of innate and acquired immunity have been implicated.[3–5] Immune stimulation and overexpression of inflammatory cytokines, particularly, tumor necrosis factor-α (TNF-α), nuclear factor kappa B, intralesional (IL)-6, and IL-8, play important roles. Furthermore, psoriasis patients with nail involvement are predisposed to fungal infections, with *Candida* onychomycosis exacerbating nail psoriasis (NP) by activating T helper 17 cells via the stimulation of cathelicidin and LL-37 in the nail bed and consequently inducing IL-23 expression by dendritic cells and macrophages.[5–7] This disease pathway is particularly relevant in older adults, in whom onychomycosis is prevalent.[8,9]

There are unique challenges in treating older adults with NP because of more frequent physical, social, and mental disabilities. Part 1 of this review summarizes topical therapies, and part 2 focuses on intralesional (IL), oral, and biologic medications in this population.[10]

INTRALESIONAL THERAPY

Treatment of NP with IL corticosteroid injections is effective, practical, and safe in patients with 3 or fewer nails affected, with no/limited skin involvement, with nail matrix features, and without the presence of psoriatic arthritis (PsA).[11] IL therapy allows for direct drug delivery to the nail matrix through a single injection into the proximal nail fold.[12] Nail bed injections may improve nail bed

Funding sources: none.
No reprints requested.
This work has not been previously published or presented.
Department of Dermatology, Weill Cornell Medicine, New York, NY, USA
* Corresponding author. 1305 York Avenue, New York, NY 10021.
E-mail address: shl9032@med.cornell.edu

Dermatol Clin 39 (2021) 195–210
https://doi.org/10.1016/j.det.2020.12.012

disease, but are technically challenging and painful, often requiring local anesthesia.[13]

The published evidence regarding IL therapies for NP with mean ages and age ranges of subjects included in each study is summarized in **Table 1**.

Triamcinolone acetonide (TAC), methotrexate, and cyclosporine have been used as IL therapy for NP, and TAC (2.5–10 mg/mL) injected monthly is the preferred therapy (**Fig. 1**).[14–16] In an open-label study of 19 NP patients (mean age = 48 years, 3 months) receiving 1 to 2 intralesional triamcinolone (ILTAC) (10 mg/mL) injections, subungual hyperkeratosis improved in all patients, with 94%, 83%, 50%, and 45% of patients showing improvement in transverse ridging, nail thickening, onycholysis, and pitting, respectively.[16] Side effects included subungual hematomas, and temporary fingertip pain and paresthesias.[16] In another open-label study of 17 NP patients comparing TAC intramatrical injections (2 injections, 6 weeks apart) with methotrexate and cyclosporine (30 nails per group), TAC and methotrexate had similar efficacy and were superior to cyclosporine.[15] Fifty percent, 56.7%, and 33.3% of nails treated with ILTAC, methotrexate, and cyclosporine, respectively, showed ≥76% improvement in the Nail Psoriasis Severity Index (NAPSI) score.[15] Patients receiving treatment with cyclosporine reported the highest rate of adverse effects, including severe pain during injection (90% of nails) despite using ring block anesthesia, postinjection pain and numbness, proximal onycholysis and nail splitting in 1 nail, and nail plate distortion in 2 nails.[15] In a randomized controlled trial (RCT), 1 to 2 treatments of ILTAC (10 mg/mL) were found to significantly improve NP, using the target NAPSI score, compared with topical 0.05% clobetasol propionate ointment applied twice daily without occlusion after 4 months (mean age = 52 years) (P = .003).[17] Subungual hyperkeratosis, pitting, discoloration, onycholysis, and crumbling showed improvement in 83%, 75%, 44%, 31%, and 20% of the nails treated with TAC, respectively, in 6 months.[17] Therefore, ILTAC is efficacious and safe for NP, with only mild side effects.

Evidence regarding the use of methotrexate as IL therapy for NP is relatively scarce. A report of 4 NP patients (mean age = 21 years; age range = 15–25 years) treated with methotrexate (5 mg/mL) nail bed injections every 3 weeks (5 treatments) showed a mean reduction of 2.34 points in the NAPSI score.[13] Mean NAPSI declined from 4.19 to 2.56 in patients with only nail bed disease, and 5.0 to 3.14 in patients with concomitant nail bed and matrix features.[13] Only mild side effects were reported, including pain during injection, injection site hyperpigmentation, and pin-point nail bed hemorrhages.[13] Thus, IL therapy with methotrexate may be used as an alternative to TAC, but RCTs in older individuals are lacking.

Despite the underrepresentation of older adults in IL NP studies, this population may benefit from this approach because it is less cumbersome compared with topical therapy. In addition, monthly injections are cost-effective compared with more costly systemic alternatives, such as biologics. The safety profile of ILTAC therapy for NP is favorable, with little to no risk of systemic toxicity. Pain on injection is the most obvious drawback when using this approach, but several techniques, including talkesthesia, using an air-cooling device, vibratory devices, applying anesthetic topical cream before surgery, ethyl chloride spray, and ice, can improve the patient experience.[18,19] Elderly individuals may have higher tolerance to mechanical pain compared with younger populations.[20] Other mild side effects include subungual hematoma, temporary paresthesia, periungual hypopigmentation, and atrophy at the injection site.[14,21]

SYSTEMIC THERAPY

Systemic therapy is considered for patients with greater than 3 nails affected, with a significant impact on QOL, concomitant PsA, or treatment failures.[11,14] Frequently used systemic medications for NP include conventional medications, such as methotrexate, cyclosporine, acitretin, newer orals, such as apremilast, and biologics, including adalimumab, etanercept, infliximab golimumab, ixekizumab, ustekinumab, and tofacitinib.

METHOTREXATE

Methotrexate has a long track record for skin psoriasis, PsA, and NP treatment. It is relatively efficacious and cost-effective (see **Fig. 1**), but a long list of potential side effects often limits its widespread use.[22] Systemic toxicity is especially concerning in older individuals, who may have other comorbidities. Potential side effects include hepatic fibrosis, cirrhosis, ulcerative stomatitis, nausea, and myelosuppression, which is particularly worrisome in older individuals, and in whom a certain degree of kidney impairment is often present.[23] Similarly, a higher prevalence of hypertriglyceridemia, elevated liver transaminase levels, obesity, and diabetes mellitus in this population increases the risk of hepatotoxicity.[23]

Studies assessing efficacy and safety of methotrexate as a treatment of NP are scarce. One RCT (mean age = 42.5) comparing oral methotrexate

Table 1
Studies on intralesional therapies for the treatment of nail psoriasis

Author, Year	Number of Patients	Age Range (y)	Mean Age (y)	Medication	Dosage, Regimen	Site	Outcome Measure	Clinical Result
De Berker and Lawrence,[16] 1998	19	Unknown	48	TAC	10 mg/mL once, and a second time after 2 mo if poor response was noted	Matrix and nail bed		Improvement in 100% of digits with hyperkeratosis, 94% with transverse ridging, 83% with thickening, 50% with onycholysis, and 45% with pitting
Boontaveeyuwat et al,[17] 2019	16	Unknown	52	TAC, clobetasol propionate	10 mg/mL, twice with a 1-mo interval; 0.05% clobetasol propionate ointment twice a day without occlusion for 6 mo	Matrix and nail bed	Target NAPSI	Improvement in 83% of nails with subungual hyperkeratosis, 75% of pitting, 44% of the discolored, 31% of onycholysis, and 20% of crumbling. After 4 mo, the reduction in the NAPSI score of the injection group was significantly higher than that of the topical ($P = .003$) and control ($P \leq .001$) groups
Mittal and Mahajan,[15] 2018	17	Unknown	Unknown	TAC, methotrexate, cyclosporine	TAC: 10 mg/mL, methotrexate: 25 mg/mL, cyclosporine: 50 mg/mL, 2 injections within a 6-wk interval	Matrix	NAPSI	50% of nails treated with TAC showed ≥76% improvement, 56.7% of nails treated with methotrexate showed ≥76% improvement, 33.3% of nails treated with cyclosporine showed ≥76% improvement

(continued on next page)

Table 1
(continued)

Author, Year	Number of Patients	Age Range (y)	Mean Age (y)	Medication	Dosage, Regimen	Site	Outcome Measure	Clinical Result
Bleeker,[55] 1974	400	Unknown	Unknown	TAC	5 mg/mL monthly for 6 mo (using a port-O-jet)	Matrix		68% improvement in pitting, 34% improvement in onycholysis
Nantel-Battista et al,[56] 2014	17	24–79	41	TAC	8 mg/mL every 4 ± 1 wk, 4 times	Matrix	Target NAPSI	46% improvement in the mean target NAPSI score, 50% and 38% improvements in nail matrix and bed target NAPSI scores
Grover et al,[13] 2017	4	15–25	21	Methotrexate	25 mg/mL at 3-wk intervals 5 times	Nail bed	NAPSI	−2.34 points

Abbreviation: target NAPSI, nail psoriasis severity index of 1 target nail.

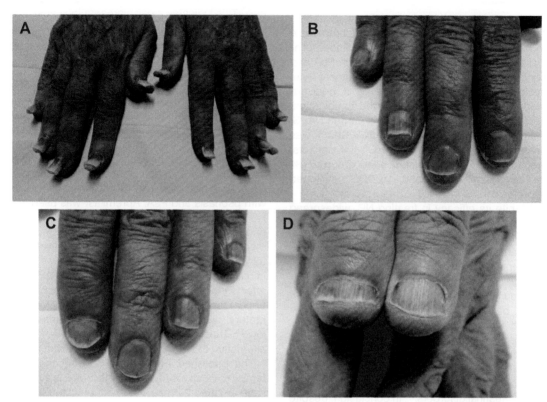

Fig. 1. (*A*) Seventy-eight-year-old woman with severe thickening, subungual hyperkeratosis, onycholysis, and yellowing of her fingernails. She also had difficulty performing activities of daily life. (*B–D*) Patient's fingernails after treatment with 7 months of oral methotrexate and ILTAC. All fingernails showed marked improvement in subungual hyperkeratosis. Residual onycholysis and splinter hemorrhages can be seen in some fingernails.

and cyclosporine (n = 17 in each group) for NP showed 43% and 37% mean reductions in NAPSI score at 24 weeks, respectively (not significant).[24] One patient had an elevated liver transaminase, and 2 patients had elevated serum creatinine in the methotrexate and cyclosporine groups, respectively.[24] In addition, 2 methotrexate-treated patients reported nausea and telogen effluvium, and 1 patient in the cyclosporine group experienced mild nail pain.[24] Another prospective controlled study of 87 psoriatic patients (mean age = 41 years) with nail involvement compared the efficacy of methotrexate (n = 20), biologic agents (n = 6; 2 etanercept, 3 infliximab, 1 adalimumab), narrowband UV-B phototherapy (n = 8), acitretin (n = 25), and no treatment (n = 25).[25] Mean improvements after 16 weeks using the NAPSI score were 13.9% with methotrexate, 78.4% with biologic agents, 30.7% with narrowband UV-B phototherapy, and 9.1% worsening with acitretin.[25] The difference among groups was significant (*P* = .008), but the only significant difference between separate groups and the control was in the biologic-treated group.[25]

No severe side effects were reported.[25] Therefore, the efficacy and safety of methotrexate for the treatment of NP are questionable; although a small number of subjects were recruited in these studies, systemic toxicity was reported.

CYCLOSPORINE

Cyclosporine is a potent immunomodulatory drug that binds cyclophilin and inhibits calcineurin, preventing activation of IL-2 and decreasing T-cell activation.[26] Use of cyclosporine for plaque psoriasis is supported by extensive evidence, but studies assessing efficacy and safety for NP are scarce. Oral cyclosporine (3.5 mg/kg/d) alone and in combination with topical calcipotriene cream was used in 54 psoriatic patients (mean age = 37 years; age range = 23–64 years) with nail involvement.[27] At 3 months, 79% of patients in the combination therapy group showed improvement in nail features (*P*≤.0004), particularly subungual hyperkeratosis, onycholysis, and pitting, whereas 47.6% of patients that received cyclosporine alone showed nail improvement, which was not statistically significant $(P \leq .15)$.[27] The efficacy of cyclosporine may be comparable to biologics. In a nonrandomized, unblinded clinical trial of 57, 58, and 55 patients with PsA and concomitant NP, who received treatment with cyclosporine alone (2.5–3.75 mg/kg/d), adalimumab (40 mg every other week), or the combination, percentage of patients achieving a (target) NAPSI improvement of at least 50% (NAPSI-50) was achieved in 44%, 56%, and 100% of patients, respectively.[28] In the cyclosporine group, 77% had any side effect, and 15.79% developed hypertension.[28]

Despite its efficacy in treating NP, widespread use of cyclosporine is limited by its relatively high rate of adverse events and increased frequency compared with methotrexate.[29] Nephrotoxicity and hypertension are the most concerning side effects.[22] Nonobese patients without hypertension and younger than 60 years may be better candidates, because older individuals may have age-related kidney impairment.[30] In addition, cyclosporine is oxidized by cytochrome P450 3A4, and drug interactions are frequent. Additional side effects include fatigue, headaches, paresthesias, hypertrichosis, gingival hyperplasia, and gastrointestinal disorders.[22] In conclusion, despite the lack of studies assessing safety of cyclosporine in elderly individuals, it should be used with extreme caution in this population.

ACITRETIN

Acitretin is a vitamin A analogue (retinoid) that modulates cellular proliferation and differentiation, keratinization, and neutrophil chemotaxis. Acitretin is unique compared with the other conventional systemic medications because it is not immunosuppressive. There is conflicting evidence regarding efficacy of acitretin for NP treatment. In an open-label study of 36 patients (mean age = 36 years; age range = 28–67 years) with moderate to severe NP treated with acitretin (0.2–0.3 mg/kg/d), there was a mean 41% reduction in NAPSI score after 6 months of treatment.[31] Only 1 patient had side effects, including severe skin dryness and pyogenic granulomas, which regressed after dose lowering.[31] Conversely, 2 prospective studies in patients taking acitretin for NP, 1 controlled (n = 25; mean age = 49 years) and 1 uncontrolled (n = 20; age range = 39–61 years), showed mean 9.1% and 2.5% worsening in the NAPSI score, respectively.[25,32] Acitretin is contraindicated in patients with hepatic or kidney impairment.[23] It often causes mucocutaneous dryness and hyperlipidemia, which may be particularly disturbing in geriatric patients,

because these conditions are already prevalent.[23] Thus, monitoring serum lipids and liver enzymes is recommended before and during treatment of older adults.

APREMILAST

Apremilast is administered orally, and its mechanism is through inhibition of phosphodiesterase-4, which targets the inflammatory cascade at an earlier stage than biologic medications.[33] It is approved in the United States by the Food and Drug Administration for the treatment of adults with psoriasis and PsA. Apremilast was used in 2 RCTs (ESTEEM 1 and 2) as treatment of NP (secondary endpoint), with 43.6% and 60% improvement in the NAPSI score, respectively, in 32 weeks.[34,35] Significant improvement was noted in nail matrix and bed psoriasis features.[34,35] Side effects included diarrhea, nausea, headache, and upper respiratory tract infections.[36] The risk of laboratory abnormalities and drug interactions is low.[36] Thus, apremilast is an effective and safe alternative to NP treatment in older individuals.

The published evidence of conventional systemic medications as treatments for NP is summarized in **Table 2**.

BIOLOGIC THERAPY

Biologic agents for NP are reserved for patients with severe nail disease with or without skin involvement, patients with PsA, and patients who have failed other treatment alternatives or have significant impact on QOL; they can be broadly classified into TNF-α inhibitors (infliximab, adalimumab, etanercept), IL-17 inhibitors (secukinumab, ixekizumab), IL-12/23 inhibitors (ustekinumab), and Janus kinase 1/3 inhibitor (tofacitinib).[22,37]

TUMOR NECROSIS FACTOR-α INHIBITORS

TNF-α is a proinflammatory cytokine that plays a role in psoriasis by promoting an inflammatory infiltrate into the skin and inducing keratinocytes proliferation, while at the same time preventing apoptosis.[22] It is found in abnormally high serum levels in psoriasis patients, particularly those with nail involvement.[38] The TNF-α inhibitors infliximab, adalimumab, and etanercept are covered in this review. Of the 3, infliximab is intravenously administered, with the other 2 injected subcutaneously. A significant improvement in the NAPSI score following treatment with TNF-α inhibitors is consistently observed among studies (**Table 3**). A retrospective study analyzed 48 patients (mean age = 46 years; age range = 15–81 years) with

Table 2
Studies on conventional systemic therapies for the treatment of nail psoriasis

Medication/Author, Year	Number of Patients	Age Range (y)	Mean Age (y)	Dosage, Regimen	Outcome Measure	Success Rate
Acitretin						
Tosti et al,[31] 2009	36	28–67	41	0.2/0.3 mg/kg/d	NAPSI, target NAPSI	NAPSI: −41%, target NAPSI: −50%
Mukai et al,[32] 2012	30 (20 completed)	39–61	Unknown	0.3 mg/kg every day for 1 mo. If improvement was noted after 1 mo, the dose would be 0.5 mg/kg every day for 4 mo in total	NAPSI	3%
Demirsoy et al,[25] 2013	25	Unknown	49	Unknown	NAPSI	9%
Methotrexate						
Gümüşel, et al,[24] 2011	17	Unknown	43	Initial dose 15 mg per week	NAPSI	−43%
Reich et al,[57] 2011	108	Unknown	43	5–15 mg per week (weeks 0–9), 20 mg per week (weeks 10–15), 25 mg per week (> week 16)	Target NAPSI	−30%
Demirsoy et al,[25] 2013	20	Unknown	41	Unknown	NAPSI	14%
Sanchez-Regana et al,[58] 2011	9	Unknown	Unknown	7.5–15 mg per week	NAPSI	−35%
Cyclosporin						
Gümüşel et al,[24] 2011	17	Unknown	38	5 mg/kg/d	NAPSI	−37%
Feliciani et al,[27] 2004	33	23–64 (including all subjects)	37 (including all subjects)	3–4.5 mg/kg/d for 3 mo	Involved area (<10/10– 50/10 > 50%)	−48%

(continued on next page)

Table 2
(continued)

Medication/Author, Year	Number of Patients	Age Range (y)	Mean Age (y)	Dosage, Regimen	Outcome Measure	Success Rate
Feliciani et al,[27] 2004	21	23–64 (including all subjects)	37 (including all subjects)	3–4.5 mg/kg/d calcipotriol cream twice a day for 3 mo	Involved area (<10/10–50/10 > 50%)	~79%
Karanikolas et al,[28] 2011	18	Unknown	Unknown	2.5–3.75 mg/kg/d	NAPSI-50	Achieved in 44% of cases
Karanikolas et al,[28] 2011	21	Unknown	Unknown	2.5–3.75 mg/kg/d, 40 mg adalimumab every other week	NAPSI-50	Achieved in 100% of cases
Apremilast						
Papp et al,[34] 2015	558	Unknown	Unknown	30 mg twice a day	Target NAPSI, NAPSI-50	~44%, NAPSI-50: 45%
Rich et al,[35] 2016	266	Unknown	Unknown	30 mg twice a day	Target NAPSI, NAPSI-50	~60%, NAPSI-50: 55%

Table 3
Studies on biologic therapies for the treatment of nail psoriasis

Medication/Name	Number of Patients	Age Range (y)	Mean Age (y)	Dosage, Regimen	Outcome Measure	Success Rate
TNF-α inhibitors						
Adalimumab						
Al-Mutairi et al,[45] 2013	105	25–65	38 (including all groups)	80 mg subcutaneous every other week for 24 wk	NAPSI	–75%
Bardazzi et al,[59] 2013	16	Unknown	50 (including all groups)	Unknown	NAPSI	–94%
Rigopoulos et al,[60] 2010	7	28–61	45	80 mg at baseline, 40 mg every 2 wk	NAPSI	–85%
Rigopoulos et al,[60] 2010	14 (nail psoriasis + psoriatic arthritis)	28–71	50	80 mg at baseline, 40 mg every 2 wk	NAPSI	–86%
Van Den Bosch et al,[61] 2010	259	Unknown	Unknown	40 mg every 2 wk	NAPSI	–57%
Kyriakou et al,[40] 2013	14	19–69	46	80 mg at baseline, 40 mg every 2 wk	NAPSI	–87%
Karanikolas et al,[28] 2011	16			40 mg every 2 wk	NAPSI-50	Achieved in 56%
Karanikolas et al,[28] 2011	21			40 mg every 2 wk, cyclosporine 2.5–3.75 mg/kg/d	NAPSI-50	Achieved in 100%
Etanercept						
Al-Mutairi et al,[45] 2013	110	22–62	38 (including all groups)	50 mg subcutaneous twice a week for 12 wk, and 50 mg subcutaneous every week for 12 wk	NAPSI	–68%
Bardazzi et al,[59] 2013	18	Unknown	50 (including all groups)	Unknown	NAPSI	–90%

(continued on next page)

Table 3
(continued)

Medication/Name	Number of Patients	Age Range (y)	Mean Age (y)	Dosage, Regimen	Outcome Measure	Success Rate
Kyriakou et al,[40] 2013	13	29–66	49	50 mg twice a week, >12 wk: 25 mg twice a week	NAPSI	~92%
Dennehy et al,[62] 2016	143	Unknown	47	50 mg twice a week	NAPSI	~28%
Luger et al,[42] 2009	564	Unknown	45	25 mg twice a week for 54 wk or 50 twice a week for 12 wk	NAPSI	~51%
Infliximab						
Al-Mutairi et al,[45] 2013	100	28–60	38 (including all groups)	5 mg/kg slow intravenous on 0, 4, 6, and then every 8 wk	NAPSI	~86%
Bardazzi et al,[59] 2013	14	Unknown	50 (including all groups)	Unknown	NAPSI	~91%
Kyriakou et al,[40] 2013	12	3–21	45	5 mg/kg weeks 0, 2, 6, +8 wk	NAPSI	~95%
Fabroni et al,[39] 2011	48	15–81	46	5 mg/kg weeks 0, 2, 6, +8 wk	NAPSI	~86%
IL-17 inhibitors						
Secukinumab						
Paul et al,[63] 2014	51	Unknown	45	150 mg week 0	Composite fingernail score (affected area)	~4%
Paul et al,[63] 2014	110	Unknown	45	150 mg weeks 0, 4, and 8		~11%
Paul et al,[63] 2014	101	Unknown	45	150 mg weeks 0, 1, 2, and 4		~19%
Reich et al,[46] 2019	67	Unknown	44	150 mg weeks 0, 1, 2, and 4, followed by every 4 wk	NAPSI	~53%

Study	N	Age range	Mean age	Dosing	Outcome measure	Result
Reich et al,[46] 2019	66	Unknown	45	300 mg weeks 0, 1, 2, and 4, followed by every 4 wk	NAPSI	−63%
Ixekizumab						
Langley et al,[48] 2015	50	Unknown	Unknown	10, 25, 75, or 150 mg, weeks 0, 2, 4, 8, 12, and 16	NAPSI	−79%
Leonardi et al,[47] 2012	13	Unknown	48	10 mg, weeks 0, 2, 4, 8, 12	NAPSI	14%
Leonardi et al,[47] 2012	10	Unknown	46	25 mg, weeks 0, 2, 4, 8, 12	NAPSI	−24%
Leonardi et al,[47] 2012	10	Unknown	46	75 mg, weeks 0, 2, 4, 8, 12	NAPSI	−57%
Leonardi et al,[47] 2012	10	Unknown	46	150 mg, weeks 0, 2, 4, 8, 12	NAPSI	−49%
Dennehy et al,[62] 2016	138	Unknown	46	80 mg every 2 wk	NAPSI	−39%
Dennehy et al,[62] 2016	139	Unknown	46	80 mg every 4 wk	NAPSI	−40%
IL-12/23 inhibitor (ustekinumab)						
Bardazzi et al,[59] 2013	6	Unknown	49.92 (including all groups)	Unknown	NAPSI	−88%
Igarashi et al,[64] 2012	44	Unknown	Unknown	45 mg (weeks 0, 4, 16, 28)	Target NAPSI	−57%
Igarashi et al,[64] 2012	40	Unknown	Unknown	90 mg (weeks 0, 4, 16, 28)	Target NAPSI	−64%
Patsatsi et al,[65] 2013	27	17–77	49	45 mg (weeks 0, 4, 16, 28)	NAPSI	−97%
Rich et al,[50] 2014	182	Unknown	46	45 mg (weeks 0, 4, 16, 28)	Target NAPSI	Target NAPSI: −47%
Rich et al,[50] 2014	187	Unknown	46	90 mg (weeks 0, 4, 16, 28)	Target NAPSI	Target NAPSI: −49%

(continued on next page)

Table 3
(continued)

Medication/Name	Number of Patients	Age Range (y)	Mean Age (y)	Dosage, Regimen	Outcome Measure	Success Rate
Janus kinase 1/3 inhibitor (tofacitinib)						
Merola et al,[52] 2017	487	18–78	Unknown	5 mg twice a day	NAPSI	–66% at week 16
Merola et al,[52] 2017	476	18–82	Unknown	10 mg twice a day	NAPSI	–75% at week 16
Abe et al,[66] 2017	22	Unknown	48	5 mg twice a day	NAPSI	–75%
Abe et al,[66] 2017	24	Unknown	48	10 mg twice a day	NAPSI	–78%

severe NP treated with infliximab and found an 86% mean reduction in the NAPSI score at week 38.[39] Another retrospective study of 12 patients treated with infliximab (mean age = 45 years; age range = 3–21 years), 14 with adalimumab (mean age = 46 years; age range = 19–69 years), and 13 with etanercept (mean age = 49 years; age range = 29–66 years) showed mean reductions of 95.1%, 89.5%, and 92.8% in NAPSI scores at week 48, respectively (P = .000).[40] Specifically, infliximab and etanercept were shown to be more effective as treatment of patients with late-onset psoriasis (age >40 years) compared with early-onset psoriasis (age ≤40 years), using data from the Psoriasis Longitudinal Assessment and Registry.[41] Similarly, in a post hoc analysis of a randomized, open-label, multicenter study (n = 720) conducted on patients with moderate to severe plaque psoriasis with nail involvement treated with etanercept (n = 564; mean age = 45 years, 54 weeks), there was a 51% improvement in the target NAPSI score.[42]

Side effects reported with TNF-α inhibitors are activation of opportunistic infections, including tuberculosis, demyelinating disease, congestive heart failure, induction of the formation of autologous antibodies, and antibodies neutralizing anti-TNF-α drugs; nonetheless, long-term safety data are still being explored.[22,43,44] The safety profile in elderly individuals is questionable, because there is a paucity of evidence in this population. In a prospective study on 187 patients aged greater than 65 years with skin psoriasis, patients treated with etanercept had a significantly lower risk of adverse events compared with patients treated with adalimumab (P = .05).[29] There were 2 cases of pneumonia, one linked to infliximab and the other to etanercept; another patient treated with infliximab had myocardial infarction.[29] Additional adverse events reported included herpes zoster, atrial fibrillation, myasthenia gravis, and pericarditis in the etanercept group, and thromboembolism in the infliximab group.[29] Furthermore, in 1 randomized controlled study of 315 NP patients treated with infliximab, etanercept, and adalimumab, a statistically positive association between onychomycosis and the use of infliximab was shown.[45]

INTERLEUKIN-17 INHIBITORS

Secukinumab and ixekizumab target IL-17, which is a critical T-cell–derived cytokine altering skin function. The limited data available have shown that these 2 medications are effective for NP, with a favorable safety profile (see **Table 3**). One RCT including 198 psoriasis patients with moderate to severe NP from the TRANSFIGURE study treated with secukinumab 300 mg (n = 66; mean age = 45 years) and secukinumab 150 mg (n = 67; mean age = 44 years) showed mean percentage NAPSI improvements of 52.6% and 63.2%, respectively, at week 32.[46] Improvement of nail features was noted in the 300-mg group as early as 2 weeks after initiation of therapy.[46] Side effects reported included headache, nasopharyngitis, upper respiratory tract infection, *Candida* infection, and neutropenia.[46] Similarly, ixekizumab has shown good efficacy for NP. In 1 phase 2, double-blind, placebo-controlled study, there was a 57% improvement in the NAPSI score in NP patients treated with ixekizumab 75 mg (weeks 0, 2, 4, 8, and 12) at week 12.[47] Mean percentage NAPSI improvement of 79% was noted in the same patients at week 48 in an open-label extension (week 68 of the original study).[48] Additional side effects with secukinumab include exacerbation of Crohn disease and urticaria.[22] Secukinumab does not increase the risk of infection in elderly individuals compared with younger populations. A post hoc analysis of 3 phase 3 trials compared 67 elderly subjects (≥65 years) treated with secukinumab for plaque psoriasis with 841younger subjects (18–64 years) and concluded that the total rates of adverse events were similar in both groups.[49]

INTERLEUKIN-12/23 INHIBITORS

Ustekinumab targets IL-12/23 and is approved for the treatment of plaque psoriasis and PsA. There are limited data assessing efficacy of ustekinumab in NP. In 1 randomized, placebo-controlled crossover study of 766 psoriasis patients (70% with NP) treated with ustekinumab (45 mg or 90 mg if >100 kg; mean age = 46 years for both groups), there was a 57% mean improvement in NAPSI score at week 24.[50] Side effects and contraindications are similar to TNF-α inhibitors. Patients should be screened for tuberculosis infection before receiving treatment with ustekinumab, and any serious active infection should be treated before initiation. Ustekinumab does not seem to increase the risk of infection in older individuals. A retrospective study (n = 24) on patients aged ≥65 years (age range = 65–88 years) with psoriasis treated with ustekinumab for 1 year showed no serious infections.[51]

JANUS KINASE INHIBITORS

Tofacitinib is an oral Janus kinase inhibitor that has been recently studied for psoriasis and NP with promising results. In 1 post hoc analysis of 2 randomized, double-blind, controlled phase 3 studies including 1196 plaque psoriasis patients with nail involvement (age range = 18–82 years), tofacitinib was found to decrease NAPSI scores up to 75% from baseline over 52 weeks.[52] Low rates of serious adverse events, infections, malignancies, and discontinuations were reported in this study. In conclusion, tofacitinib is effective and safe to use in NP.

SUMMARY

ILTAC for NP is efficacious, cost-effective, and safe to use in older individuals; its main drawback is pain on injection, but certain techniques can be used to improve the patient experience. Conversely, prescribing systemic therapy in the elderly may be questionable. Oral medications have risks of systemic toxicity. Older adults may be at a higher risk of toxicity and drug interactions than the general population because comorbidities and polypharmacy are common in this population.[53] Moreover, many of these medications are immunosuppressive, significantly increasing the risk of infection. Finally, growing evidence suggests excellent results with biologics for NP, but long-term safety is still being assessed. The main downside of biologics is price and accessibility, and biologics are more difficult to obtain for individuals with lower income and lack of insurance.[54] In conclusion, older adults are underrepresented in most studies included in this review, and conclusions may not be applicable to this population. Randomized controlled studies are needed in the elderly to draw accurate conclusions.

CLINICS CARE POINTS

- ILTAC is an efficacious, cost-effective, and safe treatment for NP in older individuals; pain may be minimized with talkesthesia and cooling.
- Systemic therapy should be prescribed cautiously in older individuals with NP, while considering potential side effects and drug-drug interactions.
- Biologics may be good options to treat NP in older individuals, but cost and accessibility are important considerations.

DISCLOSURES

Dr J.W. Ricardo and Dr S.R. Lipner have no conflicts of interest relevant to the content of the submission.

REFERENCES

1. Stern RS, Nijsten T, Feldman SR, et al. Psoriasis is common, carries a substantial burden even when not extensive, and is associated with widespread treatment dissatisfaction. J Investig Dermatol Symp Proc 2004;9(2):136–9.
2. Parisi R, Symmons DP, Griffiths CE, Ashcroft DM, et al, Identification, Management of P. Global epidemiology of psoriasis: a systematic review of incidence and prevalence. J Invest Dermatol 2013; 133(2):377–85.
3. Nestle FO, Kaplan DH, Barker J. Psoriasis. N Engl J Med 2009;361(5):496–509.
4. Mak RK, Hundhausen C, Nestle FO. Progress in understanding the immunopathogenesis of psoriasis. Actas Dermosifiliogr 2009;100(Suppl 2):2–13.
5. Ventura A, Mazzeo M, Gaziano R, et al. New insight into the pathogenesis of nail psoriasis and overview of treatment strategies. Drug Des Devel Ther 2017; 11:2527–35.
6. Kisand K, Boe Wolff AS, Podkrajsek KT, et al. Chronic mucocutaneous candidiasis in APECED or thymoma patients correlates with autoimmunity to Th17-associated cytokines. J Exp Med 2010; 207(2):299–308.
7. Taheri Sarvtin M, Shokohi T, Hajheydari Z, et al. Evaluation of candidal colonization and specific humoral responses against Candida albicans in patients with psoriasis. Int J Dermatol 2014;53(12): e555–60.
8. Lipner SR, Scher RK. Onychomycosis: clinical overview and diagnosis. J Am Acad Dermatol 2019; 80(4):835–51.
9. Gupta AK, Jain HC, Lynde CW, et al. Prevalence and epidemiology of onychomycosis in patients visiting physicians' offices: a multicenter Canadian survey of 15,000 patients. J Am Acad Dermatol 2000;43(2 Pt 1):244–8.
10. Ricardo JW, Lipner SR. Nail psoriasis in older adults: epidemiology, diagnosis and topical therapy. Dermatol Clin 2020.
11. Rigopoulos D, Baran R, Chiheb S, et al. Recommendations for the definition, evaluation, and treatment of nail psoriasis in adult patients with no or mild skin psoriasis: a dermatologist and nail expert group consensus. J Am Acad Dermatol 2019;81(1): 228–40.
12. Saleem K, Azim W. Treatment of nail psoriasis with a modified regimen of steroid injections. J Coll Physicians Surg Pak 2008;18(2):78–81.
13. Grover C, Daulatabad D, Singal A. Role of nail bed methotrexate injections in isolated nail psoriasis: conventional drug via an unconventional route. Clin Exp Dermatol 2017;42(4):420–3.
14. Tan ES, Chong WS, Tey HL. Nail psoriasis: a review. Am J Clin Dermatol 2012;13(6):375–88.

15. Mittal J, Mahajan BB. Intramatricial injections for nail psoriasis: an open-label comparative study of triamcinolone, methotrexate, and cyclosporine. Indian J Dermatol Venereol Leprol 2018;84(4):419–23.

16. de Berker DA, Lawrence CM. A simplified protocol of steroid injection for psoriatic nail dystrophy. Br J Dermatol 1998;138(1):90–5.

17. Boontaveeyuwat E, Silpa-Archa N, Danchaivijitr N, et al. A randomized comparison of efficacy and safety of intralesional triamcinolone injection and clobetasol propionate ointment for psoriatic nails. J Dermatolog Treat 2019;30(2):117–22.

18. Ricardo JW, Lipner SR. Air cooling for improved analgesia during local anesthetic infiltration for nail surgery. J Am Acad Dermatol 2019. https://doi.org/10.1016/j.jaad.2019.11.032.

19. Lipner SR. Pain-minimizing strategies for nail surgery. Cutis 2018;101(2):76–7.

20. Chakour MC, Gibson SJ, Bradbeer M, et al. The effect of age on A delta- and C-fibre thermal pain perception. Pain 1996;64(1):143–52.

21. de Berker D. Management of psoriatic nail disease. Semin Cutan Med Surg 2009;28(1):39–43.

22. Pasch MC. Nail psoriasis: a review of treatment options. Drugs 2016;76(6):675–705.

23. Di Lernia V, Goldust M. An overview of the efficacy and safety of systemic treatments for psoriasis in the elderly. Expert Opin Biol Ther 2018;18(8):897–903.

24. Gumusel M, Ozdemir M, Mevlitoglu I, et al. Evaluation of the efficacy of methotrexate and cyclosporine therapies on psoriatic nails: a one-blind, randomized study. J Eur Acad Dermatol Venereol 2011;25(9):1080–4.

25. Demirsoy EO, Kiran R, Salman S, et al. Effectiveness of systemic treatment agents on psoriatic nails: a comparative study. J Drugs Dermatol 2013;12(9):1039–43.

26. Gutfreund K, Bienias W, Szewczyk A, et al. Topical calcineurin inhibitors in dermatology. Part I: properties, method and effectiveness of drug use. Postepy Dermatol Alergol 2013;30(3):165–9.

27. Feliciani C, Zampotti A, Forlco P, et al. Nail psoriasis: combined therapy with systemic cyclosporin and topical calcipotriol. J Cutan Med Surg 2004;8(2):122–5.

28. Karanikolas GN, Koukli EM, Katsalira A, et al. Adalimumab or cyclosporine as monotherapy and in combination in severe psoriatic arthritis: results from a prospective 12-month nonrandomized unblinded clinical trial. J Rheumatol 2011;38(11):2466–74.

29. Piaserico S, Conti A, Lo Console F, et al. Efficacy and safety of systemic treatments for psoriasis in elderly patients. Acta Derm Venereol 2014;94(3):293–7.

30. Maza A, Montaudie H, Sbidian E, et al. Oral cyclosporin in psoriasis: a systematic review on treatment modalities, risk of kidney toxicity and evidence for use in non-plaque psoriasis. J Eur Acad Dermatol Venereol 2011;25(Suppl 2):19–27.

31. Tosti A, Ricotti C, Romanelli P, et al. Evaluation of the efficacy of acitretin therapy for nail psoriasis. Arch Dermatol 2009;145(3):269–71.

32. Mukai MM, Poffo IF, Werner B, et al. NAPSI utilization as an evaluation method of nail psoriasis in patients using acitretin. An Bras Dermatol 2012;87(2):256–62.

33. Keating GM. Apremilast: a review in psoriasis and psoriatic arthritis. Drugs 2017;77(4):459–72.

34. Papp K, Reich K, Leonardi CL, et al. Apremilast, an oral phosphodiesterase 4 (PDE4) inhibitor, in patients with moderate to severe plaque psoriasis: results of a phase III, randomized, controlled trial (efficacy and safety trial evaluating the effects of apremilast in psoriasis [ESTEEM] 1). J Am Acad Dermatol 2015;73(1):37–49.

35. Rich P, Gooderham M, Bachelez H, et al. Apremilast, an oral phosphodiesterase 4 inhibitor, in patients with difficult-to-treat nail and scalp psoriasis: results of 2 phase III randomized, controlled trials (ESTEEM 1 and ESTEEM 2). J Am Acad Dermatol 2016;74(1):134–42.

36. Zerilli T, Ocheretyaner E. Apremilast (Otezla): a new oral treatment for adults with psoriasis and psoriatic arthritis. P T 2015;40(8):495–500.

37. Crowley JJ, Weinberg JM, Wu JJ, et al. Treatment of nail psoriasis: best practice recommendations from the medical board of the National Psoriasis Foundation. JAMA Dermatol 2015;151(1):87–94.

38. Kyriakou A, Patsatsi A, Vyzantiadis TA, et al. Serum levels of TNF-alpha, IL-12/23 p40, and IL-17 in psoriatic patients with and without nail psoriasis: a cross-sectional study. Scientific World Journal 2014;2014:508178.

39. Fabroni C, Gori A, Troiano M, et al. Infliximab efficacy in nail psoriasis. A retrospective study in 48 patients. J Eur Acad Dermatol Venereol 2011;25(5):549–53.

40. Kyriakou A, Patsatsi A, Sotiriadis D. Anti-TNF agents and nail psoriasis: a single-center, retrospective, comparative study. J Dermatolog Treat 2013;24(3):162–8.

41. Singh S, Kalb RE, de Jong E, et al. Effect of age of onset of psoriasis on clinical outcomes with systemic treatment in the psoriasis longitudinal assessment and registry (PSOLAR). Am J Clin Dermatol 2018;19(6):879–86.

42. Luger TA, Barker J, Lambert J, et al. Sustained improvement in joint pain and nail symptoms with etanercept therapy in patients with moderate-to-severe psoriasis. J Eur Acad Dermatol Venereol 2009;23(8):896–904.

43. Pirowska MM, Gozdzialska A, Lipko-Godlewska S, et al. Autoimmunogenicity during anti-TNF therapy

in patients with psoriasis and psoriatic arthritis. Post-epy Dermatol Alergol 2015;32(4):250–4.

44. Langley RG, Saurat JH, Reich K, et al. Recommendations for the treatment of nail psoriasis in patients with moderate to severe psoriasis: a dermatology expert group consensus. J Eur Acad Dermatol Venereol 2012;26(3):373–81.

45. Al-Mutairi N, Nour T, Al-Rqobah D. Onychomycosis in patients of nail psoriasis on biologic therapy: a randomized, prospective open label study comparing etanercept, infliximab and adalimumab. Expert Opin Biol Ther 2013;13(5):625–9.

46. Reich K, Sullivan J, Arenberger P, et al. Effect of secukinumab on the clinical activity and disease burden of nail psoriasis: 32-week results from the randomized placebo-controlled TRANSFIGURE trial. Br J Dermatol 2019;181(5):954–66.

47. Leonardi C, Matheson R, Zachariae C, et al. Anti–interleukin-17 monoclonal antibody ixekizumab in chronic plaque psoriasis. N Engl J Med 2012; 366(13):1190–9.

48. Langley RG, Rich P, Menter A, et al. Improvement of scalp and nail lesions with ixekizumab in a phase 2 trial in patients with chronic plaque psoriasis. J Eur Acad Dermatol Venereol 2015;29(9):1763–70.

49. Korber A, Papavassilis C, Bhosekar V, et al. Efficacy and safety of secukinumab in elderly subjects with moderate to severe plaque psoriasis: a pooled analysis of phase III studies. Drugs Aging 2018;35(2): 135–44.

50. Rich P, Bourcier M, Sofen H, et al. Ustekinumab improves nail disease in patients with moderate-to-severe psoriasis: results from PHOENIX 1. Br J Dermatol 2014;170(2):398–407.

51. Hayashi M, Umezawa Y, Fukuchi O, et al. Efficacy and safety of ustekinumab treatment in elderly patients with psoriasis. J Dermatol 2014;41(11): 974–80.

52. Merola JF, Elewski B, Tatulych S, et al. Efficacy of tofacitinib for the treatment of nail psoriasis: two 52-week, randomized, controlled phase 3 studies in patients with moderate-to-severe plaque psoriasis. J Am Acad Dermatol 2017;77(1):79–87 e1.

53. Murdan S. Nail disorders in older people, and aspects of their pharmaceutical treatment. Int J Pharm 2016;512(2):405–11.

54. Kamangar F, Isip L, Bhutani T, et al. How psoriasis patients perceive, obtain, and use biologic agents: survey from an academic medical center. J Dermatolog Treat 2013;24(1):13–24.

55. Bleeker JJ. Intralesional triamcinolone acetonide using the Port-O-Jet and needle injections in localized dermatoses. Br J Dermatol 1974;91(1):97–101.

56. Nantel-Battista M, Richer V, Marcil I, et al. Treatment of nail psoriasis with intralesional triamcinolone acetonide using a needle-free jet injector: a prospective trial. J Cutan Med Surg 2014;18(1):38–42.

57. Reich K, Langley RG, Papp KA, et al. A 52-week trial comparing briakinumab with methotrexate in patients with psoriasis. N Engl J Med 2011;365(17): 1586–96.

58. Sanchez-Regana M, Sola-Ortigosa J, Alsina-Gibert M, et al. Nail psoriasis: a retrospective study on the effectiveness of systemic treatments (classical and biological therapy). J Eur Acad Dermatol Venereol 2011;25(5):579–86.

59. Bardazzi F, Antonucci VA, Tengattini V, et al. A 36-week retrospective open trial comparing the efficacy of biological therapies in nail psoriasis. J Dtsch Dermatol Ges 2013;11(11):1065–70.

60. Rigopoulos D, Gregoriou S, Lazaridou E, et al. Treatment of nail psoriasis with adalimumab: an open label unblinded study. J Eur Acad Dermatol Venereol 2010;24(5):530–4.

61. Van den Bosch F, Manger B, Goupille P, et al. Effectiveness of adalimumab in treating patients with active psoriatic arthritis and predictors of good clinical responses for arthritis, skin and nail lesions. Ann Rheum Dis 2010;69(2):394–9.

62. Dennehy EB, Zhang L, Amato D, et al. Ixekizumab is effective in subjects with moderate to severe plaque psoriasis with significant nail involvement: results from UNCOVER 3. J Drugs Dermatol 2016;15(8): 958–61.

63. Paul C, Reich K, Gottlieb AB, et al. Secukinumab improves hand, foot and nail lesions in moderate-to-severe plaque psoriasis: subanalysis of a randomized, double-blind, placebo-controlled, regimen-finding phase 2 trial. J Eur Acad Dermatol Venereol 2014;28(12):1670–5.

64. Igarashi A, Kato T, Kato M, et al. Efficacy and safety of ustekinumab in Japanese patients with moderate-to-severe plaque-type psoriasis: long-term results from a phase 2/3 clinical trial. J Dermatol 2012; 39(3):242–52.

65. Patsatsi A, Kyriakou A, Sotiriadis D. Ustekinumab in nail psoriasis: an open-label, uncontrolled, non-randomized study. J Dermatolog Treat 2013;24(2): 96–100.

66. Abe M, Nishigori C, Torii H, et al. Tofacitinib for the treatment of moderate to severe chronic plaque psoriasis in Japanese patients: subgroup analyses from a randomized, placebo-controlled phase 3 trial. J Dermatol 2017;44(11):1228–37.

Management of Nail Psoriasis

Dimitrios Rigopoulos, MD*, Natalia Rompoti, MD, PhD, Stamatios Gregoriou, MD, PhD

KEYWORDS

- Nail psoriasis • Nail matrix • Nail bed • Nail psoriasis treatment

KEY POINTS

- Nail psoriasis is a chronic nail disorder that commonly affects psoriatic patients and requires personalized treatment.
- General prophylactic measures to avoid Koebner phenomenon are suggested for all patients and should not be neglected.
- Topical treatment is considered when treating a few-nail disease, with involvement of 3 or fewer nails, without joint involvement and without (or with mild) skin psoriasis.
- Conventional systemic agents, biologics, and small molecules are efficacious for the treatment of nail psoriasis with significant nail involvement or impairment of quality of life.

INTRODUCTION

Nail psoriasis is a chronic nail disorder that commonly affects psoriatic patients. Regardless of the limited body surface involved, treating nail psoriasis effectively is essential not only because of the significant impact of this nail disorder on patients' quality of life (QOL)—with both psychological and functional impairment—but also because of its association as an independent prognostic factor for the development of psoriatic arthritis (PsA).[1,2]

Management of nail psoriasis is associated with several challenges and unfulfilled needs. Diagnosing and, therefore, managing nail psoriasis early on could be challenging in cases where the nail disease mimics onychomycosis, traumatic onycholysis, or other nail disorders. In order to prevent a misdiagnosis, it is essential to obtain a detailed personal and family medical history as well as to perform a thorough skin examination. If in doubt, direct microscopy, nail culture for bacterial or fungal infection, and lesional biopsy of the nail unit can be performed supplementarily. Topical therapy often is difficult due to the nail anatomy, noticeable extent of treatment, and poor adherence that often result in unsatisfactory efficacy. Moreover, topical agents effective in the treatment of nail bed lesions often have poor efficacy in nail matrix psoriasis. The introduction of biologics and small molecules resulted in rapid and highly efficacious improvement of nail psoriasis. Most of the studies, however, report results in a meta-analysis form conducted in subpopulations that primarily were recruited to assess the efficacy on the psoriatic disease of skin and joints. In addition, the presence and extent of skin and/or joint involvement should be taken under consideration. A recent consensus provided recommendations for the treatment of nail psoriasis without cutaneous involvement or with mild skin disease, suggesting that the amount of nails involved can be used as a general rule for deciding on topical or systemic therapy.[3] In cases of moderate to severe skin psoriasis or PsA, another consensus recommended systemic treatment approach according to the characteristics of skin psoriasis and/or PsA.[4] A patient's age, comorbidities, impairment of QOL, and physical and working status also might affect treatment choices (**Fig. 1**). Another

University Hospital of Venereal and Skin Diseases "A.Sygros", 5, Ionos Dragoumi str, Athens 161 21, Greece.
* Corresponding author. University Hospital of Venereal and Skin Diseases "A.Sygros", 5, Ionos Dragoumi str, Athens 161 21, Greece.
E-mail address: dimitrisrigopoulos54@gmail.com

Dermatol Clin 39 (2021) 211–220
https://doi.org/10.1016/j.det.2020.12.014

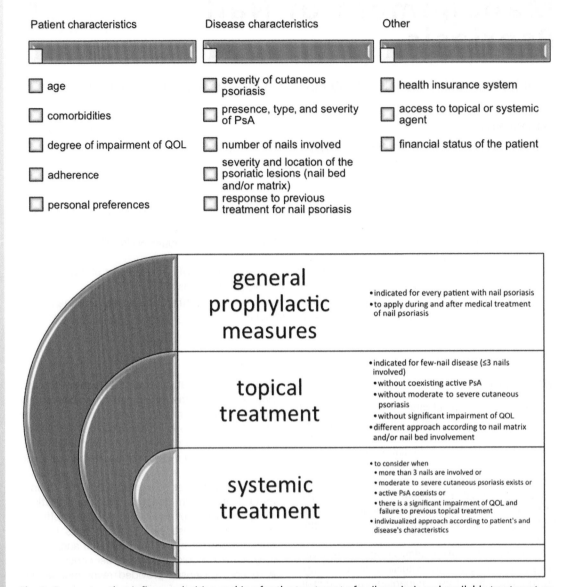

Fig. 1. Parameters that influence decision making for the treatment of nail psoriasis and available treatment options. (*Data from* Rigopoulos D, Baran R, Chiheb S, Daniel CR 3rd, Di Chiacchio N, Gregoriou S, Grover C, Haneke E, Iorizzo M, Pasch M, Piraccini BM, Rich P, Richert B, Rompoti N, Rubin AI, Singal A, Starace M, Tosti A, Triantafyllopoulou I, Zaiac M. Recommendations for the definition, evaluation, and treatment of nail psoriasis in adult patients with no or mild skin psoriasis: A dermatologist and nail expert group consensus. J Am Acad Dermatol. 2019 Jul;81(1):228-240. https://doi.org/10.1016/j.jaad.2019.01.072. Epub 2019 Feb 5. PMID: 30731172.)

challenge involves the evaluation of an effective treatment, suggestions for which are summarized in **Box 1**.[3]

GENERAL MEASURES

General prophylactic measures should be suggested to all patients with nail psoriasis (**Box 2**).[3] In cases of coexisting onychomycosis, antifungal treatment should be initiated prior or parallel to the treatment of nail psoriasis.[5,6]

TOPICAL TREATMENT OF NAIL PSORIASIS

The ideal formulation should be ointment, solution, or foam. When treating a few-nail disease (3 or fewer nails involved) with involvement of nail matrix only, topical steroids plus vitamin D analogs as well as intralesional steroid injections are suggested as first-line treatment, with different schemata in the literature.[3,7,8] Suggestions for the topical treatment with intralesional steroid injections and common adverse events (AEs) are

Box 1
Recommendations for the evaluation of response to treatment

A NAPSI reduction of 0% equals no improvement or worsening.

An index reduction of ≤25% equals minimal improvement.

An index reduction of 26% to 50% equals mild improvement.

An index reduction of 51% to 75% equals moderate improvement.

An index reduction of 76% to 99% equals great improvement.

An index reduction of 100% equals to complete improvement

Adapted from Rigopoulos D, Baran R, Chiheb S, et al. Recommendations for the definition, evaluation, and treatment of nail psoriasis in adult patients with no or mild skin psoriasis: A dermatologist and nail expert group consensus. J Am Acad Dermatol 2019;81(1):231; with permission.

Box 2
General prophylactic measures

1. Avoid
   - Biting or tearing the nails
   - Filing the nails
   - Cutting nails excessively round at the edges
   - Keeping nails long
   - Pulling skin around nails
   - Extracting debris from beneath the nail with sharp instruments
   - Frequently applying and removing nail cosmetics, including artificial or gel nails, nail polish removers with formaldehyde-acetone and toluene, etc.
   - Excessive water contact
   - Wearing tight or high heels

2. Seek
   - Wearing heavy duty cotton gloves for dry work
   - Wearing light cotton gloves underneath vinyl gloves for wet work
   - Frequent topical moisturizing on hands and nails
   - Treatment of fungal or bacterial infection of the extremities and nails

3. Remove the onycholytic part of the nail.

4. Visit an orthopedist or podiatrist for proper shoes and shoe inserts in case of anatomic problems.

Data from Rigopoulos D, Baran R, Chiheb S, et al. Recommendations for the definition, evaluation, and treatment of nail psoriasis in adult patients with no or mild skin psoriasis: A dermatologist and nail expert group consensus. J Am Acad Dermatol 2019;81(1):228-240.

summarized in **Box 3**.[3,7,8] Second-line topical treatment could include topical steroids (clobetasol propionate, 0.05% ointment), vitamin D analogs (calcipotriol, tacalcitol, and calcitriol ointment), topical retinoids (tazarotene, 0.1% gel), topical 0.1% tacrolimus ointment, or topical keratolytic agents.[3]

In cases of an isolated nail bed involvement, a variety of topical agents (intralesional steroid injections, steroid with or without vitamin D regimen, retinoids, and 0.1% tacrolimus) seem efficacious, according to several publications.[3,7,8]

Although numerous data about the use of steroids of different potency, once or twice/daily, with or without occlusion, for a period of up to 4 months to 6 months, are available, superpotent ones seem overall responsible for better results on nail psoriasis. In order to prevent any AEs from their chronic use (skin atrophy, telangiectasias, tachyphylaxis, disappearing digit, and so forth), the topical application should be restricted to once daily and in an intermittent schema. In cases of continuous daily application, treatment duration should not exceed 1 month under occlusion or 2 months without one.[3]

Other modalities that have been explored for the treatment of nail psoriasis also include 5-fluorouracil,[9,10] anthralin,[11] a solution of cyclosporine in maize oil,[12] and intralesional methotrexate injection.[13] All these topical agents, however, have either controversial results or noticeable AEs and few clinical data.

LASER AND LIGHT TREATMENT OF NAIL PSORIASIS

Pulsed dye laser (PDL),[14–17] with a wavelength of 595 nm, or intense pulsed light (IPL),[18,19] with a 550-nm filter, is employed for the treatment of nail psoriasis. Treatment with PDL once/month for 3 months resulted in a significant reduction of Nail Psoriasis Severity Index (NAPSI), especially an improvement of the subungual hyperkeratosis and onycholysis.[14]

IPL also was responsible for a NAPSI reduction of up to 82.4% in a 1-year clinical study, with remission of both nail bed and matrix lesions.[18]

The efficacy of photodynamic therapy in nail psoriasis also has been assessed, and a comparative study with PDL demonstrated improvement in nail bed and matrix features with similar response for both light treatments.[20]

The excimer laser at a wavelength of 308 nm has been approved for the treatment of cutaneous psoriasis.[21,22] In a randomized clinical trial (RCT) comparing the application of excimer laser twice/week versus PDL once/month on nail psoriasis, the results showed a superiority of PDL (38% vs 81% achieved 50% reduction of NAPSI and 55% versus 0% achieved 75% reduction of NAPSI [NAPSI75] at week 12, respectively).[23]

The efficacy of long-pulsed 1064-nm Nd:YAG laser on nail psoriasis also has been evaluated, with a recorded mean reduction of absolute NAPSI from 26 ± 7.2 at baseline to 5.7 ± 4.3 after 3 sessions of treatment once/month.[24]

SYSTEMIC TREATMENT OF NAIL PSORIASIS
Conventional Systemic Treatment

All of the conventional systemic agents indicated for cutaneous psoriasis, such as cyclosporine, methotrexate, acitretin, and fumaric acid, also have been effectively used for the treatment of nail psoriasis.

Methotrexate, in doses up to 15 mg/week, is efficacious, with a NAPSI reduction varying from 30.8% to 49.3%,[25–27] after 24 weeks of treatment. Methotrexate could be used to the lowest effective dose as a maintenance treatment.

Cyclosporine is associated with rapid improvement of nail psoriasis and recommended in doses of 3 mg/kg to 5 mg/kg for a short period of time and under monitoring. Effort should be made to use the lowest dosage that could achieve at least moderate response.[25,27–29]

Acitretin usually is initiated in a dose between 0.2 mg/kg to 0.5 mg/kg for more than 6 months due to the slow onset of action.[30,31] Treatment with this agent should be favored in cases of coexisting pustular psoriasis with nail involvement.[31] Because vitamin A derivatives could cause, in rare cases, brittle nails and paronychia, a regular assessment of the benefit-risk profile of this agent is necessary.

Fumaric acid, where available, should be initiated in a low starting dose with subsequent gradual increases according to drug tolerability.[32] Chronic use also should be monitored regularly in order to evaluate possible side effects, including the risk of lymphopenia.[33]

Continuation of treatment with the conventional systemic agents is suggested until at least moderate improvement is achieved. Because of the risk for organ toxicity, sufficient monitoring is recommended.

Biologic Treatment and Small Molecules

Anti–tumor necrosis factor (TNF)-α inhibitors infliximab,[34–37] etanercept,[38–41] adalimumab,[34,39,42–45] and golimumab[46]; interleukin (IL)-12/23 inhibitor ustekinumab[34,47–51]; IL-17 inhibitors secukinumab[52] and ixekizumab[53–55]; IL-17 receptor brodalumab[56,57]; phosphodiesterase type 4 (PDE4) inhibitor apremilast[58,59]; and tofacitinib[60,61] should be considered for systemic treatment of nail psoriasis. As literature evidence suggests, they result in rapid and significant improvement of nail psoriasis when used in patients with nail psoriasis and cutaneous disease and/or arthritis. In addition, available data document long-term maintenance of improvement of nail psoriatic signs without noteworthy AEs.[34,39,45,48,62]

Etanercept
The anti–TNF-α fusion protein etanercept demonstrated long-term efficacy, with an excellent safety profile in nail psoriasis. At week 24, 51% improvement of the initial NAPSI has been documented, and, at week 54, 100% reduction of NAPSI (NAPSI100) was reported in 30% of the patients.[41]

Infliximab
A rapid and efficacious response to the chimeric monoclonal anti–TNF-α inhibitor infliximab was demonstrated through various RCTs and case series, with a 56.3% to 94% improvement in NAPSI at weeks 22 to 24.[35,36,63,64] In another publication of 25 cases of nail psoriasis under infliximab, NAPSI75 was reached by all patients at week 22.[65]

Adalimumab
Treatment with adalimumab, a human monoclonal anti–TNF-α antibody, resulted in rapid improvement of NAPSI in patients with PsA and nail involvement, with a 57% decrease in the mean score at week 12 (n = 244) and a further reduction up to 91% by week 20 (n = 103).[42] In another study (n = 36) an improvement in NAPSI was observed as high as 54% at week 28.[66] Fingernails responded better compared with toenails (reduction of NAPSI: 85% vs 71.5%, respectively, at week 24).[43]

The good efficacy of adalimumab treatment on nail psoriasis also is reflected in the improvement of patient's QOL in a subanalysis of the BELIEVE study, with a 74.3% reduction of the initial Dermatology Life Quality Index (DLQI) after a 39.5% improvement of nail psoriasis at week 16.[44] These data prompted the conduction of a recently published phase III RCT (n = 217) investigating the efficacy and safety of adalimumab in moderate to severe nail psoriasis.[45,67] A 75% improvement of NAPSI was observed in 46.6% of the patients at week 26 and a 75% improvement of modified NAPSI of the fingernails in 25.9% at week 16, increasing to 47.4% at week 26 and to 54.5% at week 52.[45,67]

A continuing improvement of patient QoL, including pain experience associated with nail psoriasis, also was documented throughout week 52.[67] These data led to the addition of

moderate to severe fingernail psoriasis to the drug's prescribing information.

Certolizumab pegol
The effect of the PEGylated anti–TNF-α inhibitor certolizumab pegol on nail psoriasis has been investigated in patients with PsA (RAPID-PsA study).[68] A statistically significant improvement of absolute NAPSI from 50.34 (baseline) to 20.5 (at week 24) with an additional reduction to 10 (week 52) has been observed.[68,69]

Golimumab
Although golimumab, an anti–TNF-α inhibitor, is used mainly for the treatment of PsA, data extracted from RCTs reported 25% and 33% improvement of target median NAPSI at week 12 and week 24, respectively, in patients receiving 50 mg and 43% and 54% improvement at week 12 and week 24, respectively, in patients receiving 100 mg of golimumab.[70,71]

Ustekinumab
Both large RCTs[47,48] and case series[49,72,73] demonstrated promising results for the treatment of nail psoriasis with this recombinant, fully human, anti–TNF-α antibody. At week 12, a significant reduction of NAPSI was observed, varying between different studies and dosages (45 mg or 90 mg) from 24.9% to 37.6%.[47–50] At week 16, a 49% reduction of NAPSI was noted.[72] This rapid onset of success was followed by an impressive efficacy rate with a further reduction up to 88% at week 28.[72]

In another RCT (n = 158) the long-term response to ustekinumab, 45 mg and 90 mg, was evaluated and the mean improvements in NAPSI after 64 weeks of treatment were 56.6% and 67.8%, respectively.[48]

Guselkumab
A meta-analysis of the 2 multicenter RCTs VOYAGE 1 and VOYAGE 2 revealed a significant improvement in fingernail psoriasis with the use of the IL-23 antibody guselkumab compared with placebo, with results similar to the adalimumab treatment.[74,75]

Secukinumab
Secukinumab, a fully human immunoglobulin G1 kappa antagonist of IL–17A, is one of the few biologics with prospective trials designed specifically to investigate the efficacy in nail psoriasis and the influence on nail-specific QOL aspects. In the TRANSFIGURE study[76] (n = 198) 300-mg secukinumab demonstrated a positive effect as early as 2 weeks after treatment initiation. At week 16, the mean NAPSI changes were 45.3% and

37.9% for secukinumab, 300 mg and 150 mg, respectively. Fingernails showed a better response compared with toenails. A further improvement was noted at week 32 with a reduction of total fingernail NAPSI of −63.2% and −52.6% for the 300-mg and 150-mg regimens, respectively, and a noteworthy improvement of the patient's QOL.

The significant improvement in nail psoriasis also has been reported in other RCTs[52,77] and case series,[78,79] with partially more rapid and better response rates.

Ixekizumab

A post hoc analysis of a phase II study with ixekizumab (a fully humanized monoclonal IL-17A inhibitor), comprising a 20-week randomized, placebo-controlled period and a 48-week open-labeled extension phase,[53] investigated the efficacy in patients with moderate to severe psoriasis and nail involvement. The data were promising: 51.0% of the patients experienced complete resolution by week 48. Another subgroup analysis (of the UNCOVER-3 trial)[55] demonstrated an improvement of baseline NAPSI exceeding 80% with more than half of the patients reaching NAPSI100 at week 60. The positive effect seems to be sustained over a period of 156 weeks in the UNCOVER 3 study.[80] A comparison between ixekizumab and ustekinumab in the IXORA-S trial suggested superior efficacy of ixekizumab over ustekinumab in nail psoriasis during the first 24 weeks of treatment,[81] but further studies are necessary in order to establish a final conclusion.

Brodalumab

The effect of brodalumab, a monoclonal immunoglobulin G2 antibody against IL-17 receptor, on nail psoriasis recently has been explored through RCTs and case series. Psoriatic lesions on skin and nails responded rapidly to treatment with high percentage of improvement and no new safety concerns.[56,57]

Apremilast

In the RCTs responsible for the approval of this selective PDE4 inhibitor, ESTEEM 1/2, the efficacy on nail psoriasis was also evaluated, with 22.5%/29%, 43.6%/60%, and 60.2%/59.7% reduction of NAPSI at week 16, week 32, and week 52, respectively.[59] Long-term improvement of nail psoriasis also was demonstrated in the LIBERATE study with a reduction of NAPSI from baseline varying from −48.1% to −51.1% after 104 weeks of treatment.[82] Promising results recently were extracted from the multicenter APPRECIATE study, involving 250 patients with psoriasis in difficult-to-treat areas treated with apremilast for 6 months.[83] Another study in biologically naïve patients demonstrated a continuing improvement of NAPSI under treatment with apremilast, with 48.0% (24/50) achieving full remission (NAPSI100) after 52 weeks of treatment.[84] In the real-world setting, the continuing improvement of nail psoriasis also was confirmed in 100 Greek patients under apremilast, and a 50% reduction of NAPSI was observed after 24 weeks of treatment.[85]

Tofacitinib

The efficacy and safety profile of tofacitinib in nail psoriasis also have been evaluated in phase III RCTs. At week 16, this oral Janus kinase inhibitor achieved, in a dosage of 5 mg/10 mg twice/day, NAPSI75 and NAPSI100 in 16.9%/28.1% and 10.3%/18.2% of the patients, respectively.[60] A further improvement was noted through week 52, with both tofacitinib dose groups reaching NAPSI75 in 22.2% in the 5-mg and 47.6% in the 10-mg dosages.[61]

SUMMARY

As with the psoriatic disease of the skin, treatment of the nail compartment should be personalized. This should take into consideration parameters that involve a patient's characteristics, such as age, comorbidities, degree of impairment of QOL, and personal preferences. Moreover, disease characteristics, such as the severity of cutaneous psoriasis, the presence and severity of PsA, the number of nails involved, the severity and location of the psoriatic lesions (nail bed and/or matrix), and response to previous treatment of nail psoriasis, are to be taken into account. General prophylactic measures are the cornerstone of every treatment and should be followed during and after topical and/or systemic approach. The use of topical therapy should be considered in patients with few-nail disease without PsA and without or with mild skin psoriasis. Although there is no definite threshold for the initiation of systemic treatment, coexisting moderate to severe cutaneous disease, PsA, or involvement of more than 3 nails are aspects that prompt the use of systemic agents.

CONFLICT OF INTEREST

D. Rigopoulos was a speaker and has received honoraria from Celgene, Novartis, Janssen, LEO, Lilly, UCB, and Abbvie; was a consultant and has received honoraria from Celgene, Novartis, Janssen. and Abbvie; and is/was a PI for Abbvie and Genesis Pharma. N. Rompoti was a speaker and has received honoraria from Abbvie, Genesis Pharma, Janssen, Novartis, LEO, Lilly, and UCB. S. Gregoriou was a speaker and has received honoraria from Abbvie, Janssen, and Novartis. No funding has been received for this article.

CLINICS CARE POINTS

- The severity of nail psoriasis as well as the degree of skin and/or joint involvement determine the use of topical and/or systemic treatments.
- The therapeutic approach is also influenced by patients characteristics, such as age, comorbidities, personal preferences and the impairment of quality of life.
- With the introduction of biologics and small molecules a more efficacious and long-lasting disease management, with less organ toxicity, can be achieved in severe cases of nail psoriasis.

REFERENCES

1. Augustin M, Reich K, Blome C, et al. Nail psoriasis in Germany: epidemiology and burden of disease. Br J Dermatol 2010;163(3):580–5.
2. Belyayeva E, Gregoriou S, Chalikias J, et al. The impact of nail disorders on quality of life. Eur J Dermatol 2013;23(3):366–71.
3. Rigopoulos D, Baran R, Chiheb S, et al. Recommendations for the definition, evaluation, and treatment of nail psoriasis in adult patients with no or mild skin psoriasis: a dermatologist and nail expert group consensus. J Am Acad Dermatol 2019;81(1):228–40.
4. Langley RG, Saurat JH, Reich K, Nail Psoriasis Delphi Expert Panel. Recommendations for the treatment of nail psoriasis in patients with moderate to severe psoriasis: a dermatology expert group consensus. J Eur Acad Dermatol Venereol 2012; 26(3):373–81.
5. Tosti A. Nail disorders. Louis, Missouri: Elsevier Health Sciences; 2018.
6. Pasch MC. Nail psoriasis: a review of treatment options. Drugs 2016;76(6):675–705.
7. Haneke E. Nail psoriasis: clinical features, pathogenesis, differential diagnoses, and management. Psoriasis (Auckl) 2017;7:51–63.
8. Tosti A. Nail disorders 2018. Available at: https:// www.sciencedirect.com/science/book/ 9780323544337. Accessed July 28, 2018.
9. Fritz K. [Successful local treatment of nail psoriasis with 5-fluorouracil]. Z Hautkr 1989;64(12):1083–8.
10. de Jong EM, Menke HE, van Praag MC, et al. Dystrophic psoriatic fingernails treated with 1% 5-fluorouracil in a nail penetration-enhancing vehicle: a double-blind study. Dermatology 1999;199(4):313–8.
11. Yamamoto T, Katayama I, Nishioka K. Topical anthralin therapy for refractory nail psoriasis. J Dermatol 1998;25(4):231–3.
12. Cannavò SP, Guarneri F, Vaccaro M, et al. Treatment of psoriatic nails with topical cyclosporin: a prospective, randomized placebo-controlled study. Dermatology 2003;206(2):153–6.
13. Sarıcaoglu H, Oz A, Turan H. Nail psoriasis successfully treated with intralesional methotrexate: case report. Dermatology 2011;222(1):5–7.
14. Oram Y, Karincaoğlu Y, Koyuncu E, et al. Pulsed dye laser in the treatment of nail psoriasis. Dermatol Surg 2010;36(3):377–81.
15. Treewittayapoom C, Singvahanont P, Chanprapaph K, et al. The effect of different pulse durations in the treatment of nail psoriasis with 595-nm pulsed dye laser: a randomized, double-blind, intrapatient left-to-right study. J Am Acad Dermatol 2012;66(5):807–12.
16. Maranda EL, Nguyen AH, Lim VM, et al. Laser and light therapies for the treatment of nail psoriasis. J Eur Acad Dermatol Venereol 2016;30(8):1278–84.
17. Goldust M, Raghifar R. Clinical trial study in the treatment of nail psoriasis with pulsed dye laser. J Cosmet Laser Ther 2013. https://doi.org/10.3109/ 14764172.2013.854627.
18. Tawfik AA. Novel treatment of nail psoriasis using the intense pulsed light: a one-year follow-up study. Dermatol Surg 2014;40(7):763–8.
19. Wiznia LE, Quatrano NA, Mu EW, et al. A clinical review of laser and light therapy for nail psoriasis and onychomycosis. Dermatol Surg 2017;43(2):161–72.
20. Fernández-Guarino M, Harto A, Sánchez-Ronco M, et al. Pulsed dye laser vs. photodynamic therapy in the treatment of refractory nail psoriasis: a comparative pilot study. J Eur Acad Dermatol Venereol 2009;23(8):891–5.
21. Elmets CA, Lim HW, Stoff B, et al. Joint American academy of dermatology-national psoriasis foundation guidelines of care for the management and treatment of psoriasis with phototherapy. J Am Acad Dermatol 2019;81(3):775–804.
22. Abrouk M, Levin E, Brodsky M, et al. Excimer laser for the treatment of psoriasis: safety, efficacy, and patient acceptability. Psoriasis (Auckl) 2016;6:165–73.
23. Al-Mutairi N, Noor T, Al-Haddad A. Single blinded left-to-right comparison study of excimer laser versus pulsed dye laser for the treatment of nail psoriasis. Dermatol Ther 2014;4(2):197–205.
24. Kartal SP, Canpolat F, Gonul M, et al. Long-pulsed Nd: YAG laser treatment for nail psoriasis. Dermatol Surg 2018;44(2):227–33.
25. Sánchez-Regaña M, Sola-Ortigosa J, Alsina-Gibert M, et al. Nail psoriasis: a retrospective study on the effectiveness of systemic treatments (classical and biological therapy). J Eur Acad Dermatol Venereol 2011;25(5):579–86.
26. Reich K, Nestle FO, Papp K, et al. Infliximab induction and maintenance therapy for moderate-to-severe psoriasis: a phase III, multicentre, double-blind trial. Lancet 2005;366(9494):1367–74.

27. Gümüşel M, Özdemir M, Mevlitoğlu I, et al. Evaluation of the efficacy of methotrexate and cyclosporine therapies on psoriatic nails: a one-blind, randomized study. J Eur Acad Dermatol Venereol 2011;25(9):1080–4.

28. Arnold WP, Gerritsen MJ, van de Kerkhof PC. Response of nail psoriasis to cyclosporin. Br J Dermatol 1993;129(6):750–1.

29. Syuto T, Abe M, Ishibuchi H, et al. Successful treatment of psoriatic nails with low-dose cyclosporine administration. Eur J Dermatol 2007;17(3):248–9.

30. Ricceri F, Pescitelli L, Tripo L, et al. Treatment of severe nail psoriasis with acitretin: an impressive therapeutic result. Dermatol Ther 2013;26(1):77–8.

31. Piraccini BM, Tosti A, Iorizzo M, et al. Pustular psoriasis of the nails: treatment and long-term follow-up of 46 patients. Br J Dermatol 2001;144(5):1000–5.

32. Vlachou C, Berth-Jones J. Nail psoriasis improvement in a patient treated with fumaric acid esters. J Dermatolog Treat 2007;18(3):175–7.

33. Sondermann W, Rompoti N, Leister L, et al. Lymphopenia and CD4+/CD8+ Cell Reduction under Fumaric Acid Esters. Dermatology 2017;233(4):295–302.

34. Bardazzi F, Antonucci VA, Tengattini V, et al. A 36-week retrospective open trial comparing the efficacy of biological therapies in nail psoriasis. J Dtsch Dermatol Ges 2013;11(11):1065–70.

35. Rich P, Griffiths CEM, Reich K, et al. Baseline nail disease in patients with moderate to severe psoriasis and response to treatment with infliximab during 1 year. J Am Acad Dermatol 2008;58(2):224–31.

36. Rigopoulos D, Gregoriou S, Stratigos A, et al. Evaluation of the efficacy and safety of infliximab on psoriatic nails: an unblinded, nonrandomized, open-label study. Br J Dermatol 2008;159(2):453–6.

37. Reich K, Ortonne J-P, Kerkmann U, et al. Skin and nail responses after 1 year of infliximab therapy in patients with moderate-to-severe psoriasis: a retrospective analysis of the EXPRESS Trial. Dermatology 2010;221(2):172–8.

38. Ozmen I, Erbil AH, Koc E, et al. Treatment of nail psoriasis with tumor necrosis factor-alpha blocker agents: an open-label, unblinded, comparative study. J Dermatol 2013;40(9):755–6.

39. Saraceno R, Pietroleonardo L, Mazzotta A, et al. TNF-α antagonists and nail psoriasis: an open, 24-week, prospective cohort study in adult patients with psoriasis. Expert Opin Biol Ther 2013;13(4):469–73.

40. Ortonne JP, Paul C, Berardesca E, et al. A 24-week randomized clinical trial investigating the efficacy and safety of two doses of etanercept in nail psoriasis. Br J Dermatol 2013;168(5):1080–7.

41. Luger TA, Barker J, Lambert J, et al. Sustained improvement in joint pain and nail symptoms with etanercept therapy in patients with moderate-to-severe psoriasis. J Eur Acad Dermatol Venereol 2009;23(8):896–904.

42. Van den Bosch F, Manger B, Goupille P, et al. Effectiveness of adalimumab in treating patients with active psoriatic arthritis and predictors of good clinical responses for arthritis, skin and nail lesions. Ann Rheum Dis 2010;69(2):394–9.

43. Rigopoulos D, Gregoriou S, Lazaridou E, et al. Treatment of nail psoriasis with adalimumab: an open label unblinded study. J Eur Acad Dermatol Venereol 2010;24(5):530–4.

44. Thaçi D, Unnebrink K, Sundaram M, et al. Adalimumab for the treatment of moderate to severe psoriasis: subanalysis of effects on scalp and nails in the BELIEVE study. J Eur Acad Dermatol Venereol 2015;29(2):353–60.

45. Elewski BE, Okun MM, Papp K, et al. Adalimumab for nail psoriasis: efficacy and safety from the first 26 weeks of a phase 3, randomized, placebo-controlled trial. J Am Acad Dermatol 2018;78(1):90–9.e1.

46. Kavanaugh A, McInnes I, Mease P, et al. Golimumab, a new human tumor necrosis factor alpha antibody, administered every four weeks as a subcutaneous injection in psoriatic arthritis: Twenty-four-week efficacy and safety results of a randomized, placebo-controlled study. Arthritis Rheum 2009;60(4):976–86.

47. Rich P, Bourcier M, Sofen H, et al. Ustekinumab improves nail disease in patients with moderate-to-severe psoriasis: results from PHOENIX 1. Br J Dermatol 2014;170(2):398–407.

48. Igarashi A, Kato T, Kato M, et al, Japanese Ustekinumab Study Group. Efficacy and safety of ustekinumab in Japanese patients with moderate-to-severe plaque-type psoriasis: long-term results from a phase 2/3 clinical trial. J Dermatol 2012;39(3):242–52.

49. Rigopoulos D, Gregoriou S, Makris M, et al. Efficacy of ustekinumab in nail psoriasis and improvement in nail-associated quality of life in a population treated with ustekinumab for cutaneous psoriasis: an open prospective unblinded study. Dermatology 2011;223(4):325–9.

50. Vitiello M, Tosti A, Abuchar A, et al. Ustekinumab for the treatment of nail psoriasis in heavily treated psoriatic patients. Int J Dermatol 2013;52(3):358–62.

51. Rallis E, Kintzoglou S, Verros C. Ustekinumab for rapid treatment of nail psoriasis. Arch Dermatol 2010;146(11):1315–6.

52. Paul C, Reich K, Gottlieb AB, et al. Secukinumab improves hand, foot and nail lesions in moderate-to-severe plaque psoriasis: subanalysis of a randomized, double-blind, placebo-controlled, regimen-finding phase 2 trial. J Eur Acad Dermatol Venereol 2014;28(12):1670–5.

53. Langley RG, Rich P, Menter A, et al. Improvement of scalp and nail lesions with ixekizumab in a phase 2 trial in patients with chronic plaque psoriasis. J Eur Acad Dermatol Venereol 2015;29(9):1763–70.

54. Dennehy EB, Zhang L, Amato D, et al. Ixekizumab is effective in subjects with moderate to severe plaque psoriasis with significant nail involvement: results from UNCOVER 3. J Drugs Dermatol 2016;15(8): 958–61.

55. van de Kerkhof P, Guenther L, Gottlieb AB, et al. Ixekizumab treatment improves fingernail psoriasis in patients with moderate-to-severe psoriasis: results from the randomized, controlled and open-label phases of UNCOVER-3. J Eur Acad Dermatol Venereol 2016. https://doi.org/10.1111/jdv.14033.

56. Pinter A, Bonnekoh B, Hadshiew IM, et al. Brodalumab for the treatment of moderate-to-severe psoriasis: case series and literature review. Clin Cosmet Investig Dermatol 2019;12:509–17.

57. Blair HA. Brodalumab: a review in moderate to severe plaque psoriasis. Drugs 2018;78(4):495–504.

58. Nguyen CM, Leon A, Danesh M, et al. Improvement of nail and scalp psoriasis using apremilast in patients with chronic psoriasis: phase 2b and 3, 52-week randomized, placebo-controlled trial results. J Drugs Dermatol 2016;15(3):272–6.

59. Rich P, Gooderham M, Bachelez H, et al. Apremilast, an oral phosphodiesterase 4 inhibitor, in patients with difficult-to-treat nail and scalp psoriasis: Results of 2 phase III randomized, controlled trials (ESTEEM 1 and ESTEEM 2). J Am Acad Dermatol 2016;74(1): 134–42.

60. Merola JF, Elewski B, Tatulych S, et al. Efficacy of tofacitinib for the treatment of nail psoriasis: Two 52-week, randomized, controlled phase 3 studies in patients with moderate-to-severe plaque psoriasis. J Am Acad Dermatol 2017;77(1):79–87.e1.

61. Abe M, Nishigori C, Torii H, et al. Tofacitinib for the treatment of moderate to severe chronic plaque psoriasis in Japanese patients: Subgroup analyses from a randomized, placebo-controlled phase 3 trial. J Dermatol 2017;44(11):1228–37.

62. Reich K, Warren RB, Coates LC, et al. Long-term efficacy and safety of secukinumab in the treatment of the multiple manifestations of psoriatic disease. J Eur Acad Dermatol Venereol 2019. https://doi. org/10.1111/jdv.16124.

63. Torii H, Sato N, Yoshinari T, et al, Japanese Infliximab Study Investigators. Dramatic impact of a Psoriasis Area and Severity Index 90 response on the quality of life in patients with psoriasis: an analysis of Japanese clinical trials of infliximab. J Dermatol 2012; 39(3):253–9.

64. Torii H, Nakagawa H, Japanese Infliximab Study investigators. Infliximab monotherapy in Japanese patients with moderate-to-severe plaque psoriasis and psoriatic arthritis. A randomized, double-blind, placebo-controlled multicenter trial. J Dermatol Sci 2010;59(1):40–9.

65. Bianchi L, Bergamin A, de Felice C, et al. Remission and time of resolution of nail psoriasis during infliximab therapy. J Am Acad Dermatol 2005; 52(4):736–7.

66. Leonardi C, Langley RG, Papp K, et al. Adalimumab for treatment of moderate to severe chronic plaque psoriasis of the hands and feet: efficacy and safety results from REACH, a randomized, placebo-controlled, double-blind trial. Arch Dermatol 2011; 147(4):429–36.

67. Elewski BE, Baker CS, Crowley JJ, et al. Adalimumab for nail psoriasis: efficacy and safety over 52 weeks from a phase-3, randomized, placebo-controlled trial. J Eur Acad Dermatol Venereol 2019;33(11):2168–78.

68. Mease PJ, Fleischmann R, Deodhar AA, et al. Effect of certolizumab pegol on signs and symptoms in patients with psoriatic arthritis: 24-week results of a Phase 3 double-blind randomised placebo-controlled study (RAPID-PsA). Ann Rheum Dis 2014;73(1):48–55.

69. Mazzeo M, Dattola A, Cannizzaro MV, et al. Nail psoriasis treated with certolizumab pegol in patients with psoriatic arthritis: preliminary observation. Actas Dermosifiliogr 2019;110(2):169–71.

70. Kavanaugh A, van der Heijde D, McInnes IB, et al. Golimumab in psoriatic arthritis: one-year clinical efficacy, radiographic, and safety results from a phase III, randomized, placebo-controlled trial. Arthritis Rheum 2012;64(8):2504–17.

71. de Vries ACQ, Bogaards NA, Hooft L, et al. Interventions for nail psoriasis. Cochrane Database Syst Rev 2013;1:CD007633.

72. Patsatsi A, Kyriakou A, Sotiriadis D. Ustekinumab in nail psoriasis: an open-label, uncontrolled, nonrandomized study. J Dermatolog Treat 2013;24(2):96–100.

73. Kim BR, Yang S, Choi CW, et al. Comparison of NAPSI and N-NAIL for evaluation of fingernail psoriasis in patients with moderate-to-severe plaque psoriasis treated using ustekinumab. J Dermatolog Treat 2019;30(2):123–8.

74. Nakamura M, Lee K, Jeon C, et al. Guselkumab for the treatment of psoriasis: a review of phase III trials. Dermatol Ther 2017;7(3):281–92.

75. Foley P, Gordon K, Griffiths CEM, et al. Efficacy of guselkumab compared with adalimumab and placebo for psoriasis in specific body regions: a secondary analysis of 2 randomized clinical trials. JAMA Dermatol 2018;154(6):676–83.

76. Reich K, Sullivan J, Arenberger P, et al. Effect of secukinumab on clinical activity and disease burden of nail psoriasis: 32-week results from the randomized placebo-controlled TRANSFIGURE trial. Br J Dermatol 2018. https://doi.org/10.1111/ bjd.17351.

77. Augustin M, Kiedrowski R von, Rigopoulos D, et al. Effectiveness and safety of secukinumab treatment in real-world clinical settings in European countries confirms its efficacy and safety from clinical trials:

data from an interim analysis of SERENA study. J Am Acad Dermatol 2019;81(4):AB50.

78. Pistone G, Gurreri R, Tilotta G, et al. Secukinumab efficacy in the treatment of nail psoriasis: a case series. J Dermatolog Treat 2018;29(sup1):21–4.

79. Wells LE, Evans T, Hilton R, et al. Use of secukinumab in a pediatric patient leads to significant improvement in nail psoriasis and psoriatic arthritis. Pediatr Dermatol 2019;36(3):384–5.

80. Leonardi C, Maari C, Philipp S, et al. Maintenance of skin clearance with ixekizumab treatment of psoriasis: three-year results from the UNCOVER-3 study. J Am Acad Dermatol 2018;79(5): 824–30.e2.

81. Ghislain PD, Conrad C, Dutronc Y, et al. Comparison of ixekizumab and ustekinumab efficacy in the treatment of nail lesions of patients with moderate-to-severe plaque psoriasis: 24-week data from a phase 3 trial. Arthritis Rheumatol 2017;69(suppl 10). Available at: https://acrabstracts.org/abstract/comparison-of-ixekizumab-and-ustekinumab-efficacy-in-the-treatment-of-nail-lesions-of-patients-with-moderate-to-severe-plaque-psoriasis-24-week-data-from-a-phase-3-trial/. Accessed January 10, 2021.

82. Reich K, Gooderham M, Bewley A, et al. Safety and efficacy of apremilast through 104 weeks in patients with moderate to severe psoriasis who continued on apremilast or switched from etanercept treatment: findings from the LIBERATE study. J Eur Acad Dermatol Venereol 2018;32(3):397–402.

83. Real-World Experience With Apremilast: Analysis of 250 patients from the APPRECIATE study with psoriasis in difficult-to-treat areas. poster ID 9776 presented at the: 2019 AAD Annual Meeting; March 1, 2019, Washington, DC.

84. Fritzlar Stefanie, Korge Bernhard, Manasterski Maria, et al. Physician- and patient-reported outcomes for patients with plaque psoriasis treated with apremilast during routine dermatology care in Germany. J Am Acad Dermatol 2019;81(4):AB439.

85. Papakonstantis M, Georgiou S, Chasapi V, et al. Interim Results of a Nationwide, Real-World Prospective Study of the Therapeutic Effects of Apremilast on the Quality of Life and Disease Activity Parameters Among Patients With Moderate Psoriasis Treated in Greece [APRAISAL Study]. Poster ID 1641 presented at the: 28th EADV Congress 2019; September 10, 2019, Madrid.

Review of Nail Lichen Planus
Epidemiology, Pathogenesis, Diagnosis, and Treatment

Mohit Kumar Gupta, BBA[a], Shari R. Lipner, MD, PhD[b],*

KEYWORDS

- Lichen planus • Nail lichen planus • Pterygium • Anonychia • Trachyonychia • Nails • Nail bed
- Nail matrix

KEY POINTS

- Nail lichen planus (NLP) is a chronic inflammatory disorder with significant cosmetic and functional impact. Permanent scarring and nail loss may occur without prompt and effective treatment.
- In most cases, the diagnosis of NLP can be made with clinical examination and dermoscopy. Longitudinal biopsy with histopathology is recommended for more challenging cases and before starting systemic therapy.
- Although injectable and intramuscular corticosteroids are the mainstays of treatment, systemic retinoids have more recently been used with good efficacy. Controlled clinical trials are necessary to compare efficacy between therapeutic NLP options.

INTRODUCTION

Lichen planus (LP) is a chronic inflammatory disorder that may affect the skin, nails, hair, and oral mucosa with a worldwide estimated prevalence of 0.5% to 1%. Classic LP presents with flat-topped violaceous papules involving the skin, with many morphologic variants. Nail lichen planus (NLP) may occur independently or in conjunction with other forms of LP. NLP may cause significant morbidity, and it is one of the few nail diseases in which permanent nail loss may ensue with inadequate treatment. For many patients with NLP, there is a profound impact on daily activities and quality of life.

The clinical features of NLP are not specific, especially at disease onset. Thus systematically assessing symptoms and forming evidence-based diagnostic criteria is challenging. Treatment of NLP is currently guided by physician experience and evidence from case series and case reports. Treatment options are also limited by the recurrent nature of the disease. This review aims to summarize and update the current evidence guiding the epidemiology, pathogenesis, diagnosis, and management of NLP.

METHODS

Searches for peer-reviewed journal articles were conducted using the PubMed/MEDLINE database with the search terms "lichen planus" and "nail lichen planus." Reference lists from these articles were used to find additional articles. The authors included all articles published before December

Funding sources: none.
a State University of New York Downstate College of Medicine, Brooklyn, NY, USA; b Department of Dermatology, Weill Cornell Medicine, 1305 York Avenue, New York, NY 10021, USA
* Corresponding author.
E-mail address: shl9032@med.cornell.edu

Dermatol Clin 39 (2021) 221–230
https://doi.org/10.1016/j.det.2020.12.002
0733-8635/21/© 2020 Elsevier Inc. All rights reserved.

2019. Studies were not excluded based on date of publication or language.

PATHOGENESIS

The pathogenesis of LP and NLP is incompletely understood. Abnormal Toll-like receptor (TLR) activity is thought to play a role.[1] TLRs are membrane or intracellular receptor proteins that respond to pathogen-associated molecular patterns.[2] TLRs are highly expressed by sentinel cells, including plasmacytoid dendritic cells (pDC). pDCs are the most potent producers of interferons, cytokines responsible for combating viral pathogens through the recruitment of CD8+ T lymphocytes.[3] Abnormal reactivity of TLRs in pDCs may lead to excessive recruitment of CD8+ T lymphocytes. There is evidence for both accumulation of pDCs and autoreactive CD8+ T lymphocytes–mediated destruction of keratinocytes in LP.[3–6]

LP has been shown to be significantly associated with hepatitis C and herpes simplex virus.[4,5,7–9] Because both are viral pathogens, activation of the previously described pathways may be relevant to this association. An allergy to metal ions has also been linked to LP.[10–12] One study of 115 patients with LP also showed a higher prevalence of metal allergy on patch testing in patients with NLP compared with those with LP (59% vs 27%).[10] Some medications such as antimalarial drugs, nonsteroidal antiinflammatory drugs, and antihypertensive agents may trigger lichenoid drug reactions.[13] Lichenoid drug reactions typically improve or resolve with withdrawal of the offending medication. There is evidence of higher rates of pediatric LP in Indian populations, suggesting a genetic component for the disease. In a retrospective study from the United Kingdom, 80% of children with diagnosed with LP were Indian.[14,15]

EPIDEMIOLOGY

Worldwide prevalence of LP is estimated at 0.5% to 1.0%. Ten to fifteen percent of patients with LP are reported to have nail manifestations.[16,17] Some patients present with NLP without skin, mucosal, or hair involvement.[18–20] NLP is more likely to affect the fingernails compared with the toenails. In a retrospective study of 67 patients with NLP, 94% had fingernail involvement with an average of 7 fingernails affected, whereas 54% of patients had toenail involvement with an average of 3 toenails affected.[21] Adults are most often affected with only 10% to 15% of cases occurring in children.[22] The mean age of affected patients was 47 and 48.5 years in 2 retrospective

studies.[20,21] There is no gender-based predilection that is consistent in literature.[20,21,23] Often NLP affects one or a few nails initially and then involve others at different intervals. NLP differs from idiopathic trachyonychia where nails are usually affected simultaneously.[24]

CLINICAL FEATURES

Establishing criteria for clinical diagnosis of NLP is hindered by the lack of specificity and consistent chronologic pattern for many of the presenting symptoms. LP affecting the nail matrix may result in longitudinal ridging, nail plate thinning, lamina fragmentation, red or "mottled" lunula, and pterygium (**Fig. 1**). In 2 retrospective studies of patients with NLP (n = 67 and n = 24) longitudinal ridging was the most common nail finding (89.5% and 66.7%) (**Table 1**).[20,21] Erythema of the lunula, which occurs in 25.0% to 31.3% of patients, can be histopathologically correlated with distal nail matrix inflammation.[20] Lamina fragmentation, or splitting of the nail plate, is a consequence of nail plate thinning and indicates more severe disease.[25] When NLP affects the nail bed, it results in onycholysis, subungual hyperkeratosis, and splinter hemorrhages. Very few patients present with isolated nail bed involvement (10.4% and 12.5%), but onycholysis (33.3% and 43.3%) and subungual keratosis (23.8% and 37.5%) were among the most common nail findings.[20,21] Onycholysis in NLP can also result in avulsion of the nail with or without minor trauma. Trachyonychia,

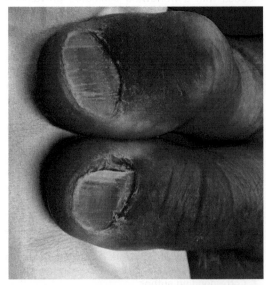

Fig. 1. A 57-year-old man with NLP presenting with 2 months of longitudinal ridging, nail plate thinning, splitting, and onycholysis of the bilateral thumbnails.

Table 1 Clinical features of nail lichen planus		
	Tosti et al,[20] 1993	Goettman et al,[21] 2011
Clinical Findings	Number of Patients (%)	Number of Patients (%)
Nail Matrix		
Longitudinal ridging	16 (66.7)	60 (89.5)
Red lunula	6 (25.0)	21 (31.3)
Thinning of nail plate	12 (50.0)	NA
Koilonychia	2 (8.3)	NA
Trachyonychia	NA	15 (22.4)
Pterygium	4 (16.7)	12 (17.9)
Anonychia	NA	24 (35.8)
Nail Bed		
Onycholysis	8 (33.3)	29 (43.3)
Subungual hyperkeratosis	9 (37.5)	16 (23.8)
Splinter hemorrhages	1 (4.2)	NA

koilonychia, paronychia, and chromonychia may also be present.[20,21,25,26] Dorsal pterygium, or scarring in the form of a "v"-shaped extension of the proximal nail fold, is more specific for NLP than other nail findings that present earlier in the disease course (**Fig. 2**). However, pterygium represents late-stage disease and is irreversible. In one study, mean duration of disease was 69 months in patients with pterygium versus 30 months in patients without scarring (n = 67).[21] Anonychia, or permanent nail loss, often results if patients fail to receive timely treatment.[27]

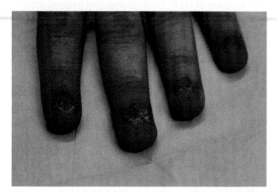

Fig. 2. A 26-year-old man with rapidly progressing NLP. Dorsal pterygia are present on the left third, fourth, and fifth fingernails.

DIAGNOSIS

Clinical examination may be sufficient for diagnosis when characteristic nail changes are present. Dermoscopy can aid in NLP diagnosis.[25] For example, NLP may present clinically with linear nail bed dyschromia, with alternating blue, brown, red, or white bands that spare the lunula. Although these bands are difficult to visualize with the naked eye, they are easily discernible with contact dermoscopy with ultrasound gel (**Fig. 3**).[26] Biopsy with histopathology is often necessary to make the diagnosis in questionable cases or when systemic therapy is being considered. Longitudinal biopsy is recommended to ensure sufficient sampling, especially because both the nail matrix and bed may be involved. In a retrospective study on 24 patients with NLP who underwent longitudinal biopsies, 79.16% had histopathological changes consistent with nail matrix involvement and 54.16% had nail bed involvement with an overlap of 37.50%. Isolated nail matrix disease was present in 41.66% of patients, with only 16.66% of patients showing isolated changes to the nail bed.[20] Histopathology consistent with NLP typically shows hyperkeratosis, acanthosis, elongation of rete ridges, a band of lymphocytes in the upper dermis and dermoepidermal junction, and necrosis of basal layer cells in the proximal nail fold, similar to cutaneous LP (**Fig. 4**).[24,28] Disappearance of the keratogenous zone and hypergranulosis is typically seen in the nail matrix.[29]

The differential diagnosis for NLP includes nail psoriasis, idiopathic trachyonychia, alopecia areata–associated nail changes, lichenoid drug reactions, trauma, onychophagia, onychotillomania, and onychomycosis.[30–32] Ruling out these other entities may prove difficult due to the nonspecific clinical findings in NLP.[33] Histopathological examination of nail clippings may reveal or rule out fungal infection or psoriatic changes. If there is relevant history of environmental exposures, metal series patch testing may be appropriate.[10,34]

There is no evidence-based grading system for NLP severity. Disease with isolated nail bed involvement (limited to onycholysis and subungual hyperkeratosis) may be considered mild disease because the nail matrix is spared. Presence of pterygium is a sign of severe or progressive disease with need of urgent management to prevent anonychia. Serial high-quality digital photography is essential in assessing patient outcomes with or without treatment.

Malignant transformation in NLP has rarely been reported. Three patients presented with ulcerating exophytic lesions at the digit tip. Two cases

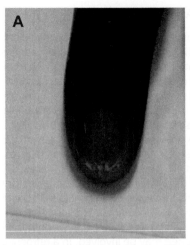
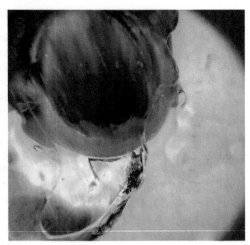

Fig. 3. A 71-year-old man with NLP of right fifth fingernail. (*A*) Clinical photograph demonstrating longitudinal ridging of the nail plate. (*B*) Contact dermoscopy revealing enhancing longitudinal nail plate ridging and subtle findings of nail plate dyschromia.

involved the left great toenail, and one patient presented with concurrent tumors of the right third and fifth fingernails. Biopsies with histopathology confirmed the presence of invasive squamous cell carcinomas. In all 3 cases patients had been diagnosed with NLP at least 10 years before presentation and had findings consistent with LP in multiple fingernails and toenails. LP was isolated to the nails, without genital, oral, or cutaneous involvement in all patients.[35,36] Squamous cell carcinoma is more common in patients with oral LP, reported as 0.8% in one retrospective study (n = 832).[37]

MANAGEMENT

Because NLP may progress to permanent nail loss, rapid and aggressive treatment is warranted.[38] However, treatment of NLP is often

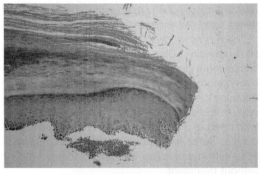

Fig. 4. Longitudinal nail biopsy and histopathological examination of a 57-year-old man with NLP shows hyperkeratosis, hypergranulosis, and focal inflammation of the dermoepidermal junction.

challenging. Efficacy of topical medications is limited by absorption through the nail plate and into the nail bed and matrix. In addition, patients may not understand the progressive nature of their disease and therefore reject systemic therapy. When diagnosis is delayed, patients may present at a stage of disease that is not treatable (ie, with pterygium and/or anonychia). Data on NLP treatment is limited to case studies and retrospective trials (**Table 2**). Finally, NLP displays a high recurrence rate. However, patients who present without a significant delay in diagnosis can benefit from treatment with improved functionality.

TOPICAL MEDICATIONS

Topical medications may be used in select patients with NLP, although they are likely only effective for mild disease and compliance may be a deterrent. Clobetasol propionate was used in 2 studies of NLP, both alone and in conjunction with tazarotene gel with limited improvement and recurrence after discontinuation.[21,39] Treatment with 0.1% topical tacrolimus ointment improved NLP in 5 patients within 6 months, although distal splitting persisted in some patients.[40] The authors recommend topical therapy only when NLP presents with isolated nail bed involvement. Clipping the onycholytic nail plate to the most proximal point allows application of topicals directly to the nail bed. Nightly application under occlusion is also recommended to maximize absorption. Localized bath psoralen and ultraviolet A (PUVA) for 4 months was shown to be effective for fingernails but not toenails in one case report.[41]

Table 2
Treatment of nail lichen planus

Medication	Dose/Strength/Frequency	Reference	Patient Data	Outcome	Level of Evidence
Topical					
Tacrolimus ointment	0.1% twice a day	40	5 pts with NLP ± OLP	Improvement after 6 mo in all patients Recurrence in 1 pt	IV
Clobetasol propionate + Tazarotene gel	0.05% + 0.1% twice a day with occlusion	39	1 pt with NLP	Cured after 7 mo Recurrence 2 mo after discontinuation	IV
Bath-PUVA	15 min soak in 5 mg/L 8-methoxypsoralen followed by 1–4 J/cm² of UVA	41	1 pt with NLP	Improved after 1 y	IV
Intralesional					
IL triamcinolone acetonide	10 mg/mL monthly	23	8 pts with NLP ± OLP	Cured after 4–7 mo in 7 patients	III
IL triamcinolone acetonide	5.0 mg/mL monthly	43	12 pts with NLP	Cured after 6 mo in 4 patients Discontinued in 5 patients due to pain Recurrence after discontinuation	IV
IL triamcinolone acetonide	10.0 mg/mL monthly	42	1 pt with NLP	Cured after 4 mo Recurrence after 2 y	IV
Systemic					
IM triamcinolone acetonide	0.5 mg/kg monthly	23	77 pts with NLP ± OLP, cutaneous LP, scalp lichen planopilaris	Cured or improved after 4 mo in 53 patients Recurrence with long-term follow-up in 11 of 16 patients	III
IM triamcinolone acetonide	IM 0.5–1.0 mg/kg monthly	42	10 pediatric pts with NLP	Cured or improved after 6–12 mo in 9 patients Recurrence with long-term follow-up in 5 of 8 patients	IV
IM/IL triamcinolone acetonide	IM 0.5–1.0 mg/kg monthly IL 5.0 mg/mL monthly	21	67 pts with NLP	Cured in 13 patients Improved in 43 patients Unchanged in 11 patients[a]	III

(continued on next page)

Table 2
(continued)

Medication	Dose/Strength/Frequency	Reference	Patient Data	Outcome	Level of Evidence
Prednisolone	40 mg daily for 2 wk, then 30 mg daily for 2 wk	18	1 pt with NLP	Improved after 4 wk	IV
Prednisolone	20 mg for 4 wk, 10 mg for 4 wk, 5 mg for 4 wk	34	1 pt with NLP	Improved after 12 wk	IV
Alitretinoin	30 mg daily	53	1 pt with NLP	Cured after 6 mo	IV
Alitretinoin	10–30 mg daily	52	2 pts with NLP	Cured after 8–9 mo	IV
Alitretinoin	30 mg daily for 3 mo, then 10 mg daily for 3 mo	51	3 pts with NLP	Improvement after 3 mo	IV
Etretinate	10–30 mg daily	19	1 pt with NLP	Cured after 12 mo	IV
Cyclosporine	100 mg twice daily for 10 mo	58	1 pt with NLP	Improvement after 10 mo Recurrence with dose reduction	IV
Griseofulvin	500 mg/d for 10 wk	61	1 pt with NLP + OLP and cutaneous LP	No effect	IV
Dapsone	1.5–2.5 mg/kg/d	60	1 pt with NLP	Slight improvement after 13 mo	IV
Chloroquine	250 mg twice daily for 30 wk	59	1 pt with NLP + OLP	Cured after 30 wk	IV

I: meta-analysis or multicenter randomized controlled trial.
II: single-center randomized controlled trial.
III: prospective or retrospective study.
IV: case series or case report.
[a] Results not reported according to intervention.

INTRALESIONAL MEDICATION

Triamcinolone acetonide (TAC) is a high-potency corticosteroid frequently used for treatment of NLP. Intralesional (IL) TAC injections into the proximal nail fold allow for targeted drug delivery to the nail matrix. This intervention has shown benefit in concentrations of 2.5 to 10 mg/mL for nail dystrophies, including NLP, nail psoriasis, and idiopathic trachyonychia.[42–45] The most common adverse effects are pain and subungual hematoma. Dilution of TAC in 1% lidocaine, use of ethyl chloride spray, application of lidocaine cream 60 minutes before injection, talkesthesia, vibratory devices, and percussive distraction techniques may all be used to increase tolerability.[38] Although, proximal nail fold atrophy is a theoretic possibility, it is rarely seen with appropriate technique and may be avoided by using lower concentrations (2.5 mg/mL).[46]

One retrospective study in patients with NLP (n = 75) compared monthly IL TAC injections (10 mg/mL, n = 8) with monthly IM TAC injections (0.5 mg/kg, n = 67). For 87.5% of patients who received 4 to 7 intralesional injections, nail findings improved compared with 65.67% of patients who received 6 intramuscular (IM) injections.[23]

In a prospective, open-label study of patients with NLP, 4 of 7 patients showed 75% to 100% improvement in nail changes with 6 months of 2.5 to 5.0 mg/mL IL TAC injections. Patients who recurred responded well to repeat treatment.[46]

SYSTEMIC MEDICATIONS

IM TAC injections into the deltoid or gluteus maximus muscle are commonly used in dermatology to treat alopecia areata, Behcet disease, and NLP.[47] Concentrations of 0.5 to 1.0 mg/kg are used for the treatment of NLP. In a prospective study of patients with steroid responsive dermatoses including LP, nummular eczema, and hand dermatitis, IM TAC did reduce mean total cortisol when compared with baseline but did not result in iatrogenic Cushing syndrome or secondary adrenal insufficiency (n = 14).[48]

Of 16 patients with NLP who received IM injections and were followed-up for greater than 5 years, 11 had recurrence of nail changes 3 months to 3 years following treatment. After repeating the IM injections in these 11 patients with recurrences, 5 improved, 2 showed no change, and 4 worsened.[23]

IM TAC has been successfully used to treat pediatric NLP.[23,49] In the previously mentioned study, 6 patients in the IM TAC group were 7 to 14 year old. All 6 were cured or improved with treatment.[23] In addition, a 3- to 6-month course

of monthly IM TAC, 0.5 mg/kg, resulted in complete reversal of nail findings in 9 of 15 patients younger than 12 years. Lipoatrophy at the site of injection occurred in 2 patients.[49]

Prednisone and prednisolone have also shown benefit for treatment of NLP.[18,34] Oral prednisolone was shown to dramatically improve NLP nail changes in one case report at a dose of 40 mg for 2 weeks followed by 30 mg for another 2 weeks.[18] In another case report, a 12-week taper of prednisolone from 20 mg to 5 mg was effective with healthy nail growing proximally even after discontinuation of treatment.[34] Systemic corticosteroids are usually only recommended for patients with involvement of greater than 3 nails.[50] However, permanent nail loss may have significant functional consequences particularly when the first 3 digits are involved. Therefore, systemic therapy should be strongly considered when initial treatments fail especially with involvement of the first 3 digits and/or significant impact on quality of life.

Retinoids have been used effectively to treat NLP. Oral alitretinoin was effective in treating NLP in 3 separate case reports. A dose of 10 to 30 mg/d was administered and improvement was observed within the first 3 to 6 months.[51–53] Etretinate has also been used with limited efficacy.[19,23] However, these medications are not available in the United States. Acitretin is readily available, though, and has been used for the treatment of other forms of LP.[54–56] In a randomized, controlled double-blind study of patients with cutaneous LP, 64% treated with acitretin 20 to 50 mg/d for 8 weeks showed remission or marked improvement compared with 13% treated with placebo (n = 65). The most common adverse effects were dry lips (84%), mouth (66%), and nose (60%). Hair loss was the least common side effect (16%).[56] Further investigation of acitretin for the treatment of NLP is necessary. Retinoids are contraindicated in women who are or may become pregnant.

Improvement in 2 patients with NLP was seen with weekly subcutaneous administration of methotrexate 10 to 20 mg.[57] Cyclosporine A, 3 mg/kg, was effective in treating NLP within the first 2 months in one case report.[58] Dapsone, chloroquine phosphate, and griseofulvin have also been used for NLP with variable efficacy.[59–61]

DISCUSSION

NLP should be treated promptly and aggressively to prevent permanent nail loss. Topical treatment is rarely effective except in patients with isolated nail bed involvement and few nails involved.

Intralesional triamcinolone is a safe and efficacious treatment of NLP that avoids systemic side effects while depositing medication directly at the site of inflammation. However, for patients with low pain tolerance and multiple nails involved, IM triamcinolone or oral corticosteroids are acceptable alternatives. IM triamcinolone is preferred over oral corticosteroids at typically used dosages due to the more favorable side-effect profile. When few nails are affected, systemic therapy should not be withheld if the first 3 digits are involved and/or with a significant impact on quality of life. Acitretin, either alone or in conjunction with systemic corticosteroids, is reasonable for recalcitrant disease. Tofacitinib, a janus kinase 1 and janus kinase 3 inhibitor, may be a future treatment option. There is evidence for its effectiveness in the treatment of various dermatoses including psoriasis, alopecia areata, and lichen planopilaris.[62,63] Long-term follow-up for patients NLP is necessary due to high rates of recurrence.

SUMMARY

Early recognition of NLP and appropriately aggressive therapy is necessary to prevent irreversible nail changes and loss. A comprehensive method for grading severity is also needed for the evaluation of superiority between treatment options. IL TAC matrix injections are an underutilized therapy for NLP that provides the antiinflammatory effect of corticosteroids without adverse systemic effects. Acitretin may be reasonable in recalcitrant cases, and tofacitinib is a promising more directed approach. There is a need for randomized controlled trials for improved efficacy and outcomes for patients with NLP.

CLINICS CARE POINTS

- Nail lichen planus should be treated promptly and aggressively to prevent permanent nail loss.
- Intralesional triamcinolone is a safe and efficacious treatment of NLP and well tolerated by many patients.
- Alternatives are intramuscular triamcinolone, oral corticosteroids, and acitretin.

DISCLOSURE

M.K. Gupta and Dr S.R. Lipner have no conflicts of interest relevant to the content of the submission.

REFERENCES

1. Domingues R, de Carvalho GC, da Silva Oliveira LM, et al. The dysfunctional innate immune response triggered by Toll-like receptor activation is restored by TLR7/TLR8 and TLR9 ligands in cutaneous lichen planus. Br J Dermatol 2015;172(1):48–55.
2. Jimenez-Dalmaroni MJ, Gerswhin ME, Adamopoulos IE. The critical role of toll-like receptors–From microbial recognition to autoimmunity: a comprehensive review. Autoimmun Rev 2016;15(1):1–8.
3. Wenzel J, Scheler M, Proelss J, et al. Type I interferon-associated cytotoxic inflammation in lichen planus. J Cutan Pathol 2006;33(10):672–8.
4. De Vries HJ, van Marle J, Teunissen MB, et al. Lichen planus is associated with human herpesvirus type 7 replication and infiltration of plasmacytoid dendritic cells. Br J Dermatol 2006;154(2):361–4.
5. de Vries HJ, Teunissen MB, Zorgdrager F, et al. Lichen planus remission is associated with a decrease of human herpes virus type 7 protein expression in plasmacytoid dendritic cells. Arch Dermatol Res 2007;299(4):213–9.
6. Santoro A, Majorana A, Roversi L, et al. Recruitment of dendritic cells in oral lichen planus. J Pathol 2005;205(4):426–34.
7. Shengyuan L, Songpo Y, Wen W, et al. Hepatitis C virus and lichen planus: a reciprocal association determined by a meta-analysis. Arch Dermatol 2009;145(9):1040–7.
8. Sanchez-Perez J, De Castro M, Buezo GF, et al. Lichen planus and hepatitis C virus: prevalence and clinical presentation of patients with lichen planus and hepatitis C virus infection. Br J Dermatol 1996;134(4):715–9.
9. Chuang TY, Stitle L, Brashear R, et al. Hepatitis C virus and lichen planus: a case-control study of 340 patients. J Am Acad Dermatol 1999;41(5 Pt 1):787–9.
10. Nishizawa A, Satoh T, Yokozeki H. Close association between metal allergy and nail lichen planus: detection of causative metals in nail lesions. J Eur Acad Dermatol Venereol 2013;27(2):e231–4.
11. Kato Y, Hayakawa R, Shiraki R, et al. A case of lichen planus caused by mercury allergy. Br J Dermatol 2003;148(6):1268–9.
12. Yokozeki H, Niiyama S, Nishioka K. Twenty-nail dystrophy (trachyonychia) caused by lichen planus in a patient with gold allergy. Br J Dermatol 2005;152(5):1087–9.
13. Husein-ElAhmed H, Gieler U, Steinhoff M. Lichen planus: a comprehensive evidence-based analysis of medical treatment. J Eur Acad Dermatol Venereol 2019;33(10):1847–62.
14. Kanwar AJ, De D. Lichen planus in children. Indian J Dermatol Venereol Leprol 2010;76(4):366–72.
15. Balasubramaniam P, Ogboli M, Moss C. Lichen planus in children: review of 26 cases. Clin Exp Dermatol 2008;33(4):457–9.
16. Samman PD. The nails in lichen planus. Br J Dermatol 1961;73:288–92.

17. Bhattacharya M, Kaur I, Kumar B. Lichen planus: a clinical and epidemiological study. J Dermatol 2000;27(9):576–82.

18. Evans AV, Roest MA, Fletcher CL, et al. Isolated lichen planus of the toe nails treated with oral prednisolone. Clin Exp Dermatol 2001;26(5):412–4.

19. Kato N, Ueno H. Isolated lichen planus of the nails treated with etretinate. J Dermatol 1993;20(9):577–80.

20. Tosti A, Peluso AM, Fanti PA, et al. Nail lichen planus: clinical and pathologic study of twenty-four patients. J Am Acad Dermatol 1993;28(5 Pt 1):724–30.

21. Goettmann S, Zaraa I, Moulonguet I. Nail lichen planus: epidemiological, clinical, pathological, therapeutic and prognosis study of 67 cases. J Eur Acad Dermatol Venereol 2012;26(10):1304–9.

22. Halteh P, Scher RK, Brinster NK, et al. A 10-year-old boy with dystrophy of the fingernails. Pediatr Dermatol 2017;34(2):193–4.

23. Piraccini BM, Saccani E, Starace M, et al. Nail lichen planus: response to treatment and long term follow-up. Eur J Dermatol 2010;20(4):489–96.

24. Joshi RK, Abanmi A, Ohman SG, et al. Lichen planus of the nails presenting as trachyonychia. Int J Dermatol 1993;32(1):54–5.

25. Nakamura R, Broce AA, Palencia DP, et al. Dermatoscopy of nail lichen planus. Int J Dermatol 2013;52(6):684–7.

26. Grover C, Kharghoria G, Bhattacharya SN. Linear nail bed dyschromia: a distinctive dermoscopic feature of nail lichen planus. Clin Exp Dermatol 2019;44(6):697–9.

27. Pall A, Gupta RR, Gulati B, et al. Twenty nail anonychia due to lichen planus. J Dermatol 2004;31(2):146–7.

28. Jellinek NJ, Lipner SR. Longitudinal Erythronychia: Retrospective Single-Center Study Evaluating Differential Diagnosis and the Likelihood of Malignancy. Dermatol Surg 2016;42(3):310–9.

29. Fanti PA, Tosti A, Cameli N, et al. Nail matrix hypergranulosis. Am J Dermatopathol 1994;16(6):607–10.

30. Chelidze K, Lipner SR. Nail changes in alopecia areata: an update and review. Int J Dermatol 2018;57(7):776–83.

31. Halteh P, Scher RK, Lipner SR. Onychotillomania: diagnosis and Management. Am J Clin Dermatol 2017;18(6):763–70.

32. Halteh P, Scher RK, Lipner SR. Onychophagia: a nail-biting conundrum for physicians. J Dermatolog Treat 2017;28(2):166–72.

33. Grover C, Khandpur S, Reddy BS, et al. Longitudinal nail biopsy: utility in 20-nail dystrophy. Dermatol Surg 2003;29(11):1125–9.

34. Takeuchi Y, Iwase N, Suzuki M, et al. Lichen planus with involvement of all twenty nails and the oral mucous membrane. J Dermatol 2000;27(2):94–8.

35. Costa C, Villani A, Russo D, et al. Squamous cell carcinomas in two cases of nail lichen planus: is there a real association? Dermatol Ther (Heidelb) 2018;8(3):491–4.

36. Okiyama N, Satoh T, Yokozeki H, et al. Squamous cell carcinoma arising from lichen planus of nail matrix and nail bed. J Am Acad Dermatol 2005;53(5):908–9.

37. Rajentheran R, McLean NR, Kelly CG, et al. Malignant transformation of oral lichen planus. Eur J Surg Oncol 1999;25(5):520–3.

38. Lipner SR. Nail lichen planus: a true nail emergency. J Am Acad Dermatol 2019;80(6):e177–8.

39. Prevost NM, English JC 3rd. Palliative treatment of fingernail lichen planus. J Drugs Dermatol 2007;6(2):202–4.

40. Ujiie H, Shibaki A, Akiyama M, et al. Successful treatment of nail lichen planus with topical tacrolimus. Acta Derm Venereol 2010;90(2):218–9.

41. Pita da Veiga G, Perez-Feal P, Moreiras-Arias N, et al. Treatment of nail lichen planus with localized bath-PUVA. Photodermatol Photoimmunol Photomed 2019;36(3):241–3.

42. Gerstein W. Psoriasis and lichen planus of nalis. Treatment with triamcinolone. Arch Dermatol 1962;86:419–21.

43. Khoo BP, Giam YC. A pilot study on the role of intralesional triamcinolone acetonide in the treatment of pitted nails in children. Singapore Med J 2000;41(2):66–8.

44. Gupta MK, Geizhals S, Lipner SR. Intralesional triamcinolone matrix injections for treatment of trachyonychia. J Am Acad Dermatol 2019;82(4):e121–2.

45. Brauns B, Stahl M, Schon MP, et al. Intralesional steroid injection alleviates nail lichen planus. Int J Dermatol 2011;50(5):626–7.

46. Grover C, Bansal S, Nanda S, et al. Efficacy of triamcinolone acetonide in various acquired nail dystrophies. J Dermatol 2005;32(12):963–8.

47. Thomas LW, Elsensohn A, Bergheim T, et al. Intramuscular steroids in the treatment of dermatologic disease: a systematic review. J Drugs Dermatol 2018;17(3):323–9.

48. Reddy S, Ananthakrishnan S, Garg A. A prospective observational study evaluating hypothalamic-pituitary-adrenal axis alteration and efficacy of intramuscular triamcinolone acetonide for steroid-responsive dermatologic disease. J Am Acad Dermatol 2013;69(2):226–31.

49. Tosti A, Piraccini BM, Cambiaghi S, et al. Nail lichen planus in children: clinical features, response to treatment, and long-term follow-up. Arch Dermatol 2001;137(8):1027–32.

50. Le Cleach L, Chosidow O. Clinical practice. Lichen planus. N Engl J Med 2012;366(8):723–32.

51. Iorizzo M. Nail lichen planus - a possible new indication for oral alitretinoin. J Eur Acad Dermatol Venereol 2016;30(3):509–10.

52. Alsenaid A, Eder I, Ruzicka T, et al. Successful treatment of nail lichen planus with alitretinoin: report of 2 cases and review of the literature. Dermatology 2014;229(4):293–6.

53. Pinter A, Patzold S, Kaufmann R. Lichen planus of nails - successful treatment with Alitretinoin. J Dtsch Dermatol Ges 2011;9(12):1033–4.

54. Rallis E, Liakopoulou A, Christodoulopoulos C, et al. Successful treatment of bullous lichen planus with acitretin monotherapy. Review of treatment options for bullous lichen planus and case report. J Dermatol Case Rep 2016;10(4):62–4.

55. Kolb-Maurer A, Sitaru C, Rose C, et al. Treatment of lichen planus pemphigoides with acitretin and pulsed corticosteroids. Hautarzt 2003;54(3):268–73.

56. Laurberg G, Geiger JM, Hjorth N, et al. Treatment of lichen planus with acitretin. A double-blind, placebo-controlled study in 65 patients. J Am Acad Dermatol 1991;24(3):434–7.

57. Manousaridis I, Manousaridis K, Peitsch WK, et al. Individualizing treatment and choice of medication in lichen planus: a step by step approach. J Dtsch Dermatol Ges 2013;11(10):981–91.

58. Florian B, Angelika J, Ernst SR. Successful treatment of palmoplantar nail lichen planus with cyclosporine. J Dtsch Dermatol Ges 2014;12(8):724–5.

59. Mostafa WZ. Lichen planus of the nail: treatment with antimalarials. J Am Acad Dermatol 1989;20(2 Pt 1):289–90.

60. Basak PY, Basak K. Generalized lichen planus in childhood: is dapsone an effective treatment modality? Turk J Pediatr 2002;44(4):346–8.

61. Haldar B. Lichen planus with pterygium unguis treated by grisiofulvin (F.P.). Indian J Dermatol 1976;21(3):53.

62. Ismail FF, Sinclair R. JAK inhibition in the treatment of alopecia areata - a promising new dawn? Expert Rev Clin Pharmacol 2020;13(1):43–51.

63. Kvist-Hansen A, Hansen PR, Skov L. Systemic treatment of psoriasis with JAK inhibitors: a review. Dermatol Ther (Heidelb) 2020;10(1):29–42.

Pediatric Nail Disorders

Jane Sanders Bellet, MD

KEYWORDS

- Congenital malalignment • Chevron nail • Onychomadesis • Congenital hypertrophy
- Parakeratosis pustulosa • Trachyonychia • Pachyonychia congenita • Ectodermal dysplasia

KEY POINTS

- Many common pediatric nail findings are normal variants that require no treatment, just reassurance.
- Examination of children's nails can help to diagnose genodermatoses.
- Some abnormal pediatric nail findings are amenable to therapy and should be treated.

INTRODUCTION

Abnormal-appearing nails in children cause fear and anxiety among parents and physicians. Many pediatric nail findings are normal variants and are no cause for alarm. Others represent congenital abnormalities or genetic syndromes for which there is no cure. Still others are inflammatory or infectious entities that require treatment. Pediatric nail disorders are reviewed, along with management.

NORMAL VARIANTS
Koilonychia (Spoon Nails)

Key features
• Physiologic in children
• Thin, concave nails
• Great toenails most commonly affected

Koilonychia or "spoon nails" are a normal finding in infants and young children. The nail plate is thinner than usual and has upward curvature, so that a drop of water would stay in place and not roll off. The curvature is usually more pronounced proximal to distal, but can be lateral, so that the edges are more elevated. The great toenails are most commonly affected and noticed; however, other

nails can be involved as well. In young children whose feet are growing very rapidly, shoes may quickly become too small, and koilonychia can develop. As children grow older, the nails become thicker and the curvature resolves. Iron deficiency can also cause koilonychia; however, the American Academy of Pediatrics recommends iron deficiency screening at age 1,[1] so unless there is significant concern due to unusual diet, or the child develops koilonychia at an older age, no investigations or treatment is required.[2,3]

Chevron Nail (Herringbone Nail, V-Shaped Ridging)

Key features
• Oblique ridges
• Involvement of all fingernails
• Resolves by adulthood

Diagonal ridges that extend from the side of the nail and converge in the center lead to a "herringbone" or "chevron" appearance. This is a normal variant that presents between the ages of 5 and 7 years and will resolve in young adulthood, without treatment. One hypothesis of etiology is incomplete formation of the central dorsal matrix.[4,5] No tests are required for diagnosis.

Duke University School of Medicine, 5324 McFarland Drive, Suite 410, Durham, NC 27707, USA
E-mail address: Jane.bellet@duke.edu

Dermatol Clin 39 (2021) 231–243
https://doi.org/10.1016/j.det.2020.12.005
0733-8635/21/© 2020 Elsevier Inc. All rights reserved.

Beau's Lines

Key features

- Transverse depressions
- Single-digit involvement most likely due to trauma
- Multiple-digit involvement most likely due to systemic causes

---

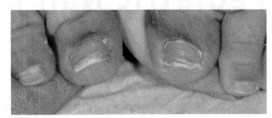

Fig. 1. Beau's lines. Note the transverse depressions of nail plates.

Transverse depressions in one or more nails are termed Beau's lines (**Fig. 1**) and occur in 1 nail due to trauma or multiple nails due to systemic cause of temporary cessation of nail matrix growth. When seen in young infants, this is thought to represent the "stress of birth and adapting to extrauterine life." Viral infections, especially with prolonged or high fever are often causative. Hand, foot, mouth disease caused by coxsackievirus is a common culprit,[6] as are chemotherapeutic agents.[7] Beau's lines can be considered a *forme fruste* of onychomadesis, as the plate has not developed complete separation from the bed.[8] Resolution occurs with time.

Onychomadesis (Nail Shedding)

Key features

- Complete detachment of the nail
- Single-digit involvement most likely due to trauma
- Multiple-digit involvement most likely due to systemic causes

---

Shedding of nails can occur after trauma, as well as with other insults to the nail matrix, such as viral infection or medications. Temporary cessation of nail matrix growth that is more severe than with Beau's lines leads to proximal detachment of the nail plate from the bed, which can then progress to full detachment. Reassurance can be provided that a normal nail is growing right behind the one being shed.

Congenital Malalignment of the Great Toenail

Key features

- Lateral deviation of the nail plate
- Often bilateral
- Discolored, thickened, ridged plates develop with time

Lateral deviation of the great toenails (**Fig. 2**A) is commonly seen in young children. Often, both great toenails are affected. The nail becomes triangular in shape, thickened, with transverse ridges and develops brown-gray discoloration (**Fig. 2**B). Onycholysis often develops with time. Resolution can occur, with reports of up to 50% in the literature; however, can remain persistent into adulthood.[9,10]

Congenital Hypertrophy of the Nail Folds

Key features

- Infants
- Hypertrophic lateral nail folds
- Can be seen concomitantly with congenital malalignment

Commonly affecting the great toenails of infants, the lateral nail folds are hypertrophied, which grow up and over the lateral nail plate (**Fig. 3**). Usually asymptomatic, topical steroids and/or topical antibiotics are all that is needed to manage the inflammation and sometimes secondary infection. This most often resolves within the first year of life.[11] No surgery is needed, unless a true ingrown nail with erythema, edema, and pain develop.[12] Concomitant koilonychia and congenital malalignment can be seen.

Syndromes Anonychia/Micronychia

Some people are born with no nail plate or a very small or rudimentary nail. Multiple etiologies can cause this finding. Isolated anonychia is caused by a mutation in the RSPO4 gene, which causes a defect in the Wnt signaling pathway. For a normal nail to develop, normal bone must be present, therefore if the bone is abnormal under the nail bed, the nail plate also will be abnormal. Epidermolysis bullosa can present at birth with anonychia or develop anonychia after persistent blistering and subsequent scarring of the nail bed/unit. DOORS syndrome (Deafness-Onycho-Osteodystrophy-mental Retardation-Seizures),[13] as well as

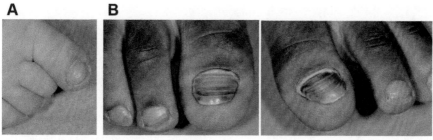

Fig. 2. (*A*) Congenital malalignment of the great toenail in a 4-month-old. (*B*) Congenital malalignment of the great toenails in a 3-year-old. Note lateral deviation and thickened nail plate with ridging and brown-gray discoloration.

fetal teratogens, such as alcohol, anticonvulsants,[14] and warfarin,[15,16] also can present with anonychia or micronychia.

Congenital Onychodysplasia of the Index Finger

A rudimentary nail plate is seen on the index fingers in this condition (**Fig. 4**). A radiograph of the affected digits will show a bifurcated distal phalanx. No treatment is required.[17,18] Some patients prefer to ablate small nail plates, while other young patients prefer to use them as a platform for application of artificial nails.

Pachyonychia Congenita

Key features
• Thickened, yellow-brown nails
• Palmoplantar keratoderma
• Plantar pain

Thickened, discolored nails become evident at approximately age 2 to 3 years, often with increased transverse curvature.[19] Usually all 20 nails are affected; however, sometimes only a few nails are abnormal. The thumb and index fingernails can be more severely affected; however, for some patients, the toes are more involved, perhaps because of the trauma of wearing shoes.[20] Hyperkeratosis of the nail bed leads to distal nail plate thickening. Palmoplantar keratoderma, associated with severe plantar pain, oral leukokeratosis, natal teeth and cysts, including steatocystomas, also are features of this disorder.[21] Pachyonychia congenita is caused by mutations in certain keratin genes and is inherited in an autosomal dominant fashion. The previously used eponyms of Jadassohn-Lewandowsky and Jackson-Lawler

are now classified based on these keratin mutations: 6a, 6b, 16, 17. PC-6a signifies a mutation in keratin 6a.[19] Biopsy is not required for diagnosis.

Treatment is focused on managing both pain and the appearance of the nails, and can be challenging. Urea preparations, including creams, gels, ointments, and pastes can be used to help soften the nail plates.[22] This usually is followed by paring or grinding of the nail plates, either with clippers or a device such as a Dremel (Robert Bosch Tool Corporation, Racine, WI) drill, marketed as a Pet Nail Grooming Tool.[23] Surgical approaches, including curettage of the nail matrix or nail avulsion with chemical ablation, can be used to decrease the amount of hyperkeratosis.[24] However, recovery

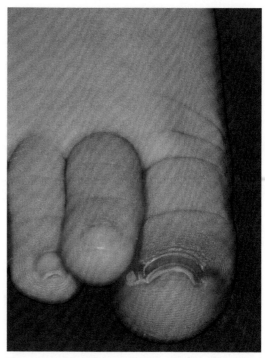

Fig. 3. Congenital hypertrophy of the lateral nail folds.

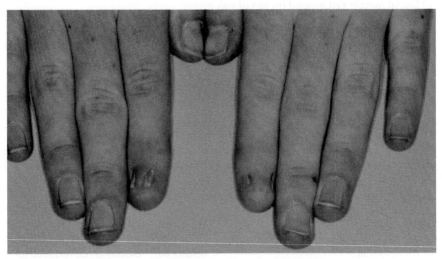

Fig. 4. Congenital onychodysplasia of the index fingernails.

can be very painful and such procedures are usually not recommended for children or adolescents, especially as they cannot appropriately comprehend the fact that they will never have nails if the postprocedural results are as expected.

Ectodermal Dysplasia

> **Key features**
>
> - Small, short, thickened nail plates
> - Nail hypoplasia
> - Hair and teeth abnormalities

The ectodermal dysplasias are a heterogeneous group of genetic disorders that all have defects in the ectoderm leading to abnormalities of hair, skin, teeth, nails, and sweat glands. The diagnosis is often made due to the constellation of findings, not just abnormal nails. The nail findings can be relatively mild or more severe and can consist of small, thick dystrophic nails or fragile, thin nails. The shape is often abnormal, along with discoloration, brittleness, and ridging. Nails are very slow-growing, requiring trimming only infrequently; paronychia can be seen.

Nail-Patella Syndrome

> **Key features**
>
> - Triangular lunula
> - Patellar abnormalities
> - Kidney involvement

An autosomal dominant disorder, triangular lunula is the hallmark of this condition. Either micronychia or complete anonychia is seen, with the thumb and index fingers most commonly affected. The distal interphalangeal joints do not have the usual creases present.[25] A number of bone findings can be seen: complete absence of the patella, or luxation, bilateral iliac horns, or arthrodysplasia of the elbow. Kidney involvement can be severe, in some cases requiring transplantation. Diagnosis can be made via genetic testing for LMX1B gene mutations or pelvis radiograph showing the iliac horns.

Dyskeratosis Congenita

> **Key features**
>
> - Longitudinal ridging, splitting
> - Fingernails > toenails
> - Can develop complete nail loss

The classic triad of nail dystrophy, reticulated pigmentation, and leukoplakia of the tongue are seen in dyskeratosis congenita; however, patients may not present with all 3. A very rare disorder, the nails develop longitudinal ridging and splitting during childhood. Subsequently, pterygium and complete nail loss can occur. A genetic condition, dyskeratosis congenita is usually transmitted in an X-linked fashion; however, both autosomal dominant and autosomal recessive inheritance has been reported. The following genes have been implicated: *DKC1, TERC, TERT, NOP10, NHP2,* and shelterin (*TINF2*).[26,27] Bone marrow failure is caused by telomere maintenance defects, which is fatal unless a bone marrow transplant is successful. A predisposition to other malignancies, in addition to pulmonary fibrosis, is also seen.

Epidermolysis Bullosa

> **Key features**
>
> - Periungual blistering
> - Thick, short nails develop
> - Certain forms develop complete atrophy

Nail findings can be observed in all forms of epidermolysis bullosa (EB), with abnormal nails sometimes preceding blistering. In certain forms of EB, nail findings are the only manifestation of the condition (dominant dystrophic EB-nails only).[28] The most severe nail abnormalities are seen in junctional and recessive forms of EB, usually correlating with the severity of disease.

Blistering of periungual or subungual skin leads to onycholysis and subsequent onychomadesis; granulation tissue of the nail bed; short, yellow, thickened nails (pachyonychia) (**Fig. 5**); onychogryphosis of the great toenails; as well as nail atrophy (very short, thin, brittle nail) and anonychia

secondary to frequent blistering leading to scarring all can be seen. In severe recessive dystrophic EB, complete loss of all nails, along with fusion of the digits leads to the "mitten hand" deformity.

With the elucidation of genetic mutations and refinement of the phenotypes of EB, classification of the subtypes has recently been updated.[28] Diagnosis is usually made via biopsy for immunofluorescence mapping; however, in families in which the diagnosis is already known, this is not necessary. Management is focused on minimizing trauma and blistering of the digits, caring for any wounds to prevent infection, and delaying fusion of digits (particularly in recessive dystrophic EB) as best as possible.

MECHANICAL/TRAUMA
Onychophagia/Onychotillomania

> **Key features**
>
> - Cuticle often absent
> - Inflammation of proximal nail fold
> - Nail plate surface changes (ridging)

Biting or picking at the nail plates or nail folds is a common behavior in children and adolescents. Up to 60% will have onychophagia at some point

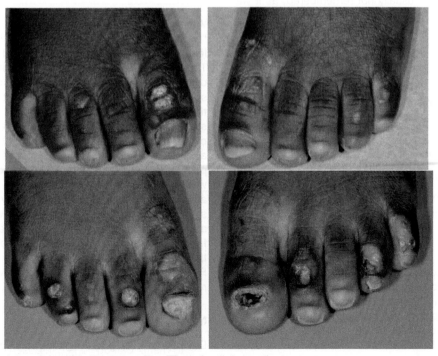

Fig. 5. Dominant dystrophic EB. Note progression of nail dystrophy.

during their childhood. Infants do not bite their nails, and if that specific behavior is seen, should raise concerns for congenital absence of pain syndrome or Lesch-Nyhan syndrome. Nail biting is part of the obsessive-compulsive spectrum, and often anxiety or low self-esteem may be present. On examination, the nail plates are often very short with jagged edges. The cuticle may be absent. Chronic paronychia can develop due to constant exposure to moisture that penetrates the now-breached barrier between skin and nail. Infections such as periungual verrucae also can develop. Permanent shortening of the affected nails can occur if the damage is long-standing. Management is challenging, as the habit is hard to alter. Various approaches, including bad tasting nail lacquers or devices to prevent placing the digit in the mouth, or cognitive behavioral therapy can be used.

Onychotillomania can include picking of the nail plate, as well as the periungual skin. This can lead to transverse ridges of the nail plate (habit tic deformity, washboard nails, median canaliform dystrophy). Even just rubbing the nail plate itself can lead to these findings, if applied with sufficient vigor.

Punctate/Striate Leukonychia

Parents are often extremely concerned by the new appearance of white spots on their child's nail or nails. This is caused by trauma to the distal nail matrix and is usually not remembered, as it was likely relatively minor. These are frequently seen in basketball players, as they chronically dribble the ball. The white spot will grow out as the nail grows out, without any permanent change to the nail plate.

Onychocryptosis (Ingrown Nail)

Key features
• Painful inflammation of lateral fold(s)
• Usually great toenails
• Congenital malalignment can be concomitant

Ingrown toenails are most often seen in adolescents who experience trauma and also clip the toenails in a "rounded" fashion, which often leads to development of a nail spicule and then inflammation and pain of the lateral nail fold. Tight shoes and hyperhidrosis of the feet likely facilitate development of ingrown toenails. Isotretinoin also increases the risk of developing onychocryptosis. Younger, pediatric patients with congenital malalignment of the great toenail also can develop ingrown toenails. As inflammation worsens, granulation tissue eventually develops, along with hypertrophy of the nail fold. Multiple staging classification systems have been proposed by different investigators, including Mozena in 2002,[29] Martinez-Nova and colleagues in 2007,[30] and Kline in 2008.[31] Each system delineates worsening of erythema, edema, development of granulation tissue, purulent drainage, and an embedded nail covered by the hypertrophic nail fold, with some degree of onycholysis. Conservative management of onychocryptosis in children and adolescents is preferred, if possible. Surgical approaches, including partial nail avulsion with phenol ablation, are otherwise the same as they would be for adults, except that general anesthesia may be required for young children (usually younger than 12 years), in addition to standard anesthetic blocks.

Retronychia

Key features
• Backward nail plate growth
• Chronic trauma
• Multiple stacked nails

When the nail plate starts to grow backward "retro," it pushes into the proximal nail fold and leads to chronic paronychia, pain, and drainage. This usually occurs in the setting of chronic, ongoing trauma, particularly in the setting of sports, dance, or wearing either tight shoes or those that exert excess pressure on the toes, such as occurs with high-heeled shoes.[32] More common in young female patients, this finding also has been observed in much younger pediatric patients who have abnormal gait (such as toe walking) due to neurologic problems (personal anecdote). Multiple nail plates may become stacked on one another, leading to a very thick, abnormal-appearing nail (**Fig. 6**). For early, mild forms, treatment with topical steroids can halt the process, leading to reversal and healing.[33] For chronic, severe forms, nail avulsion is required.[34]

MELANOCYTIC ACTIVATION

Development of gray longitudinal stripes of the nails (**Fig. 7**) can occur with chronic manipulation

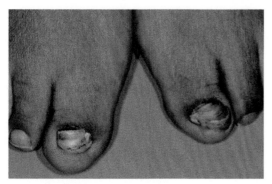

Fig. 6. Retronychia.

of any part of the nail unit, including biting, picking, and rubbing.[35] This is usually seen in patients of darker skin tone. If secondary to chronic trauma, such as rubbing of the shoe on the fifth toe, this is called frictional melanonychia.[36]

Melanonychia

> **Key features**
>
> - Most common cause: congenital melanocytic nevus or nail matrix nevus
> - Melanoma of the nail unit is very rare in children

Melanonychia is seen in young children as well as adolescents. This can present as a very thin longitudinal brown or black stripe (**Fig. 8**), or as involvement of the entire nail plate. In children, melanonychia is most often due to a nail matrix nevus,[37] and in some cases a congenital

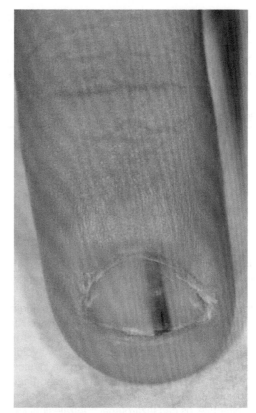

Fig. 8. Longitudinal melanonychia.

melanocytic nevus, which frequently presents with pigmentation of the periungual skin (nail folds and hyponychium). Nail unit melanoma in children is exceedingly rare and therefore observation is often a reasonable course.[38–40] Nail matrix biopsy can be done for confirmation, with either a 3-mm punch trephine for a thin band, or a nail matrix shave for a wider band.

INFLAMMATORY
Atopic Dermatitis

> **Key features**
>
> - Inflammation surrounding nail plate
> - Cuticle often absent
> - Atopic dermatitis findings elsewhere on the skin

The proximal nail fold (cuticle) is often missing in atopic dermatitis, due to chronic picking, rubbing, and inflammation. The surrounding periungual skin can be edematous and erythematous. When the

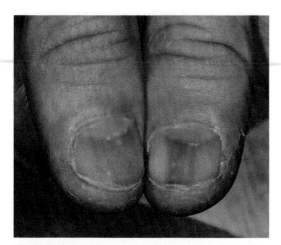

Fig. 7. Melanocytic activation secondary to biting in a 10-year-old boy.

nail matrix is involved, the plate can develop large pits and transverse grooves, in addition to Beau's lines. Treatments for atopic dermatitis, such as topical steroids and emollients, are used. As the inflammation resolves, the nail plate will slowly return to a normal appearance.

Psoriasis

> **Key features**
>
> - Wide, irregular pits
> - Usually multiple nails involved
> - Psoriasis elsewhere on the skin

Nail psoriasis is more common in adults than children, but does occur; 40% of pediatric patients with psoriasis have nail involvement.[41] Large, deep, irregular pits are the most common finding, but onycholysis, subungual hyperkeratosis, and salmon patches (yellow-red discoloration) can all be seen. Keeping the nails short and avoiding trauma, such as biting or sucking the digits, is important to avoid the Koebner phenomenon. Topical steroids and calcipotriene can sometimes be effective, as can tazarotene.[42] Intralesional steroid injections can work well; however, injections are usually not well tolerated in children. Systemic treatments are often very efficacious in treating severe nail psoriasis. Acitretin should be cautiously used in women of child-bearing age. Biologics such as secukinumab have been reported to completely clear nail psoriasis, when other agents such as methotrexate and adalimumab have been unsuccessful.[43]

Parakeratosis Pustulosa

> **Key features**
>
> - Young girls
> - Usually 1 finger
> - Improves with time

Seen in girls aged 5 to 7 years, often of a solitary digit, parakeratosis pustulosa presents with erythema, scale, subungual hyperkeratosis, and onycholysis. Acute pain with pustules can be seen. Pitting and nail dystrophy can develop with time. Resolution often occurs with time; however, topical steroids can help ameliorate pain and inflammation. This condition is thought to be a symptom of an inflammatory disorder such as psoriasis or atopic dermatitis, so more characteristic findings may develop over time.[44]

Trachyonychia

> **Key features**
>
> - 1 to 20 nails can be involved
> - Rough nails

Longitudinal ridging leading to roughness of the entire nail plate is seen (**Fig. 9**). The nail plate becomes thin and brittle, and the proximal nail folds can become thickened. This condition can affect 1 or all 20 nails, therefore the term "20 nail dystrophy" is incorrect. Idiopathic trachyonychia is a pediatric condition, whereas the forms caused by psoriasis or lichen planus can be seen in children or adults.[45] Approximately 50% of cases will spontaneously regress. Usual treatments for psoriasis or lichen planus do not help this condition.[46]

Alopecia Areata: Nail Findings

> **Key features**
>
> - Geometric pitting
> - Trachyonychia can be seen
> - Severity of nail disease can correlate with severity of hair loss

A wide variety of nail findings can be seen in patients with alopecia areata, including pitting and trachyonychia. The more diffuse the hair loss, the higher likelihood of having nail findings, and ones that are more severe.[47] Shallow geometric pitting is commonly seen.[48] Immediately after the onset of hair shedding, Beau's lines or onychomadesis can develop.

Lichen Planus

> **Key features**
>
> - Thinned nails, onycholysis, splitting
> - Depending on type, scarring can result

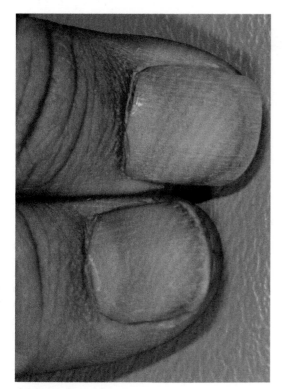

Fig. 9. Trachyonychia.

Nail lichen planus is an inflammatory disorder. Boys are reportedly more often affected than girls. Because a biopsy confirms the diagnosis, this diagnosis may be underreported, as biopsy is frequently avoided in children. Four subtypes of lichen planus can be seen in children: (1) typical (as seen in adults with nail lichen planus), with nail plate thinning, ridging, distal onycholysis, and splitting; (2) trachyonychia (see earlier in this article); (3) idiopathic atrophy, in which destruction of the nail plate occurs, with or without pterygium formation. This is a rare variant, usually seen in those of Asian background.[49] (4) Hypertrophic, in which the nail plate becomes very thickened and discolored (**Fig. 10**). This is also a rare variant in children.

Treatment of typical lichen planus is often difficult. Topical steroids can rarely help. Intralesional steroids can be helpful; however, in children, injections are not well tolerated. Systemic steroids, such as intramuscular triamcinolone acetonide given as 0.5 to 1 mg/kg 1 time per month for 6 months can be very effective.[50] Some patients require retreatment. Other treatment options, such as systemic retinoids or dapsone, have not yet been studied in children for nail lichen planus. No treatment is required for the trachyonychia variant. Unfortunately, the idiopathic atrophic form represents permanent damage of the nail plate. For hypertrophic lichen planus, sometimes

resolution occurs without treatment. Topical steroids, retinoids, and urea have been used with some success.

Lichen Striatus

> **Key features**
>
> - Linear papules along the digit often point to the affected, dystrophic nail
> - Resolves with time

Usually seen in children and adolescents younger than 15, lichen striatus can occur at any age. Small, flat-topped hypopigmented or hyperpigmented papules are seen in a linear array following the lines of Blaschko. When this is present along a digit that involves the nail plate, the plate can become very dystrophic, with longitudinal ridging, splitting, onycholysis, and the appearance of a "pseudo-growth" under the nail plate[51] (**Fig. 11**). If linear papules are seen on the skin near the nail, this supports the diagnosis.[52–55] No treatment is required, as this condition will resolve with time, usually over 6 to 12 months. Topical steroids can be used to alleviate any pruritus.[56] Topical tacrolimus has been reported to hasten resolution.[57]

Verruca Vulgaris

> **Key features**
>
> - Periungual hyperkeratotic papules
> - Often will resolve spontaneously

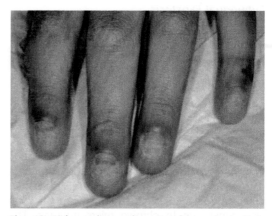

Fig. 10. Lichen planus, hypertrophic variant. Note thickened proximal nail plate with distal thinned, crumbled plate.

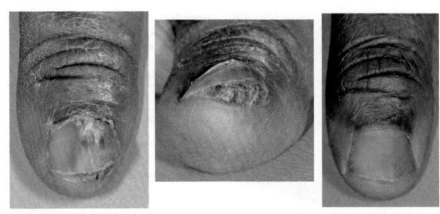

Fig. 11. Lichen striatus. Note hyperkeratotic subungual papule. Resolution after 6 months.

Periungual verruca vulgaris is commonly seen in children due to transmission via picking, biting, and/or sucking of their fingers. Hyperkeratotic, flesh-colored papules of the periungual skin and subungual locations can be very painful, bleed, and cause onycholysis, with subsequent nail dystrophy. Spontaneous resolution can occur; however, this is unpredictable, and patients and parents are often eager to treat to avoid both pain and stigma at school. Treatment is often challenging in this location. Many different topical treatments are available: salicylic acid lacquers (17%–28%), imiquimod 5% cream,[58] sinecatechins cream (Veregen), and 5-fluorouracil cream. Cantharidin, candida antigen injections, and topical immunotherapy (squaric acid dibutylester or diphenylcyclopropenone)[59] are also options. Care must be taken with any injected treatment, as vascular compromise and significant pain due to edema in this tight location can occur.[60] Regimens that combine multiple treatments are usually required. Surgical excision is not recommended, as this leads to permanent scarring.[61]

Subungual Exostosis

> **Key features**
>
> - Due to trauma
> - Bony growth
> - Surgical excision required

Caused by trauma, subungual exostoses are bony growths from the distal phalanx that present as a painful, firm, subungual nodule (**Fig. 12**). Often precipitated by a single traumatic event, they can also occur due to chronic micro-traumas. The great toe is most commonly affected; however, involvement of other toes can be seen. The nodule

is not attached to the nail plate, as it is growing from the bone. Surrounding inflammation, infection, and an ingrown toenail appearance can obfuscate the diagnosis. In addition, this entity is often misdiagnosed as subungual verrucae. A plain film of the toe confirms the diagnosis; definitive treatment is surgical.[62,63]

Pyogenic Granuloma

> **Key features**
>
> - Commonly due to trauma
> - Glistening, erythematous, friable papule

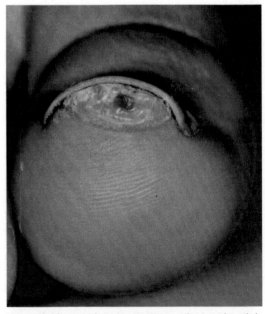

Fig. 12. Subungual exostosis. Note subungual nodule that is not attached to the nail plate.

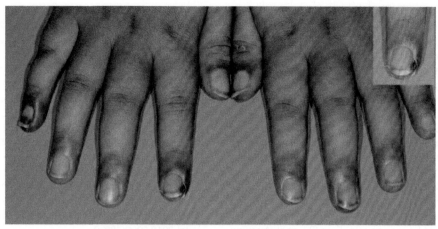

Fig. 13. Pyogenic granulomas secondary to methotrexate for lymphoma.

Frequently seen in children, pyogenic granulomas are most commonly found on the head and neck; however, can occur elsewhere, including periungually. They seem to develop after minor trauma in healthy children. Medication-induced pyogenic granulomas are caused by a number of different drugs, including cyclosporine, systemic retinoids, chemotherapeutic agents, particularly the epidermal growth factor inhibitors and taxanes, as well as antiretrovirals.[64,65] A pyogenic granuloma presents as an erythematous, friable, vascular papule that easily bleeds (**Fig. 13**) and hemostasis can be difficult to achieve. If caused by a medication, the papule will self-resolve approximately 6 weeks after discontinuation. If the agent cannot be stopped, as in the case of chemotherapy, management with antiseptic warm soaks, topical steroids to treat inflammation, and sometimes systemic antibiotics are needed. For idiopathic pyogenic granulomas around the nail, treatment with potent topical steroids or topical timolol under occlusion can be enough; if not, laser or surgical treatment is needed.

SUMMARY

Pediatric nail conditions are common and almost always benign, although they may cause concern regarding appearance, or pain, in certain instances. Carefully examining the nails and skin, and sometimes the hair and teeth as well, will often provide a clinical diagnosis. A biopsy is rarely needed. Management of pediatric nail conditions is similar to that in adults, with some exceptions.

DISCLOSURE

The author has nothing to disclose.

REFERENCES

1. Baker RD, Greer FR, Committee on Nutrition American Academy of Pediatrics. Diagnosis and prevention of iron deficiency and iron-deficiency anemia in infants and young children (0-3 years of age). Pediatrics 2010;126(5):1040–50.
2. Barth JH, Dawber RP. Diseases of the nails in children. Pediatr Dermatol 1987;4(4):275–90.
3. de Berker D. Childhood nail diseases. Dermatol Clin 2006;24(3):355–63.
4. Delano S, Belazarian L. Chevron nails: a normal variant in the pediatric population. Pediatr Dermatol 2014;31(1):e24–5.
5. Zaiac MN, Glick BP, Zaias N. Chevron nail. J Am Acad Dermatol 1998;38(5 Pt 1):773.
6. Ventarola D, Bordone L, Silverberg N. Update on hand-foot-and-mouth disease. Clin Dermatol 2015; 33(3):340–6.
7. Chen W, Yu YS, Liu YH, et al. Nail changes associated with chemotherapy in children. J Eur Acad Dermatol Venereol 2007;21(2):186–90.
8. Shah KN, Rubin AI. Nail disorders as signs of pediatric systemic disease. Curr Probl Pediatr Adolesc Health Care 2012;42(8):204–11.
9. Samman PD. Great toe nail dystrophy. Clin Exp Dermatol 1978;3(1):81–2.
10. Wulkan AJ, Tosti A. Pediatric nail conditions. Clin Dermatol 2013;31(5):564–72.
11. Cambiaghi S, Pistritto G, Gelmetti C. Congenital hypertrophy of the lateral nail folds of the hallux in twins. Br J Dermatol 1997;136(4):635–6.
12. Piraccini BM, Parente GL, Varotti E, et al. Congenital hypertrophy of the lateral nail folds of the hallux: clinical features and follow-up of seven cases. Pediatr Dermatol 2000;17(5):348–51.
13. Campeau PM, Hennekam RC, Group Dsc. DOORS syndrome: phenotype, genotype and comparison with Coffin-Siris syndrome. Am J Med Genet C Semin Med Genet 2014;166C(3):327–32.

14. Babu S, Agarwal N. Anonychia due to prenatal phenytoin exposure. J Assoc Physicians India 2012;60:64.

15. Ruthnum P, Tolmie JL. Atypical malformations in an infant exposed to warfarin during the first trimester of pregnancy. Teratology 1987;36(3):299–301.

16. Sathienkijkanchai A, Wasant P. Fetal warfarin syndrome. J Med Assoc Thai 2005;88(Suppl 8): S246–50.

17. Baran R, Stroud JD. Congenital onychodysplasia of the index fingers. Iso and Kikuchi syndrome. Arch Dermatol 1984;120(2):243–4.

18. Di Chiacchio N, Jasso-Olivares JC, Di Chiacchio NG, et al. Syndrome in question. An Bras Dermatol 2015;90(3):423–5.

19. Eliason MJ, Leachman SA, Feng BJ, et al. A review of the clinical phenotype of 254 patients with genetically confirmed pachyonychia congenita. J Am Acad Dermatol 2012;67(4):680–6.

20. McLean WH, Hansen CD, Eliason MJ, et al. The phenotypic and molecular genetic features of pachyonychia congenita. J Invest Dermatol 2011; 131(5):1015–7.

21. Wallis T, Poole CD, Hoggart B. Can skin disease cause neuropathic pain? A study in pachyonychia congenita. Clin Exp Dermatol 2016;41(1):26–33.

22. El-Darouti MA, Marzouk SA, Nabil N, et al. Pachyonychia congenita: treatment of the thickened nails and palmoplantar circumscribed callosities with urea 40% paste. J Eur Acad Dermatol Venereol 2006;20(5):615–7.

23. Rohold AE, Brandrup F. Pachyonychia congenita: therapeutic and immunologic aspects. Pediatr Dermatol 1990;7(4):307–9.

24. Thomsen RJ, Zuehlke RL, Beckman BI. Pachyonychia congenita: surgical management of the nail changes. J Dermatol Surg Oncol 1982;8(1):24–8.

25. Sweeney E, Fryer A, Mountford R, et al. Nail patella syndrome: a review of the phenotype aided by developmental biology. J Med Genet 2003;40(3): 153–62.

26. Bessler M, Wilson DB, Mason PJ. Dyskeratosis congenita. FEBS Lett 2010;584(17):3831–8.

27. Walne AJ, Dokal I. Advances in the understanding of dyskeratosis congenita. Br J Haematol 2009;145(2): 164–72.

28. Fine JD, Bruckner-Tuderman L, Eady RA, et al. Inherited epidermolysis bullosa: updated recommendations on diagnosis and classification. J Am Acad Dermatol 2014;70(6):1103–26.

29. Mozena JD. The Mozena classification system and treatment algorithm for ingrown hallux nails. J Am Podiatr Med Assoc 2002;92(3):131–5.

30. Martinez-Nova A, Sanchez-Rodriguez R, Alonso-Pena D. A new onychocryptosis classification and treatment plan. J Am Podiatr Med Assoc 2007; 97(5):389–93.

31. Kline A. Onychocryptosis: a simple classification system. The Foot and Ankle Online Journal 2008;1(5):6.

32. Piraccini BM, Richert B, de Berker DA, et al. Retronychia in children, adolescents, and young adults: a case series. J Am Acad Dermatol 2014;70(2): 388–90.

33. Lencastre A, Iorizzo M, Caucanas M, et al. Topical steroids for the treatment of retronychia. J Eur Acad Dermatol Venereol 2019;33(9):e320–2.

34. Poveda-Montoyo I, Vergara-de Caso E, Romero-Perez D, et al. Retronychia a little-known cause of paronychia: a report of two cases in adolescent patients. Pediatr Dermatol 2018;35(3):e144–6.

35. Anolik RB, Shah K, Rubin AI. Onychophagia-induced longitudinal melanonychia. Pediatr Dermatol 2012;29(4):488–9.

36. Baran R. Frictional longitudinal melanonychia: a new entity. Dermatologica 1987;174(6):280–4.

37. Goettmann-Bonvallot S, Andre J, Belaich S. Longitudinal melanonychia in children: a clinical and histopathologic study of 40 cases. J Am Acad Dermatol 1999;41(1):17–22.

38. Cooper C, Arva NC, Lee C, et al. A clinical, histopathologic, and outcome study of melanonychia striata in childhood. J Am Acad Dermatol 2015; 72(5):773–9.

39. Bonamonte D, Arpaia N, Cimmino A, et al. In situ melanoma of the nail unit presenting as a rapid growing longitudinal melanonychia in a 9-year-old white boy. Dermatol Surg 2014;40(10):1154–7.

40. Tosti A, Baran R, Piraccini BM, et al. Nail matrix nevi: a clinical and histopathologic study of twenty-two patients. J Am Acad Dermatol 1996;34(5 Pt 1):765–71.

41. Mercy K, Kwasny M, Cordoro KM, et al. Clinical manifestations of pediatric psoriasis: results of a multicenter study in the United States. Pediatr Dermatol 2013;30(4):424–8.

42. Diluvio L, Campione E, Paterno EJ, et al. Childhood nail psoriasis: a useful treatment with tazarotene 0.05%. Pediatr Dermatol 2007;24(3):332–3.

43. Wells LE, Evans T, Hilton R, et al. Use of secukinumab in a pediatric patient leads to significant improvement in nail psoriasis and psoriatic arthritis. Pediatr Dermatol 2019;36(3):384–5.

44. Tosti A, Peluso AM, Zucchelli V. Clinical features and long-term follow-up of 20 cases of parakeratosis pustulosa. Pediatr Dermatol 1998;15(4):259–63.

45. Tosti A, Bardazzi F, Piraccini BM, et al. Idiopathic trachyonychia (twenty-nail dystrophy): a pathological study of 23 patients. Br J Dermatol 1994;131(6): 866–72.

46. Kumar MG, Ciliberto H, Bayliss SJ. Long-term follow-up of pediatric trachyonychia. Pediatr Dermatol 2015;32(2):198–200.

47. Kasumagic-Halilovic E, Prohic A. Nail changes in alopecia areata: frequency and clinical presentation. J Eur Acad Dermatol Venereol 2009;23(2):240–1.

48. Finner AM. Alopecia areata: clinical presentation, diagnosis, and unusual cases. Dermatol Ther 2011;24(3):348–54.

49. Tosti A, Piraccini BM, Fanti PA, et al. Idiopathic atrophy of the nails: clinical and pathological study of 2 cases. Dermatology 1995;190(2):116–8.

50. Tosti A, Piraccini BM, Cambiaghi S, et al. Nail lichen planus in children: clinical features, response to treatment, and long-term follow-up. Arch Dermatol 2001;137(8):1027–32.

51. Brys AK, Bellet JS. Pediatric dermatology photoquiz: persistent lesion of the thumbnail of a 3-year-old boy. Lichen striatus. Pediatr Dermatol 2016;33(1):95–6.

52. Patrizi A, Neri I, Fiorentini C, et al. Lichen striatus: clinical and laboratory features of 115 children. Pediatr Dermatol 2004;21(3):197–204.

53. Tosti A, Peluso AM, Misciali C, et al. Nail lichen striatus: clinical features and long-term follow-up of five patients. J Am Acad Dermatol 1997;36(6 Pt 1): 908–13.

54. Vozza A, Baroni A, Nacca L, et al. Lichen striatus with nail involvement in an 8-year-old child. J Dermatol 2011;38(8):821–3.

55. Kavak A, Kutluay L. Nail involvement in lichen striatus. Pediatr Dermatol 2002;19(2):136–8.

56. Youssef SM, Teng JM. Effective topical combination therapy for treatment of lichen striatus in children: a case series and review. J Drugs Dermatol 2012; 11(7):872–5.

57. Kim GW, Kim SH, Seo SH, et al. Lichen striatus with nail abnormality successfully treated with tacrolimus ointment. J Dermatol 2009;36(11):616–7.

58. Micali G, Dall'Oglio F, Nasca MR. An open label evaluation of the efficacy of imiquimod 5% cream in the treatment of recalcitrant subungual and periungual cutaneous warts. J Dermatolog Treat 2003; 14(4):233–6.

59. Upitis JA, Krol A. The use of diphenylcyclopropenone in the treatment of recalcitrant warts. J Cutan Med Surg 2002;6(3):214–7.

60. Perman M, Sterling JB, Gaspari A. The painful purple digit: an alarming complication of Candida albicans antigen treatment of recalcitrant warts. Dermatitis 2005;16(1):38–40.

61. Tosti A, Piraccini BM. Warts of the nail unit: surgical and nonsurgical approaches. Dermatol Surg 2001; 27(3):235–9.

62. Calligaris L, Berti I. Subungual exostosis. J Pediatr 2014;165(2):412.

63. Lokiec F, Ezra E, Krasin E, et al. A simple and efficient surgical technique for subungual exostosis. J Pediatr Orthop 2001;21(1):76–9.

64. Richert B, Lecerf P, Caucanas M, et al. Nail tumors. Clin Dermatol 2013;31(5):602–17.

65. Piraccini BM, Alessandrini A. Drug-related nail disease. Clin Dermatol 2013;31(5):618–26.

Bacterial and Viral Infections of the Nail Unit

Matilde Iorizzo, MD, PhD[a],*, Marcel C. Pasch, MD, PhD[b]

KEYWORDS

- Nail disorders • Bacterial infections • Syphilis • Viral infections • Paronychia • Herpes simplex virus
- Warts • Papilloma virus

KEY POINTS

- With suspected acute paronychia, always perform culture to confirm the microorganism and ask for antibiotic sensitivity.
- A viral cause should be considered when suspected acute paronychia is unresponsive to antibiotics.
- With paronychia unresponsive to treatment or with a high rate of recurrences, consider performing imaging or biopsy to exclude osteomyelitis or another underlying disorder.
- Viral paronychia is often self-limiting, but treatment may reduce severity, duration, and postinfective sequelae.

BACTERIAL INFECTIONS OF THE NAIL UNIT

Bacterial infections of the nail unit may involve not only the proximal and lateral nail folds (paronychia) but also the nail plate and the underlying nail bed. Staphylococcus aureus or pyogenes and Pseudomonas species are the typical etiologic agents, but Streptococci and gram-negative bacteria are possible culprits.[1,2] Fingernails are more commonly affected than toenails. Any digit may be involved and even more than one at the same time. The infection is more common in women than in men, with a ratio of 3:1.[3]

A minor trauma (mechanical or chemical as nail and cuticle picking, overzealous manicuring with cuticle removal, a neglected wound, onycholysis) is usually the trigger that allows infiltration of micro-organisms.[4,5] Artificial nails are also a possible cause of bacterial infections due to their ability to harbor microorganisms inaccessible to routine hand hygiene practices.[6]

In general, the affected digit is painful, with erythema, tenderness, swelling, and sometimes purulent drainage (**Fig. 1**). If the infection spreads to the nail bed, it may generate enough pressure to lift the nail plate and damage the nail matrix: Beau lines and onychomadesis may occur as a consequence (**Figs. 2** and **3**).[7,8] When Pseudomonas is the responsible agent, the clinical picture is typical: green discoloration of the nail plate associated with onycholysis (**Fig. 4**).

If left untreated, a bacterial infection of the paronychium may spread not only to the fingertip (felon) but also to the underlying bone (osteomyelitis). The degree of host immune competence is responsible for the severity of clinical manifestations.

Bacterial infections of the nail unit can occur as isolated infections or complicate other nail disorders. This is the reason why it is always useful to rule out underlying predisposing conditions, such as chronic eczema, psoriasis, lichen planus, ingrown nail/retronychia, and onychomycosis among others. The patient's history is fundamental in these cases. Clinical examination is usually sufficient for diagnosis, but sometimes dermoscopy

Financial Disclosures: None.
Conflict of Interests: None.
[a] Private Dermatology Practice, Viale Stazione 16, Bellinzona 6500, Switzerland; [b] Department of Dermatology, Radboud University Medical Center, Rene Descartesdreef 1, Nijmegen 6525GL, The Netherlands
* Corresponding author.
E-mail address: matildeiorizzo@gmail.com

Dermatol Clin 39 (2021) 245–253
https://doi.org/10.1016/j.det.2020.12.001

derm.theclinics.com

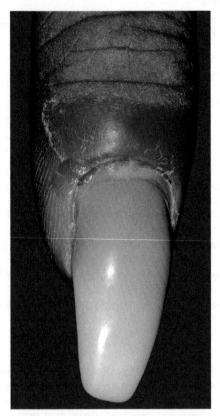

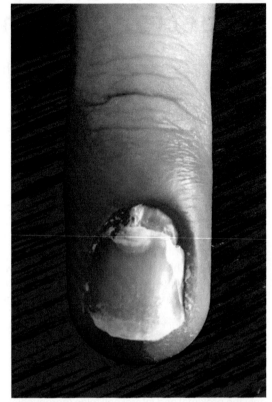

Fig. 1. Acute bacterial paronychia: erythema, tenderness, swelling, and pus discharge.

Fig. 2. Onychomadesis as a consequence of bacterial infection in the nail matrix area.

is helpful to exclude other conditions such as warts, nail plate spicules, and exogenous bodies that might be not visible with the naked eye.

More rarely the nail unit may be affected by other bacteria, such as Treponema pallidum, Neisseria gonorrhoeae, and Bacillus anthracis. In the case of syphilis, although uncommon, the nail unit may be affected in primary, secondary, and tertiary phases. In primary syphilis, not only painful paronychia with onychomadesis but also periungual erosions or ulcerations (chancre) may be present. The nail bed may also be involved with various degrees of onycholysis. Regional lymphadenopathy is generally associated. Secondary and tertiary syphilis may also involve the nail unit, with secondary syphilis involving the nail matrix with various degrees of inflammation and tertiary syphilis involving the entire nail apparatus with tissue necrosis and permanent nail loss.[9] Because of the broad clinical spectrum it is almost impossible to make a diagnosis just through the clinical findings, and laboratory tests or biopsy are mandatory.[10,11]

In the case of gonorrhea, the presence of nail unit lesions and more general skin lesions is a sign of disseminated disease. When this happens,

vesico-pustules with a hemorrhagic to necrotic center are typical (embolic focus of the gonococcus). Acute high temperature and arthritis are generally associated. Culture is always mandatory to make the diagnosis.[12]

Finally, in the case of anthrax, the clinical picture is more specific because the affected part shows, 1 to 7 days after cutaneous contact with the anthrax spores, itchy red bumps sometimes surrounded by swelling. Soon after, the center of the bumps is replaced by a painless black eschar and regional lymphadenopathy ensues. Clinical examination must be confirmed by culture.

Management[13]:
- Avoidance of wet environment, chronic microtraumas, and contact with irritants or allergens (during treatment and for at least 3 months after the condition is solved).
- Wear cotton gloves under rubber gloves during manual work.
- No aggressive/overzealous manicuring and nail cosmetics of any kind.
- Stop nail/cuticle picking, nail biting, finger sucking.

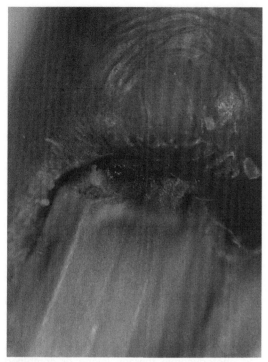

Fig. 3. Dermoscopy of onychomadesis showing purulent discharge.

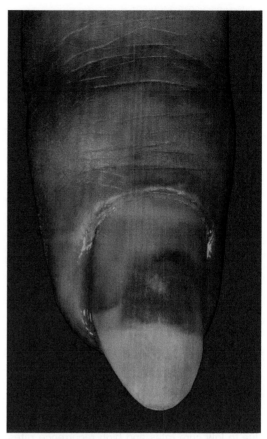

Fig. 4. Onycholysis with Pseudomonas colonization: note the typical green staining.

- Mycological, atypical mycobacterium, and viral culture/radiography/biopsy in recalcitrant or not responding cases. Note that most herpetic paronychias are initially misdiagnosed as bacterial infections.

More specifically:

- Local medications with antiseptics (4% thymol in chloroform twice a day) and warm saline soaks 20 minutes 4 times a day to obtain relief of inflammation and pain.[14]
- Sodium hypochlorite 2% solution, one drop twice a day to remove Pseudomonas green stain when present.[15]
- Drainage of the abscess when present.
- A topical combination of fusidic acid and bethamethasone-17-valerate cream once or twice a day to reduce swelling.[16] Mupirocin cream in the morning and 0.05% clobetasol cream in the evening are alternative options.
- Systemic antibiotics only for severe cases not responding to topical therapy or in frequent recurrences, as well as in populations at risk (diabetes, immunosuppression, peripheral vascular impairment, presence of prosthetic heart valve). Always obtain sensitivities provided by the laboratory after culture. Systemic antibiotic treatment is always mandatory in the presence of osteomyelitis,[17,18] syphilis, gonorrhea, and anthrax.

- A broad-spectrum antibiotic such as amoxicillin/clavulanate or clindamycin is advisable when sensitivities are not feasible.

VIRAL INFECTIONS OF THE NAIL UNIT

A viral infection of the nail unit may present as a chronic dermatosis such as a wart or as an acute paronychia. In antibiotic-resistant acute paronychia, in fact, a viral infection should always be ruled out.[19] Viral paronychia is often self-limiting, but treatment may reduce severity, duration, and postinfective sequelae.

Human Papilloma Virus

Human papilloma virus (HPV) is the etiologic agent for common warts. In addition, in ungual Bowen disease and squamous cell carcinoma several HPV subtypes can be found.

Warts

Periungual and subungual warts involve fingernails more often than toenails and are caused by HPV 1,

2, 4, 27, and 57 infection of abraded or macerated skin.[20]

Biting, picking, and tearing of the nail and nail walls are common habits in subjects with periungual warts. Because the virus is very resistant to heat, desiccation, and detergents, warts can also be acquired by indirect contact and not only by direct contact in a susceptible host.

Clinical warts develop in a few weeks to many months after viral inoculation of the skin. Most frequently they are localized to the lateral nail folds (**Fig. 5**), but other locations are possible (**Fig. 6**). Subungual warts initially affect the hyponychium, growing slowly toward the nail bed and finally elevating the nail plate. Usually, ungual warts are cosmetically disturbing but otherwise asymptomatic, although fissuring or subungual localization may cause pain. In rare cases, a wart may develop underneath the proximal nail fold and swelling may ensue. Multiple warts distorting the nail unit are commonly seen in immunosuppressed patients.

Generally, the diagnosis of warts is clinical. Histopathology can be useful to rule out other verrucous disorders, such as Bowen disease, squamous cell carcinoma, tuberculosis cutis verrucosa, onycholemmal horn, or mucinous syringometaplasia involving the distal nail bed.

Treatment of warts of the nail unit is challenging due to low cure rates and high recurrence rates. Most warts disappear spontaneously with a natural life span of about 4 to 5 years, especially in healthy children, but treatment is generally advised because of social embarrassment. However, aggressive measures are not recommended.[20]

Cryotherapy with liquid nitrogen is often the first choice for a small wart. When treating the proximal nail fold, freezing must not be prolonged because one may easily damage the matrix, which may result in temporary or permanent nail dystrophy. Available topical therapies that may help to control the growth of the warts are keratolytic agents (containing salicylic acid, lactic acid, dichloroacetic acid, or trichloroacetic acid), virucidal agents (containing glutaraldehyde or formaldehyde), cidofovir,[21] and saturated monochloroacetic acid. Subungual warts are treated similarly, after cutting away the overlying part of the nail plate.

Topical immunotherapy with squaric acid dibutylester[22] or 2% diphenylcyclopropenone (diphencyprone)[23] is a more time-consuming, but effective and painless, approach for recalcitrant warts. Many other treatments are also reported effective to treat periungual warts, including vaccines,[24] 0.007% cantharidin, 5% imiquimod, and 5-fluorouracil.[25] Also, intralesional treatment with

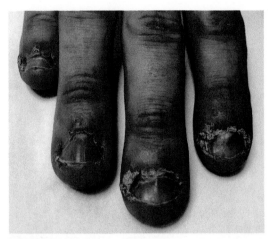

Fig. 5. Periungual warts in a patient with onychophagia.

bleomycin has been used[26] but nail dystrophy and even complete nail loss have been reported.[27] Physical treatments for ungual warts are laser treatment (CO_2, pulsed dye, and Nd-Yag laser) and photodynamic therapy (alone or combined with CO_2 laser), but in daily practice efficacy is not always convincing and permanent nail dystrophy is possible. Systemic treatments are not indicated in periungual warts, despite some positive anecdotal reports with cimetidine.

Bowen disease and squamous cell carcinoma

The main differential diagnosis of an ungual wart is Bowen disease, which frequently is also HPV induced. HPV 16, 18, 52, 56, 58, and 73 are associated with malignant transformation to squamous cell carcinoma.[20,28] Any single verrucous lesion of the nail unit in men older than 40 years should raise the suspicion of squamous carcinoma in situ and should be biopsied. Histopathology and treatment of Bowen disease and squamous cell carcinoma are not discussed here but have been discussed extensively elsewhere.[29,30]

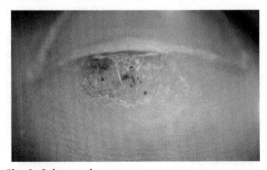

Fig. 6. Subungual wart.

Herpes Simplex Virus

Both herpes simplex virus (HSV) type 1 and type 2 may cause nail unit infections if the virus is able to enter a disrupted epidermis in the nail region. Women and children, especially finger suckers and nail biters, are more frequently affected than adult men.[31] Medical and dental personnel are particularly at risk.[32] Fingernails, especially the index finger, are more frequently affected than toenails. Any finger may be involved, even more than one at the same time.[33]

Clinically, the two HSV subtypes give an identical clinical picture: defining the subtype with a diagnostic test is important to identify the presumed source of contagion. The infection may be due to autogenous inoculation from another affected area, exogenous inoculation from close contact with a person actively shedding the virus, or due to virus that remained viable on surfaces. HSV may affect the periungual skin of the terminal phalanx with the typical vesicles, but alternatively it may cause an acute and extremely painful paronychia often confused with bacterial paronychia. After a prodromal period (up to 20 days, but <6 hours in recurrent infections) of local tenderness, erythema, and swelling, clusters of small and tense vesicles appear around the perionychium.[34] More rarely the vesicles develop within the nail bed producing onycholysis. Lymphangitis, axillary/inguinal adenopathy, and flu-like symptoms are rare but may be observed. In the early vesicular phase, the patient is extremely contagious due to viral shedding. In the next days the vesicles increase in size and sometimes also coalesce into a large bulla, which may lead to a misdiagnosis (**Fig. 7**). Vesicular liquid, clear at the beginning, becomes then turbid and, in rare cases, also purulent or hemorrhagic. After this acute phase, dry crusts are formed. Healing generally occurs in 15 to 20 days in primary infections, less in recurrences. Scars of periungual skin or permanent nail dystrophies may occur but are rare. The clinical presentation of recurrences is generally less severe.

The diagnosis of HSV infection is generally clinical, so a biopsy is never required. A Tzanck smear, culture, polymerase chain reaction (PCR), or serum analysis could, however, be performed for confirmation.

The Tzanck test reveals the characteristic acantholytic and multinucleate giant cells ("balloon" giant cells). This test is fast and cheap but cannot distinguish between HSV1, HSV2, and herpes zoster virus.[19] Differentiation between HSV subtypes 1 and 2 and herpes zoster virus is possible with

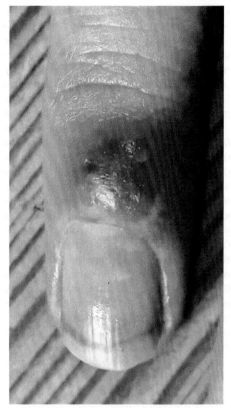

Fig. 7. HSV paronychia: vesicles increased in size and coalesced into a large bulla.

PCR, culture, and serologic testing. Culture is the gold standard, but PCR is faster and more sensitive. Culture results take 3 to 7 days and preferably sampling should be taken within 24 to 48 hours after appearance of the vesicles. However, treatment should be started earlier than culture results are available. Serum analysis for HSV antibodies is helpful to differentiate between HSV type 1 or type 2 and also helpful when the vesicles are localized to inaccessible areas such as the nail bed.

Treatment of HSV infections is primarily aimed at symptomatic relief to reduce pain and to accelerate healing. Treating the primary infection, even if done within 24 to 48 hours, does not prevent recurrences but could reduce number per year and severity.[35] It is very important, contrary to acute bacterial paronychia, not to incise vesicles to avoid spreading of the virus and to facilitate bacterial superinfection.[36] No specific guidelines exist for medical treatment of HSV of the nail unit, but because HSV type 2 is the most common causative agent of HSV infections in the nail unit, treatment guidelines for this specific virus are generally followed.[37]

In adult patients and children older than 12 years, oral acyclovir, 400 mg, 3 times a day for 10 days is the first-line treatment (acyclovir, 200 mg, 5 times a day is an alternative). Other options are valacyclovir, 500 mg, 2 times a day for 10 days and famciclovir, 250 mg, 3 times a day for 10 days. Shorter treatments are enough in recurrences: acyclovir, 400 mg, orally thrice daily for 5 days, 800 mg twice daily for 5 days, or 800 mg thrice daily for 2 days; valaciclovir, 500 mg, orally twice daily for 3 days; or famciclovir, 250 mg, orally twice daily for 5 days. Patients who have frequent recurrences (>4–6 times a year), severe symptoms, or distressing episodes will likely elect suppressive therapy over episodic therapy: acyclovir, 400 mg, orally twice daily; valaciclovir, 500 mg, orally once daily; or famciclovir, 250 mg, orally twice daily, all for at least 6 months. For patients younger than 12 years oral acyclovir, 400 mg, suspension (2,5 mL every 4 hours) is generally used for 5 to 20 days. Although widely used, topical acyclovir and topical famciclovir provide no relevant benefit in reducing the duration of symptoms. Moreover, the topical application will not reach the site of reactivation and does not influence the host immune response.[38]

Herpes Zoster Virus

Herpes zoster of the nail unit occurs in the context of reactivation of the varicella zoster virus in the dorsal root ganglion of that particular dermatome. Grouped vesicles may be seen around the proximal nail fold. In case of subungual involvement severe pain is present, and subungual roundish hemorrhagic spots slowly grow out with the nail. Inflammation in the matrix area may result in temporary parakeratosis of the onychocytes, clinically presenting as transverse leukonychia weeks after the infection.[39] In patients with AIDS, verrucous lesions may also be present.[40] The most common complication is bacterial superinfection, most often caused by Staphylococcus aureus or pyogenes. Herpes zoster can almost always be diagnosed clinically. To differentiate herpes zoster from HSV, PCR, immunohistochemistry, or cultures may be helpful. Postherpetic neuralgia is the most common complication and is more likely in older patients, where it can take 6 months or more to resolve. Treatment should be considered particularly in patients older than 50 years and started preferably within 72 hours after the onset of symptoms. A 7-day course of an oral antiviral drug such as acyclovir (800 mg 5 times a day), famciclovir (500 mg twice a day), or valaciclovir (1 g thrice a day) is recommended.[41]

Hand-Foot-and-Mouth Disease

Hand-foot-and-mouth disease (HFMD) is most often caused by coxsackie viruses (CVA) 16 and 6, but enterovirus 71 may also be responsible. Postsyndrome findings, occurring 3 to 12 weeks after the initial clinical presentation, are the development of Beau lines or onychomadesis in about a quarter of patients (**Fig. 8**). Nail abnormalities are more frequent in patients older than 5 years and following CVA6 infection.[42] Familial cases have also been described. In general, multiple nails are involved, and nail changes are caused by direct cytopathic effects to the matrix from the virus.[43] The diagnosis of HFMD can be made clinically, but histology can also be helpful: this shows ballooning and vesicles common to HSV infection. However, in HFMD, there is no acantholysis, viral inclusions, or giant multinucleated cells, but there may be necrotic keratinocytes and shadow cells. Within several months and without any specific treatment HFMD-induced nail dystrophies recover completely.

Molluscum Contagiosum

Molluscum contagiosum (MC) is a common infectious dermatosis caused by a DNA poxvirus. MC of the nail unit is very rare[44] and may present as a tender brownish oval lesion. The lesion may grow over weeks and simultaneously a keratotic papule can be formed on the hyponychium. Dermoscopic examination is useful for the diagnosis and reveals whitish, amorphous structure in the

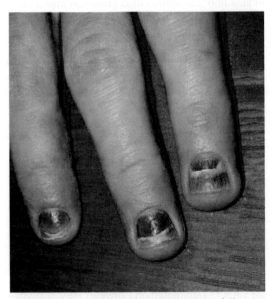

Fig. 8. Onychomadesis of multiple digits following hand-foot-and-mouth disease.

center of the lesion with a surrounding crown of linear, blurred, and branching vessels.[44,45] To avoid spread of the infection it is important to avoid scratching, rubbing, picking, or squeezing the lesion because the central plugs are laden with MCV particles that can easily spread to uninfected skin. Watchful waiting is an option, but mechanical treatments (eg, cryotherapy with liquid nitrogen or curettage) are also quite effective.[46] Chemical methods (including cantharidin, podophyllotoxin, tretinoin, salicylic acid) and the immunomodulatory agent imiquimod may also be effective. Histologic examination reveals the presence of intracytoplasmic hyaline eosinophilic inclusion bodies (Henderson-Paterson bodies), confirming the clinical suspect.

Orf

Orf (ecthyma contagiosum) is a highly contagious zoonotic parapoxvirus infection that may be spread in patients handling sheep and goats but can also be transmitted to humans by indirect contact. It usually occurs on the dorsal aspect of hands and fingers, including the nail folds.

After an incubation period of 3 to 7 days, the disease passes through several stages during the next 6 to 12 weeks. In the maculopapular stage there is an erythematous macule/papule. The lesion then acquires a reddish center with an outer halo (target stage). In the acute stage it starts to weep, and then it becomes dry (regenerative stage). The papillomatous stage is then characterized by a papilloma-like lesion, which forms a dry crust and then undergoes spontaneous resolution, with little or no residual scarring.[47] Orf mainly is a clinical diagnosis and based on history of contact with animals. Biopsy is rarely indicated and will suggest a viral infection. Keratinocytes that are infected with the orf virus have eosinophilic cytoplastic inclusion and irregularly shaped nuclei. The benign course justifies conservative management awaiting spontaneous resolution. Many other approaches such as imiquimod, cidofovir, curettage, shave excision, cryotherapy, and electrocautery have, however, been reported to be successful.[48]

Chikungunya

Chikungunya (CHK) is a reemerging mosquito-borne infectious disease prevalent in Africa, Asia, and the Indian subcontinent and caused by a Togavirus. A few days after the mosquito bite, patients suffer from polyarthralgia, high fever, myalgia, headache, and often skin involvement.[49] Coexistent nail involvement is rare and has been reported as subungual hemorrhage,[50] black

lunula, diffuse and longitudinal melanonychia, transverse pigmented leukonychia, and onychomadesis.[51] Isolated and persistent nail pigmentation occurring weeks after a CHK infection without skin lesions has also been observed.[49] Diagnosis is often clinical but should be confirmed by serologic tests. In early phases reverse transcriptase–PCR may detect the viral nucleic acid in serum, and ELISA shows the presence of IgM and IgG anti-CHK antibodies. CHK is a self-limiting disease in which the treatment focuses only on relieving the symptoms.

SUMMARY

Bacterial and viral infections of the nail unit are very common, but they can be superinfections complicating other nail disorders. For this reason, it is very important to check for hidden conditions or predisposing factors before making a definitive diagnosis.

A thorough understanding of the infection is always necessary for appropriate management, especially the causative microorganism to determine the appropriate medication.

CLINICS CARE POINTS

- Isolated Beau's lines or onychomadesis are common sequelae of acute nail infections.
- Treatment of periungual warts should be performed carefully to prevent permanent damage to the nail unit.
- Hand-foot-and-mouth disease is a common cause of onychomadesis of multiple nails in children over the age of five.

REFERENCES

1. Brook I. Aerobic and anaerobic microbiology of paronychia. Ann Emerg Med 1990;19(9):994–6.
2. Maes M, Richert B, de la Brassinne M. [Green nail syndrome or chloronychia]. Rev Med Liege 2002; 57(4):233–5.
3. Fowler JR, Ilyas AM. Epidemiology of adult acute hand infections at an urban medical center. J Hand Surg 2013;38(6):1189–93.
4. Rockwell PG. Acute and chronic paronychia. Am Fam Physician 2001;63(6):1113–6.
5. Shafritz AB, Coppage JM. Acute and chronic paronychia of the hand. J Am Acad Orthop Surg 2014; 22(3):165–74.
6. Boyce JM, Pittet D. Healthcare Infection Control Practices Advisory C, Force HSAIHHT. Guideline for Hand Hygiene in Health-Care Settings. Recommendations of the Healthcare Infection Control Practices Advisory Committee and the HIPAC/SHEA/

APIC/IDSA Hand Hygiene Task Force. Am J Infect Control 2002;30(8):S1–46.

7. Daniel CR 3rd. Paronychia. Dermatol Clin 1985;3(3): 461–4.

8. Rigopoulos D, Larios G, Gregoriou S, et al. Acute and chronic paronychia. Am Fam Physician 2008; 77(3):339–46.

9. Noriega L, Gioia Di Chiacchio N, Cury Rezende F, et al. Periungual Lesion due to Secondary Syphilis. Skin Appendage Disord 2017;2(3–4):116–9.

10. Starzycki Z. Primary syphilis of the fingers. Br J Vener Dis 1983;59(3):169–71.

11. Anemuller W, Brauninger W, Krahl D, et al. [Chancre of the finger. A circuitous route to diagnosis]. Hautarzt 2008;59(6):499–502.

12. Silva J Jr, Wilson K. Disseminated gonococcal infections (DGI). Cutis 1979;24(6):601–6.

13. Iorizzo M. Tips to treat the 5 most common nail disorders: brittle nails, onycholysis, paronychia, psoriasis, onychomycosis. Dermatol Clin 2015;33(2): 175–83.

14. Ritting AW, O'Malley MP, Rodner CM. Acute paronychia. J Hand Surg 2012;37(5):1068–70 [quiz: 1070].

15. Baran R. Common-sense advice for the treatment of selected nail disorders. J Eur Acad Dermatol Venereol 2001;15(2):97–102.

16. Wollina U. Acute paronychia: comparative treatment with topical antibiotic alone or in combination with corticosteroid. J Eur Acad Dermatol Venereol 2001; 15(1):82–4.

17. Tosti R, Samuelsen BT, Bender S, et al. Emerging multidrug resistance of methicillin-resistant Staphylococcus aureus in hand infections. J Bone Joint Surg Am 2014;96(18):1535–40.

18. Pierrart J, Delgrande D, Mamane W, et al. Acute felon and paronychia: Antibiotics not necessary after surgical treatment. Prospective study of 46 patients. Hand Surg Rehabil 2016;35(1):40–3.

19. Durdu M, Ruocco V. Clinical and cytologic features of antibiotic-resistant acute paronychia. J Am Acad Dermatol 2014;70(1):120–6.e1.

20. Herschthal J, McLeod MP, Zaiac M. Management of ungual warts. Dermatol Ther 2012;25(6):545–50.

21. Padilla Espana L, Del Boz J, Fernandez Morano T, et al. Successful treatment of periungual warts with topical cidofovir. Dermatol Ther 2014;27(6): 337–42.

22. Lee AN, Mallory SB. Contact immunotherapy with squaric acid dibutylester for the treatment of recalcitrant warts. J Am Acad Dermatol 1999;41(4):595–9.

23. Choi Y, Kim DH, Jin SY, et al. Topical immunotherapy with diphenylcyclopropenone is effective and preferred in the treatment of periungual warts. Ann Dermatol 2013;25(4):434–9.

24. Iorizzo M, Marazza G. Measles, mumps, and rubella vaccine: a new option to treat common warts? Int J Dermatol 2014;53(4):e243–5.

25. De Anda MC, Dominguez JG. Melanonychia induced by topical treatment of periungual warts with 5-fluorouracil. Dermatol Online J 2013;19(3):10.

26. Sardana K, Garg V, Relhan V. Complete resolution of recalcitrant periungual/subungual wart with recovery of normal nail following "prick" method of administration of bleomycin 1%. Dermatol Ther 2010;23(4): 407–10.

27. Urbina Gonzalez F, Cristobal Gil MC, Aguilar Martinez A, et al. Cutaneous toxicity of intralesional bleomycin administration in the treatment of periungual warts. Arch Dermatol 1986;122(9):974–5.

28. Kato M, Shimizu A, Hattori T, et al. Detection of human papillomavirus type 58 in periungual Bowen's disease. Acta Derm Venereol 2013;93(6): 723–4.

29. Starace M, Alessandrini A, Dika E, et al. Squamous cell carcinoma of the nail unit. Dermatol Pract Concept 2018;8(3):238–44.

30. Lecerf P, Richert B, Theunis A, et al. A retrospective study of squamous cell carcinoma of the nail unit diagnosed in a Belgian general hospital over a 15-year period. J Am Acad Dermatol 2013;69(2): 253–61.

31. Muller SA, Herrmann EC Jr. Association of stomatitis and paronychias due to herpes simplex. Arch Dermatol 1970;101(4):396–402.

32. Herbert AM, Bagg J, Walker DM, et al. Seroepidemiology of herpes virus infections among dental personnel. J Dent 1995;23(6):339–42.

33. Pechere M, Friedli A, Krischer J. [Multiple herpes simplex type 1 whitlow lesions]. Ann Dermatol Venereol 1999;126(8–9):646.

34. Gill MJ, Arlette J, Buchan KA. Herpes simplex virus infection of the hand. J Am Acad Dermatol 1990; 22(1):111–6.

35. Cernik C, Gallina K, Brodell RT. The treatment of herpes simplex infections: an evidence-based review. Arch Intern Med 2008;168(11):1137–44.

36. Feder HM Jr, Long SS. Herpetic whitlow. Epidemiology, clinical characteristics, diagnosis, and treatment. Am J Dis Child 1983;137(9):861–3.

37. In: WHO Guidelines for the Treatment of Genital Herpes Simplex Virus. Geneva2016. Available at: https://www.who.int/publications/i/item/978924154987.

38. Cunningham A, Griffiths P, Leone P, et al. Current management and recommendations for access to antiviral therapy of herpes labialis. J Clin Virol 2012;53(1):6–11.

39. Zizmor J, Deluty S. Acquired leukonychia striata. Int J Dermatol 1980;19(1):49–50.

40. Cohen JI, Brunell PA, Straus SE, et al. Recent advances in varicella-zoster virus infection. Ann Intern Med 1999;130(11):922–32.

41. Bader MS. Herpes zoster: diagnostic, therapeutic, and preventive approaches. Postgrad Med 2013; 125(5):78–91.

42. Wei SH, Huang YP, Liu MC, et al. An outbreak of cox-sackievirus A6 hand, foot, and mouth disease associated with onychomadesis in Taiwan, 2010. BMC Infect Dis 2011;11:346.

43. Ventarola D, Bordone L, Silverberg N. Update on hand-foot-and-mouth disease. Clin Dermatol 2015; 33(3):340–6.

44. Elmas OF, Kilitci A. Subungual molluscum contagiosus: a rare presentation. Skin Appendage Disord 2020;6(1):55–7.

45. Lacarrubba F, Verzi AE, Dinotta F, et al. Dermatoscopy in inflammatory and infectious skin disorders. Dermatol Venereol 2015;150(5):521–31.

46. Leung AKC, Barankin B, Hon KLE. Molluscum contagiosum: an update. Recent Pat Inflamm Allergy Drug Discov 2017;11(1):22–31.

47. Al-Qattan MM. Orf infection of the hand. J Hand Surg 2011;36(11):1855–8.

48. Bergqvist C, Kurban M, Abbas O. Orf virus infection. Rev Med Virol 2017;27(4).

49. Singal A, Pandhi D. Isolated nail pigmentation associated with chikungunya: a hitherto unreported manifestation. Skin Appendage Disord 2018;4(4): 312–4.

50. Inamadar AC, Palit A, Sampagavi VV, et al. Cutaneous manifestations of chikungunya fever: observations made during a recent outbreak in south India. Int J Dermatol 2008;47(2):154–9.

51. Riyaz N, Riyaz A, Rahima, et al. Cutaneous manifestations of chikungunya during a recent epidemic in Calicut, north Kerala, south India. Indian J Dermatol Venereol Leprol 2010;76(6):671–6.

Diagnosis of Melanonychia

Aurora Alessandrini, MD*, Emi Dika, MD, PhD, Michela Starace, MD, PhD,
Marco Adriano Chessa, MD, Bianca Maria Piraccini, MD, PhD

KEYWORDS

• Nail pigmentation • Nail melanoma • Melanonychia • Dermoscopy • Histopathology

KEY POINTS

- The term melanonychia describes the presence of melanin in the nail plate.
- It is caused by an activation or a proliferation of the nail matrix melanocytes that is benign or malignant.
- Dermoscopy of the nail is useful, adding data to history and clinical signs, revealing aspects not visualized by the naked eye.
- A definitive diagnosis of nail pigmentation can be made exclusively with histopathology.

INTRODUCTION

The term melanonychia describes the presence of melanin in the nail plate, which appears in most cases as a longitudinal brown-black band of nail pigmentation, also known as longitudinal melanonychia (LM). Less commonly, the pigmentation presents as a transverse band (transverse melanonychia) or can involve the whole nail plate (total melanonychia). Pigmented lesions in the nail bed usually do not cause LM and are viewed through the nail as grayish brown or black spots.[1] Melanocytes are present in low density in the nail matrix and nail bed and they are usually quiescent in Whites.[2,3] They possess enzymes that are necessary for melanin production and may become activated by a large number of physiologic and pathologic conditions, inducing the pigmentation of the nail plate.[4]

Melanonychia can involve one digit or several digits, in fingernails and toenails, and appear at any age. The clinical presentation depends on the color of the bands, edges, and width. In any patient with LM involving one digit it is always important to exclude a melanoma. The causes of LM are difficult to differentiate clinically, and the

use of nail dermoscopy (onychoscopy) has become over the years a useful addition to traditional examination for the evaluation and the management of such lesions. The real problem, even today, is to distinguish if the lesion is benign or malignant, because an early diagnosis of melanoma is crucial for prognosis, which in late diagnoses is poor with a high mortality. Biopsy for histopathologic examination is recommended when an LM occurs in an adult and it is localized in a single digit, in the absence of local or systemic causes that may explain its onset.

From a histologic point of view, LM may result either from simple activation of nail matrix melanocytes, the most common cause, or from benign (lentigo or nevus) or malignant (melanoma) melanocyte proliferation.[1]

At the first examination of a melanonychia, three steps should be followed:

1. Establish if the nail pigmentation is melanin or not.
2. Determine if melanin is produced by activated or proliferated nail matrix melanocytes.
3. Determine if the melanocyte proliferation is benign or malignant. For the examination of

Department of Specialised Experimental and Diagnostic Medicine, Dermatology Alma Mater Studiorum - Università di Bologna, Via Massarenti 1, Bologna 40138, Italy
* Corresponding author. Dermatology, Department of Experimental, Diagnostic and Specialty Medicine, University of Bologna, Via Massarenti 1, Bologna 40138, Italy.
E-mail address: aurora.alessandrini3@unibo.it

Dermatol Clin 39 (2021) 255–267
https://doi.org/10.1016/j.det.2020.12.004

the pigmented lesions using nail dermoscopy, gel is recommended to observe the color alterations, because it increases visibility through the nail plate, even though application of gel increases the tendency of the lens to slide off the plate. Onychoscopy permits differentiation of melanocytic from nonmelanocytic pigmentation. Generally, melanic pigmentation is brown-black in color and resides within the nail plate forming a longitudinal band running from the proximal nail fold to the distal edge of the nail, whereas exogenous pigmentation includes different types of color of the substance, which adhere to the nail plate or is beneath it and does not always have a longitudinal appearance.

NONMELANOCYTIC PIGMENTATION

Common causes of nonmelanocytic pigmentation are subungual hematoma, fungal melanonychia, and green nails.[5]

Green Nails

Green nails are a variety of chromonychia, where the green-black color is caused by the presence of the pigment pyocyanin produced by *Pseudomonas aeruginosa*, a gram-negative bacterium. In nails affected by paronychia and onycholysis, *Pseudomonas* grows in the humid environment and produces its pigments, turning the nail color into yellow-green to dark green. The appearance of a deep green-black pigmentation is often misdiagnosed as melanin pigmentation and worries the clinician. The exogenous deposition is above the nail plate, usually on one side, or beneath it in case of onycholysis and may resemble a band of melanonychia. A careful observation of the pigmentation with a magnifying lens or a dermatoscope and examination of the nail apparatus allows an easy and quick discrimination between the two entities. Onychoscopy typically

shows a bright green color that fades to yellow and its localization on or under the nail plate (**Fig. 1**).[6,7]

Subungual Hematomas

These are commonly caused by trauma to the fingers or toes. The affected nail shows a patchy or diffuse red-brown-black pigmentation that migrates distally with nail growth and does not fade in a few days or weeks, because the extravasated blood is entrapped between the nail plate and the nail bed. Acute hematoma is easily recognized by the patient, because it follows an acute trauma, has a rapid onset, and is associated with pain. However, the most common "chronic" subungual hematoma is caused by chronic trauma that the patient is not aware of. In this case, the patient or the doctor notices a deep-red or black nail pigmentation and is not able to explain its appearance, hence becoming anxious thinking that the pigment is melanin. This occurs especially when the discoloration does not have a round shape and is black. Subungual hematoma appears as a dark band or an irregularly shaped purple to brown-black round area. Onychoscopy is characteristic, showing a red-purple color that fades in the periphery, round dark-red spots at the periphery, and a "filamentous" distal end (**Fig. 2**).[8–10]

Fungal Melanonychia

Another diagnosis to consider facing a brown-black partial nail discoloration is fungal melanonychia. This indicates a nail pigmentation caused by dematiaceous molds or, most commonly, by *Trichophyton rubrum* variant *melanoides*.[11] The nail appears black because subungual scales are pigmented, as is easily appreciated by onychoscopy.[12,13] Dermoscopy of fungal melanonychia reveals that the band is not running longitudinally from start to tip of the nail plate, but starts distally;

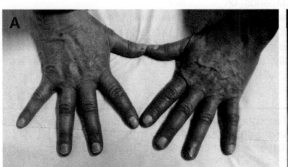
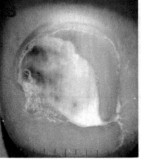

Fig. 1. Clinical (*A*) and dermoscopic image (*B*) of onycholysis with a green discoloration caused by *Pseudomonas aeruginosa* colonization.

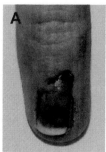
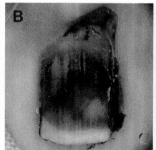
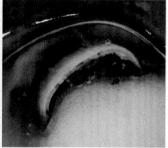

Fig. 2. Clinical (*A*) and dermoscopic (*B–C*) photographs of a subungual hematoma with brown-red nail pigmentation caused by blood deposition irregularly shaped.

it does not have visible inclusions of melanin and has multiple colors, including black, orange, white, and yellow. Onychoscopy of the distal margin reveals the presence of subungual yellow and brown-black scales (**Fig. 3**).

MELANIC PIGMENTATION

If melanonychia is caused by melanin produced by nail matrix melanocytes, the second step is to identify whether the pigmentation is caused by activation or proliferation of these cells. Melanin produced by matrix melanocytes is transferred to onychocytes during nail plate production: melanonychia therefore appears as a longitudinal band that runs from the cuticle region to the free margin of the nail plate. Overall, the thumbs, index fingers, and great toes are the

most commonly affected. Onychoscopy of melanonychia should consider[9]

- The shape of the band, which usually is rectangular.
- The color of the background, which varies to gray to brown to black.
- The aspect of the borders, which is blurred of sharp.
- The longitudinal lines that compose the band: they can be of different width, color, parallel or not, interrupted, or continuous.
- Presence of pigmented dots within the band.
- Presence of melanic pigmentation in the periungual tissues (Hutchinson and micro-Hutchinson signs). Hutchinson sign describes a periungual pigmentation not detected with the naked eye (**Fig. 4**).

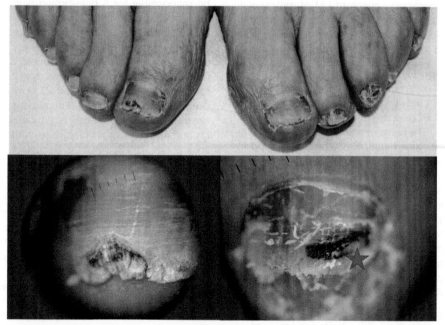

Fig. 3. Clinical and dermoscopic pictures of fungal melanonychia of the toenail, with thick subungual hyperkeratosis with yellow and brown scales. Subungual hematoma is also visible (*asterisk*).

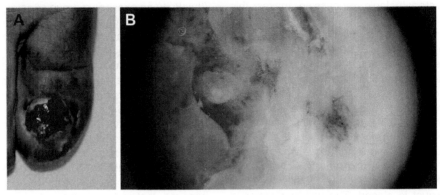

Fig. 4. Clinical (*A*) and dermoscopic (*B*) photographs of a 55-year-old patient with invasive melanoma presenting as an eroded nodule with micro-Hutchinson sign.

- Upper or lower, or total pigmentation of the free margin of the nail corresponding to the band. Pigmentation of the lower nail plate indicates that the melanocytes producing melanin reside in the distal nail matrix, whereas pigment localized in the upper nail plate indicates that the melanocytes producing melanin reside in the proximal mail matrix. Evaluation of these parameters is a useful addition to clinical data.

Activation of Nail Matrix Melanocytes

The number of digits involved is an important diagnostic clue. If more than one digit is involved, the first thought should be melanocytic activation. The most common causes of LM of melanocytic activation are: racial/ethnic, drugs, systemic diseases, mechanical factors, inflammatory nail diseases, and keratinocyte nail tumors.

Racial melanonychia

Racial melanonychia typically involves several/all nails and occurs in dark-skinned individuals, especially with Fitzpatrick phototypes IV, V, and VI (**Fig. 5**).[14,15] The number and width of the bands increases with age: nearly 100% of the black population develops one or more pigmented bands by the age of 50 years.[15,16] Racial melanonychia in mainly seen in the most used digits (ie, thumb, index finger, and middle finger), or in traumatized digits (eg, the great toe). Additionally, patients with darker phototypes develop LM because of melanocytic activation by other causes more easily than patients with light skin phototypes.[15] Onychoscopy shows multiple grey-black band with parallel thin lines.

Drug-induced melanonychia

Among drugs able to induce melanonychia the most common causes are chemotherapeutic agents. A long list of cancer chemotherapeutic agents may activate clusters of nail matrix melanocytes inducing melanin production, giving rise to the development of melanonychia in multiple longitudinal or transverse bands. Generally, several nails are affected with multiple grey-brown bands (**Fig. 6**). Among chemotherapeutic agents, a high risk to develop melanonychia is associated with cyclophosphamide, doxorubicin, and capecitabine.[17–19] Antiretrovirals, especially azidothymidine, and antibiotics, mainly tetracyclines, can induce melanonychia that most commonly appears 3 to 8 weeks after drug intake. Pigmentation is usually reversible within 6 to 8 weeks but may persist for months after drug interruption.[20,21] The antimalarial drug hydroxychloroquine could be responsible for a blue-brown pigmentation of the nail bed but also for LM.[22] Calcium channel blockers, such as amlodipine, have been reported as responsible for LM.[23] Psoralens and also psoralen plus ultraviolet A therapy could cause melanonychia.[24] Fortunately, when melanonychia is drug-related, it typically fades slowly following drug withdrawal. In drug-induced melanonychia, onychoscopy may show a typical gray background or a more brow-black one, with thin regular lines.

Melanonychia in systemic diseases

Systemic factors causing LM because of melanocytic activation include specific syndromes, pregnancy, or endocrine disorders. The syndromes often cited with melanonychia are Peutz-Jeghers syndrome and Laugier-Hunziker syndrome (LHS).

LHS is an acquired pigmentary condition affecting the lips, oral mucosa, and acral area, frequently associated with LM, without any malignant predisposition or underlying systemic abnormality. The cause of this disorder is still unknown, and no familiar factor seems to be present. The

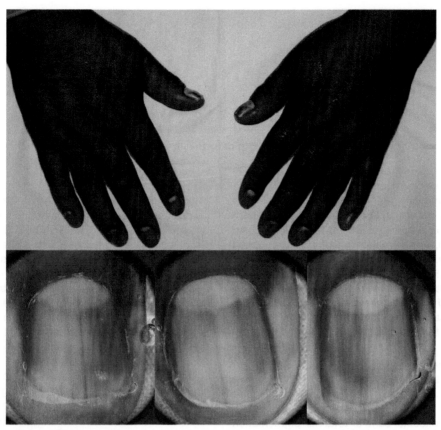

Fig. 5. Clinical and dermoscopic photographs of racial melanonychia involving all fingernails.

most important differential diagnosis is with Peutz-Jeghers syndrome, an autosomal-dominant inherited disease characterized by mucocutaneous pigmentation associated with hamartomatous gastrointestinal polyposis. In LHS, gastrointestinal hamartomatous polyposis is not observed, nor is a familial history. In addition, the pigmented macules of Peutz-Jeghers syndrome usually occur in infancy or early childhood, reaching a maximum at puberty, unlike those of LHS, which progressively appear later. Finally, the pigmentary macules in Peutz-

Jeghers syndrome can also be present around the mouth, nose, and eyes and pigmented nail bands rarely occur.[25] Nail involvement is seen in two-thirds of cases and is divided into four types based on the extent of pigmentation: (1) single 1 to 2 mm longitudinal bands, (2) double 2 to 3 mm longitudinal bands on the lateral parts, (3) homogenous pigmentation involving radial or ulnar half, and (4) total pigmentation. However, one or all types may be seen in the same patient. A nail fold pigmentation termed pseudo-Hutchinson sign can be also present.[26]

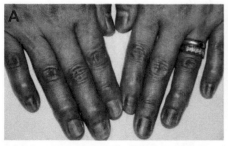
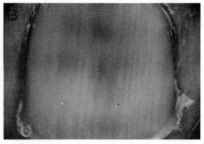

Fig. 6. Clinical (*A*) and dermoscopic (*B*) photographs of longitudinal melanonychia involving multiple digits caused by melanocytic activation in a patient under chemotherapy.

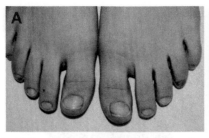
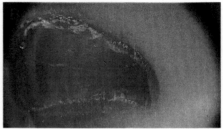

Fig. 7. Clinical (*A*) and dermoscopic (*B*) photographs of frictional melanonychia involving the fourth toe caused by ill-fitting shoes.

Endocrine diseases that cause skin and nail hyperpigmentation are those associated with increased circulating levels of corticotropin, such as Addison disease, Nelson syndrome, Cushing syndrome, and ectopic corticotropin production by tumors.[27] Cutaneous hyperpigmentation is present in 98% of patients with chronic primary adrenal insufficiency, such as Addison disease. In 20% to 40% of cases hyperpigmentation could be the first clinical manifestation and could be useful to diagnose this disease.[28]

Melanonychia cause by mechanical trauma

Mechanical causes of activation of nail matrix melanocytes are frictional melanonychia and onychotillomania. Frictional melanonychia presents as a brown longitudinal band or total nail pigmentation of the fifth and/or fourth toenails, often symmetric, and is caused by an activation of nail matrix melanocytes caused by chronic friction of these digits with the shoe (**Fig. 7**).[29] Onychoscopy shows a brown background of the band with parallel thin lines.[5] Other skin and nail abnormalities because of chronic trauma may be associated, including calluses of the dorsum of the digits and small red spots or splinter hemorrhages, reinforcing the diagnosis of a traumatic-induced nail

pigmentation. In onychophagia, the mechanical trauma of the teeth to the proximal nail folds of fingernails induces an activation of matrix melanocytes (**Fig. 8**). In onychotillomania, the patient periodically cuts, trims, pulls off, or files the nail and periungual tissues, using various instruments, and severely damages all components of the nail apparatus. In these cases, it is frequent to observe nail abnormalities involving several fingernails with different types of signs, including periungual scaling, hemorrhagic crusts and wounds, nail plate fragility and shortening, and LM and splinter hemorrhages.[30–32]

Onychoscopy permits to better observe a shorter and irregular nail plate, with irregular distal margin and exposure of the nail bed epithelium; the dilated proximal nail fold capillaries, scaling and crusts, wounds, and diffuse inflammation of the periungual folds, associated with hemorrhages. One or more bands of melanonychia is associated with melanocytic activation caused by trauma of the nail matrix. A recent study[33] noted that the absence of the nail plate with multiple obliquely oriented nail bed hemorrhages, nail bed gray pigmentation, and presence of wavy lines are characteristic findings of onychotillomania and not seen in others nail disease.

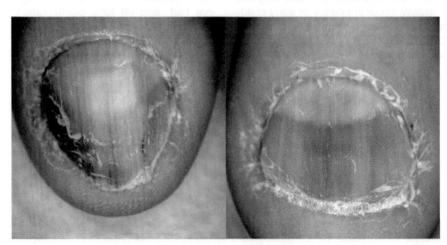

Fig. 8. Dermoscopic magnification (×10) of melanonychia caused by onychophagia.

Postinflammatory melanonychia

Melanocytes are also activated by inflammatory skin diseases of the nail unit, such as nail psoriasis, in particular Hallopeau acrodermatitis, chronic paronychia, and nail lichen planus.[34,35] Beside presence of melanin in the nail, onychoscopy in these cases shows other specific signs of the diseases, allowing the diagnosis.

Melanonychia associated with keratinocyte nail tumors

Nonmelanocytic benign and malignant nail tumors often cause melanonychia by stimulation of melanocytes; these include Bowen disease, squamous cell carcinoma, onychopapilloma, and rarely onychomatricoma.[1]

In 1988, Baran and Simon[36] described LM as one of the clinical features of Bowen disease of the nail. The pigmentation is caused by melanocytic activation induced by the tumor (**Fig. 9**). At onychoscopy, the pigmented band is composed of small brownish dots distributed along thin lines that vary in color from greyish to light/dark brown.[37–39]

Occurrence of squamous cell carcinoma in the nail is rare, although it is the most common epithelial malignancy of the nail apparatus. Ishida and colleagues[40] demonstrated the presence of melanocytes and melanin pigment within the tumor cells of neoplastic squamous cells. It has been hypothesized that cancer epithelial cells may produce factors that simulate the proliferation and differentiation of melanocytes, such as stem cell factors and endothelin-1.[40]

Onychopapilloma is a benign neoplasm of the distal matrix and the nail bed described by Baran and Perrin in 1995.[41] It typically presents with a red longitudinal band (erythronychia) associated with splinter hemorrhages and a distal subungual nodule. The first case of onychopapilloma presenting as LM was reported in 2015,[42] but a recent review of 47 cases of onychopapilloma showed that 8.5% of the cases presented as LM (pigmented onychopapilloma).[43] In case of pigmented onychopapilloma, a diagnostic clue for diagnosis is the frontal observation of the nail distal margin with a dermatoscope, showing a small subungual mass. Onychomatricoma can also present with LM, where the pigmentation is probably caused by the activation of the matrix melanocytes. Onychoscopy of the nail distal margin is helpful in the diagnosis, showing the typical honeycomb aspect of the tumor.[44]

Benign Melanocytic Proliferation

When faced with melanonychia of a single nail, not associated with a history that could explain its appearance, and having excluded causes of matrix melanocyte activation, the differential diagnosis includes benign and malignant proliferation of nail matrix melanocytes.[35]

Melanocytic hyperplasia is defined as an increase in the number of nail matrix melanocytes. Benign melanocytic hyperplasia is subdivided into lentigo, when nests are absent, and nevus, when at least one nest is present. Both of them appear as an asymptomatic band of LM, with a width rarely greater than 5 mm, involving a single digit, either a fingernail or a toenail. The distinction between nail matrix lentigo and melanocyte and nevus is clinically impossible and requires dermoscopy of the nail matrix or even biopsy with histopathologic examination.

Nail matrix nevi in Whites are uncommon, but not exceptional and usually appear in childhood as a band of LM of a single digit. They may be congenital or acquired and occur more frequently in fingernails than in toenails, the thumb being affected in about half of the cases. A striking

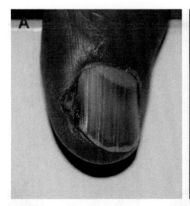
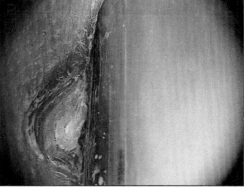

Fig. 9. Clinical (*A*) and dermoscopic (*B*) photographs of longitudinal melanonychia involving one digit caused by Bowen disease.

feature of nail matrix nevi is that they have a clinical and dermoscopic appearance that in a band with adult onset would be worrisome. Dermoscopic patterns that suggest a nevus are the presence of a brown background with longitudinal brown to black regular and parallel lines with regular spacing and thickness and, more important in children, black dots, regular in size and shape (less than 0.1 mm), because of pigment accumulation in the nail plate (**Fig. 10**).[1] In most young patients, the disappearance of the dots occurs over time and accompanies the fading of melanonychia. This phenomenon, which has been exclusively reported in children, may be erroneously interpreted as a benign clinical sign, but it indicates only a decreased activity of the nevus cells and not a regression of the nevus itself.[45]

Some clinical features of nail matrix nevi in children can, however, be alarming. The band may be wide and involve the whole nail plate. The color may be dark brown to black, and in this case, it is associated with the pseudo-Hutchinson sign, that is, an apparent pigmentation of the cuticle, because the dark nail plate color is homogeneously visible through the transparent nail fold (illusory phenomenon).[5] The band may be even associated with a true Hutchinson sign because of presence of nevus nets in the periungual skin. Color and size changes are also common in children nail matrix nevi. A gradual darkening and enlargement of the band with the proximal part broader than the distal (triangular shape) is observed; thinning, fissuring, and gradual fading of the pigmented band may also occur.[46,47] Dermoscopic appearance of these bands shows parallel irregular changes, with line not evident because of the dark background or not parallel and of irregular thickness.

The previously mentioned features, if seen in a band in adulthood, would be strongly suggestive for nail matrix melanoma. In children, however, they should be considered as a sign of the nevus cell behavior in young age. We usually do not excise surgically pigmented bands in White children, because we consider them benign. The decision to make a surgical procedure in a younger child with melanonychia is taken either when the parents are anxious, or when the band presents the following features: rapid enlargement to involve the whole nail and/or severe darkening of the pigmentation.

Malignant Melanocytic Proliferation: Nail Apparatus Melanoma

Nail apparatus melanoma (NAM) is considered as a subgroup of acral lentiginous melanomas, comprising only 0.7% to 3.5% of all forms of melanoma.[48] It affects patients older than 50 years, being exceptional in children, and it is commonly located at the first digits of hands and feet.[49,50] NAM represents 20% of all melanoma cases in African-Americans and 1.5% to 2% of all melanomas in Whites.[49] The literature is unclear about which gender is more affected. According to Lee and colleagues,[48] in Japan, Korea, and Taiwan, there is a male predominance, whereas in Western countries a female predominance is observed. A preceding trauma is reported by half of the patients.[51]

Nail melanoma in children is exceptional. In literature only 12 cases of nail melanoma in children have been described: eight of these reports are in Asian children (from Japan),[52] two cases are from South America (from Argentina and Brazil),[53] and the last two cases are in Whites.[54]

NAM may have two clinical presentations:

1. *Melanonychia*: A band of LM of one digit that appears in adulthood, with a variable width that may progressively enlarge to involve the

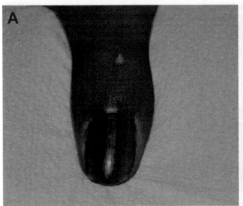
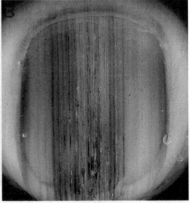

Fig. 10. Clinical (*A*) and dermoscopic (*B*) photographs of nail matrix nevi in a 7-year-old female patient.

whole plate. The color may vary from pale brown to black. Signs suggestive for nail melanoma are: width of 3 mm or more; irregular or blurred borders; homogenous black pigmentation; and presence of multiple shades of brown, black, and gray color.[48] The nail plate may present a longitudinal fissure in correspondence of the band, indicating wide matrix invasion. More advanced cases of NAM may show partial or complete nail plate destruction.[55] Hutchinson sign (ie, the pigmentation of the proximal or lateral nail folds and/or the hyponychium) represents the clinical sign of the radial growth phase of melanoma.[1] This sign is, however, not exclusive of melanoma.

2 .*Achromic melanoma*: This is a diagnostic challenge, often leading to a poor prognosis related to a delayed diagnosis. It represents 20% to 33% of NAMs,[56] and appears as an ulcerated bleeding nail bed mass that may resemble a pyogenic granuloma or a squamous cell carcinoma.

The diagnostic accuracy of LM in adults has improved over the years, first because of the use of the ABCDEF rule for nail pigmentation, and second because of the use of onychoscopy.[9,57,58]

The ABCDEF rule for diagnosing nail melanoma

This rule includes the following criteria, suggestive for a malignant lesion[59]:

- A, for age and Asian, African, American, or Native American race/ethnicity
- B, brown-black pigment, breadth of at least 3 mm, or blurred border
- C, change in the nail band or lack of change subsequent to adequate treatment
- D, digit affected or involving the dominant hand
- E, extension of pigment into the proximal or lateral nail folds
- F, family or personal history of melanoma or dysplastic nevus

The most important clinical clue is age, that is, appearance of the band in adulthood, in a single digit, with no causes that can explain its onset. NAM generally involves more than two-thirds of the nail plate. Considering the width of the pigmentation, lesions could be classified into three different groups: less than one-third, between one-third and two-thirds, and more than two-thirds of the nail plate. Melanonychia with a diameter less than one-third is generally a benign nevus.[51] A width of the pigmentation between 3 mm and 6 mm or width percentage greater

than 40% should be used as cutoff suggestive for a malignant origin of LM.[60]

Onychoscopy of nail melanoma

Nail dermoscopy adds data to clinical signs, revealing aspects not visualized by the naked eye, because it permits seeing with high magnification the details of the pigmentation. In some conditions, however, such as thickened nails and a black pigmentation that involves the whole nail, onychoscopy is not performable.[61]

Dermoscopic features suggestive of nail melanoma include a brown to black background of the band with longitudinal lines irregular in their thickness, spacing, color, or parallelism.[58] However, this rule is not always reliable, because it is possible to find lines that are irregular in width or color also in benign lesions. The result of dermoscopy should therefore be used together with the clinical features and the history of the nail pigmentation. A recent study demonstrated a strong association between clinical and onychoscopy findings in nail band pigmentation, helping to distinguish if the band is benign or malignant. The authors identified three important dermoscopic patterns that could increase three times the possibility of detecting a nail melanoma: (1) width of the band, which involves more than two-thirds of the nail plate; (2) the presence of gray to black color; and (3) the presence of nail dystrophy (**Fig. 11**).[62]

In case of amelanotic melanoma, dermoscopic images show an eroded nail bed nodule, with a vascular pattern characterized by a red discoloration with a milky-red veil and different patterns of the vessels: some appear as dots and others as irregular lines. The color in younger lesion is white in the center and red in the periphery with hairpin, linear, or dotty vessels, whereas in older lesions, the predominant color is dark red with dotted vessels.[63] Distinguishing this tumor from pyogenic granuloma is difficult and a biopsy should always be performed in nonhealing nail bed lesions.

Onychoscopy also allows to identify other important features. According to Starace and colleagues[64] onychoscopy is useful for the diagnosis of NAM particularly in two situations:

- When an ulcerated nodule of the nail bed is present, dermoscopy can show micro-Hutchinson sign, not visible to the naked eye.
- When a band of LM is present, not associated with periungual pigmentation and/or nail plate changes.

A useful step-by-step algorithm is also provided by the authors in case of suspected nail melanoma.

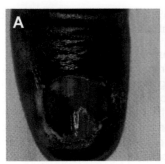
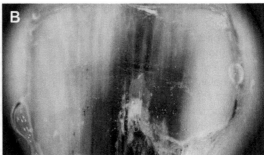

Fig. 11. Clinical (*A*) and dermoscopic (*B*) photographs of a 48-year-old woman with a longitudinal melanonychia caused by melanoma, characterized by the presence of gray to black color with interrupted lined and nail plate dystrophy.

Intraoperative dermoscopy, which permits the direct observation of the matrix after removal of the overlaying proximal nail fold and plate, is more reliable and accurate than nail plate dermoscopy.[65] Four dermoscopic patterns of the nail matrix seen by intraoperative dermoscopy have been recognized, all with high sensitivity and specificity in differentiating pigmented nail lesions:

- Regular gray pattern, typical of hypermelanosis
- Regular brown pattern, typical of benign melanocytic hyperplasia
- Regular brown pattern with globules or blotches, typical of melanocytic nevi
- Irregular pattern, typical of melanoma

Nail matrix dermoscopy is, however, an invasive technique that cannot be performed in all cases of melanonychia. The use of intraoperative procedure may facilitate vitalization of the matrix site to biopsy.[62]

Histopathology of nail melanoma

A definitive diagnosis of nail pigmentation can be made exclusively with histopathology. The most important histopathologic features to considered for prognosis of nail melanoma are: Breslow thickness, infiltration depth, number of mitosis, regression, and ulceration. The most important value is actually the Breslow thickness, but because the subungual space is narrow, the interpretation of tumor thickness of more than 1 to 1.5 mm has to be guarded.[64]

The second step is the presence of irregular crowding of melanocytes, mostly in the basal and suprabasal layers, with multinucleated cells and a lichenoid infiltrate even when only focal. The epithelium may be hyperplastic or atrophic.[66,67] The last step is positivity to antibodies against protein S-100 (95%), HMB45% (80%), and anti-Mart1/MelaninA antibodies (79%).[68–71]

Ulceration and number of mitoses are other prognostic signs.

Starace and colleagues[64] performed a correlation study between dermoscopic and histopathologic features in 23 patients, with interesting findings. Based on Breslow thickness, the thicker melanomas were amelanotic melanoma, with regression and the highest number of mitosis. Ulceration was present in 7/23 cases, which were all invasive nail melanoma. According to Kim and colleagues,[72] another important predictor factor is proximal nail plate destruction. The authors stated that it is a predictor of invasion thicker than 1.25 mm.

When suspecting nail melanoma, the whole lesion should be biopsied and observed at histopathology. The best technique should be chosen according to site and width of the band: (1) a laterally based LM may be excised with a lateral longitudinal excision; (2) a band smaller than 3 mm of the proximal or distal nail matrix is biopsied using a 3-mm punch; and (3) a band with 3 mm or more width requires tangential matrix excision.[73,74] Nail surgery needs an experienced histologic technician and pathologist to follow the specimen processing and for a histopathologic diagnosis.[75]

CLINICS CARE POINTS

- The first step in the evaluation of melanonychia is to establish if the nail pigmentation is due to melanin. For this aim, dermoscopy is the best tool in clinical practice.
- The second step is to determine if melanin is produced by activated or proliferated nail matrix melanocytes: for this aim dermoscopy is very useful, together with clinical information such as number of affected digit, race of the patient, drug intake, other systemic disease.
- The third step is to determine if the melanocyte proliferation is benign or malignant: for

this aim the age of the patient and clinical history is critical. Dermoscopy should be performed in every case and it's fundamental when an ulcerated nodule of the nail bed is present, as dermoscopy can show micro-Hutchinson's sign, and when a band of longitudinal melanonychia is present, not associated with periungual pigmentation and/or nail plate changes.

- Nail biopsy should be performed in doubtful cases, especially in an adult with a recent onset of melanonychia due to melanocyte proliferation.
- Nail biopsy is mandatory when a nail apparatus melanoma is suspected.
- A definitive diagnosis of nail pigmentation can be made exclusively with histopathology.

DISCLOSURE

Conflict of interest: none.

REFERENCES

1. Tosti A, Piraccini BM, de Farias DC. Dealing with melanonychia. Semin Cutan Med Surg 2009;28(1):49–54.
2. Tosti A, Cameli N, Piraccini BM, et al. Characterization of nail matrix melanocytes with anti-PEP1, anti-PEP8, TMH-1, and HMB-45 antibodies. J Am Acad Dermatol 1994;31(2 Pt 1):193–6.
3. Perrin C, Michiels JF, Pisani A, et al. Anatomic distribution of melanocytes in normal nail unit: an immunohistochemical investigation. Am J Dermatopathol 1997;19(5):462–7.
4. Braun R, Baran R, Saurat J, et al. Surgical pearls: dermatoscopy of the free edge of the nail to determinate the level of the nail plate pigmentation and the location of its probable origin in the proximal or distal nail matrix. J Am Acad Dermatol 2006;58:714–5.
5. Starace M, Alessandrini A, Brandi N, et al. Use of nail dermoscopy in the management of melanonychia: review. Dermatol Pract Concept 2019;9(1):38–43.
6. Maes M, Richert B, de la Brassinne M. Green nail syndrome or chloronychia. Rev Med Liege 2002;57:233–5.
7. Chiriac A, Brzezinski P, Foia L, et al. Chloronychia: green nail syndrome caused by Pseudomonas aeruginosa in elderly persons. Clin Interv Aging 2015;14(10):265–7.
8. Lencastre A, Lamas A, Sà D, et al. Onychoscopy. Clin Dermatol 2013;31(5):587–93.
9. Ronger S, Touzet S, Ligeron C, et al. Dermoscopic examination of nail pigmentation. Arch Dermatol 2002;138:1327–33.
10. Haas N, Henz BM. Pitfall in pigmentation: pseudopods in the nail plate. Dermatol Surg 2002;28(10):966–7.
11. Finch J, Arenas R, Baran R. Fungal melanonychia. J Am Acad Dermatol 2012;66(5):830–41.
12. Kilinc Karaarslan I, Acar A, Aytimur D, et al. Dermoscopic features in fungal melanonychia. Clin Exp Dermatol 2015;40(3):271–8.
13. Ohn J, Choe YS, Park J, et al. Dermoscopic patterns of fungal melanonychia: a comparative study with other causes of melanonychia. J Am Acad Dermatol 2017;76(3):488–93.e2.
14. Astur Mde M, Farkas CB, Junqueira JP, et al. Reassessing melanonychia striata in phototypes IV, V, and VI patients. Dermatol Surg 2016;42:183–90.
15. Andre J, Lateur N. Pigmented nail disorders. Dermatol Clin 2006;24(3):329–39.
16. Baran R, Kechijian P. Longitudinal melanonychia (melanonychia striata): diagnosis and management. J Am Acad Dermatol 1989;21(6):1165–75.
17. Piraccini BM, Alessandrini A. Drug-related nail disease. Clin Dermatol 2013;31(5):618–26.
18. Dana Ranta MD, Caroline Bonmati MD. Acquired melanonychia. N Engl J Med 2009;361:12.
19. Paravar T, Hymes SR. Longitudinal melanonychia induced by capecitabine. Dermatol Online J 2009;15:11.
20. Calista D, Boschini A. Cutaneous side effects induced by indinavir. Eur J Dermatol 2000;10(4):292–6.
21. Criado PR, Cosenza FD, Junior WB, et al. Longitudinal melanonychia due to voriconazole therapy during treatment of chromoblastomycosis. Clin Exp Dermatol 2018;43:75–6.
22. Zhang S, Liu X, Cai L, et al. Longitudinal melanonychia and subungual haemorrhage in a patient with systemic lupus erythematosus treated with hydroxychloroquine. Lupus 2019;28(1):129–32.
23. Sladden MJ, Mortimer NJ, Osborne JE. Longitudinal melanonychia and pseudo-Hutchinson sign associated with amlodipine. Br J Dermatol 2005;153:219–20.
24. Parkins GJ, Burden AD, Makrygeorgou A. Psoralen ultraviolet A-induced melanonychia. Clin Exp Dermatol 2015;40(3):331–2.
25. Piraccini BM, Iorizzo M, Starace M, et al. Drug-induced nail diseases. Dermatol Clin 2006;24(3):387–91.
26. Aboobacker S, Gupta G. Laugier-Hunziker syndrome. In: statPearls. Treasure Island (FL): StatPearls Publishing. 2020. Available at: https://www.ncbi.nlm.nih.gov/books/NBK534300/.
27. Schepis C, Siragusa M, Palazzo R, et al. Multiple melanonychia as a sign of pituitary adenoma. Clin Exp Dermatol 2013;38(6):689–90.
28. Prat C, Vinas M, Marcoval J, et al. Longitudinal melanonychia as the first sign of Addison's disease. J Am Acad Dermatol 2008;58:522–4.

29. Baran R. Frictional longitudinal melanonychia: a new entity. Dermatologica 1987;174(6):280–4.

30. Baran R. Nail biting and picking as a possible cause of longitudinal melanonychia: a study of 6 cases. Dermatologica 1990;181:126–8.

31. Anolik RB, Shah K, Rubin AI. Onychophagia-induced longitudinal melanonychia. Pediatr Dermatol 2012;29:488–9.

32. Diani M, Frigerio E, Clemente C, et al. Post-traumatic melanonychia with pseudo-Hutchinson's sign. G Ital Dermatol Venereol 2017;152(1):96–7.

33. Maddy AJ, Tosti A. Dermoscopic features of onychotillomania: a study of 36 cases. J Am Acad Dermatol 2018;79(4):702–5.

34. Baran R, Jancovici E, Sayag J, et al. Longitudinal melanonychia in lichen planus. Br J Dermatol 1985;113(3):369–70.

35. Piraccini BM, Dika E, Fanti PA. Nail disorders: practical tips for diagnosis and treatment. Dermatol Clin 2015;33:185–95.

36. Baran R, Simon C. Longitudinal melanonychia: a symptom of Bowen's disease. J Am Acad Dermatol 1988;18:1359–60.

37. Ragi G, Turner MS, Klein LE, et al. Pigmented Bowen's disease and review of 420 Bowen's disease lesions. J Dermatol Surg Oncol 1988;14:765–9.

38. Russo T, Piccolo V, Panarese I, et al. A challenging toenail melanonychia. J Dtsch Dermatol Ges 2019; 17(1):85–8.

39. Saito T, Uchi H, Moroi Y, et al. Subungual Bowen disease revealed by longitudinal melanonychia. J Am Acad Dermatol 2012;67(5):e240–1.

40. Ishida M, Iwai M, Yoshida K, et al. Subungual pigmented squamous cell carcinoma presenting as longitudinal melanonychia: a case report with review of the literature. Int J Clin Exp Pathol 2014;7: 844–7.

41. Baran R, Perrin C. Localized multinucleate distal subungual keratosis. Br J Dermatol 1995;133(1):77–82.

42. Ito T, Uchi H, Yamada Y, et al. Onychopapilloma manifesting longitudinal melanonychia: a mimic of subungual malignancy. J Dermatol 2015;42(12): 1199–201.

43. Tosti A, Schneider SL, Ramirez-Quizon MN, et al. Clinical, dermoscopic, and pathologic features of onychopapilloma: a review of 47 cases. J Am Acad Dermatol 2016;74(3):521–6.

44. Fayol J, Baran R, Perrin C, et al. Onychomatricoma with misleading features. Acta Derm Venereol 2000;80(5):370–2.

45. Murata Y, Kumano K. Dots and lines: a dermoscopic sign of regression of longitudinal melanonychia in children. Cutis 2012;90:293–6.

46. Tosti A, Baran R, Morelli R, et al. Progressive fading of a longitudinal melanonychia due to a nail matrix melanocytic nevus in a child. Arch Dermatol 1994; 130(8):1076–7.

47. Kikuchi I, Inoue S, Sakaguchi E, et al. Regressing nevoid nail melanosis in childhood. Dermatology 1993;186:88–93.

48. Lee DJR, Arbache ST, Quaresma MV, et al. Nail apparatus melanoma: experience of 10 years in a single institution. Skin Appendage Disord 2018; 5(1):20–6.

49. Haenssle HA, Blum A, Hofmann-Wellenhof R, et al. When all you have is a dermatoscope: start looking at the nails. Dermatol Pract Concept 2014;4(4): 11–20.

50. Benati E, Ribero S, Longo C, et al. The incidence and prognosis of nail apparatus melanoma. Clinical and dermoscopic clues to differentiate pigmented nail bands: an International Dermoscopy Society study. J Eur Acad Dermatol Venereol 2017;31(4):732–6.

51. Braun RP, Baran R, Le Gal FA, et al. Diagnosis and management of nail pigmentations. J Am Acad Dermatol 2007;56(5):835–47.

52. Uchiyama M, Minemura K. Two cases of malignant melanoma in young persons. Nihon Hifuka Gakkai Zasshi 1979;89:668.

53. Iorizzo M, Tosti A, Di Chiacchio N, et al. Nail melanoma in children: differential diagnosis and management. Dermatol Surg 2008;34:974–8.

54. Tosti A, Piraccini BM, Cagalli A, et al. In situ melanoma of the nail unit in children: report of two cases in fair-skinned Caucasian children. Pediatr Dermatol 2012;29:79–83.

55. Banfield CC, Dawber RP. Nail melanoma: a review of the literature with recommendations to improve patient management. Br J Dermatol 1999;141:628–32.

56. Ishii L, Richmond NA, Carstens SJ, et al. An amelanotic nail bed melanoma presenting as persistent onychodystrophy. Dermatol Online J 2018;24(3). 13030/qt3jj8z264.

57. Levit EK, Kagen MH, Scher RK, et al. The ABC rule for clinical detection of subungual melanoma. J Am Acad Dermatol 2000;42(2):269–74.

58. Thomas L, Dalle S. Dermoscopy provides useful information for the management of melanonychia striata. Dermatol Ther 2007;20(1):3–10.

59. Ko D, Oromendia C, Scher R, et al. Retrospective single-center study evaluating clinical and dermoscopic features of longitudinal melanonychia, ABCDEF criteria, and risk of malignancy. J Am Acad Dermatol 2019;80(5):1272–83.

60. Koga H, Saida T, Uhara H. Key point in dermoscopic differentiation between early nail apparatus melanoma and benign longitudinal melanonychia. J Dermatol 2011;38(1):45–52.

61. Di Chiacchio N, Hirata AH, Daniel R, et al. Consensus on melanonychia nail plate dermoscopy. An Bras Dermatol 2013;88(2):309–13.

62. Hirata SH, Yamada S, Almeida FA, et al. Dermoscopic examination of the nail bed and matrix. Int J Dermatol 2006;45(1):28–30.

63. Phan A, Dalle S, Touzet S, et al. Dermoscopic features of acral lentiginous melanoma in a large series of 110 cases in a white population. Br J Dermatol 2010;162(4):765–71.

64. Starace M, Dika E, Fanti PA, et al. Nail apparatus melanoma: dermoscopic and histopathologic correlations on a series of 23 patients from a single centre. J Eur Acad Dermatol Venereol 2018;32(1):164–73.

65. Hirata SH, Yamada S, Enokihara MY, et al. Patterns of nail matrix and bed of longitudinal melanonychia by intraoperative dermatoscopy. J Am Acad Dermatol 2011;65(2):297–303.

66. Amin B, Nehal KS, Jungbluth AA, et al. Histologic distinction between subungual lentigo and melanoma. Am J Surg Pathol 2008;32:835–43.

67. Tan KB, Moncrieff M, Thompson JF, et al. Subungual melanoma: a study of 124 cases highlighting features of early lesions, potential pitfall in diagnosis, and guidelines for histologic reporting. Am J Surg Pathol 2007;31:1902–12.

68. Phan A, Touzet S, Dalle S, et al. Acral lentiginous melanoma: histopathological prognostic features of 121 cases. Br J Dermatol 2007;157:311–8.

69. Stalkup JR, Orengo IF, Katta R. Controversies in acral lentiginous melanoma. Dermatol Surg 2002;28:1051–9.

70. Möhrle M, Lichte V, Breuninger H. Operative therapy of acral melanomas. Hautarzt 2011;62:362–7.

71. Theunis A, Richert B, Sass U, et al. Immunohistochemical study of 40 cases of longitudinal melanonychia. Am J Dermatopathol 2011;33:27–34.

72. Kim JY, Kim MB, Park BC, et al. Proximal nail plate destruction in subungual melanoma could be a possible predictor of invasiveness thicker than 1.25 mm. J Dermatol 2018;45(1):83–6.

73. Jellinek N. Nail matrix biopsy of longitudinal melanonychia: diagnostic algorithm including the matrix shave biopsy. J Am Acad Dermatol 2007;56:803–10.

74. Dika E, Piraccini BM, Fanti PA. Management and treatment of nail melanoma. G Ital Dermatol Venereol 2017;152(3):197–202.

75. Chiacchio N, Loureiro WR, Michalany NS, et al. Tangential biopsy thickness versus lesion depth in longitudinal melanonychia: a pilot study. Dermatol Res Pract 2012;2012:353864.

Management of Nail Unit Melanoma

Junqian Zhang, MD[a,1], Sook Jung Yun, MD, PhD[b,1], Stacy L. McMurray, MD[c],
Christopher J. Miller, MD[c],*

KEYWORDS

• Melanoma • Nail unit • Amputation • Functional surgery • Mohs micrographic surgery

KEY POINTS

• Nail unit melanoma is often diagnosed at a late stage.
• Diagnosis of nail unit melanoma requires targeted biopsies.
• Digit-sparing surgery is preferred over amputation for thin melanomas.

INTRODUCTION

Nail unit melanoma (NUM) accounts for an estimated 0.7% to 3.5% of cutaneous melanomas in Whites,[1] and up to 20% of melanomas in dark-skinned and Asian populations.[2,3] Diagnosis is often delayed, and the median Breslow thickness at the time of diagnosis has been reported to be between 3.2 and 4.0 mm with 5-year survival ranging from 18% to 58%.[2,4,5] Compared with similarly staged nonacral melanomas, acral melanomas have higher rates of locoregional recurrence and worse survival.[6] Surgical techniques for NUM are evolving. This article reviews the clinical presentation, diagnosis, and surgical treatment of NUM to promote early diagnosis and rational surgery.

CLINICAL PRESENTATION

NUM occurs most frequently in patients aged 50 to 70 years, and has a predilection for the thumb and hallux.[4] Risk factors are undetermined. It is uncertain whether ultraviolet radiation increases risk for NUM, and trauma is a proposed risk factor.[7]

NUM most commonly presents as a pigmented longitudinal band in a single nail plate.[4] Longitudinal melanonychia that occupies more than 40% of the width of the nail plate is concerning for NUM.[8] Radial growth phase NUM may not affect integrity of the nail plate, but vertical growth phase can cause nail dystrophy and ulceration.[9,10] Extension of pigment to the nail folds (Hutchinson sign) is a helpful clue but is not pathognomonic for malignancy (**Fig. 1**).[10,11] One-quarter of NUM lack pigment (**Fig. 2**).[2,5]

The ABCDEF mnemonic summarizes the classic clinical presentation of NUM.[1] "A" stands for peak incidence in *a*ges 40 to 70 years and in *A*frican-Americans, Native *A*mericans, and *A*sians. "B" stands for *b*and with *b*rown-*b*lack color, *b*readth greater than or equal to 3 mm, and *b*lurred borders. "C" stands for *c*hange in size or color of

J. Zhang and S.J. Yun contributed equally to all aspects of this article and are co-first authors.
Funding Sources: None.
Conflict of Interest Disclosures: No authors involved in the production of this article have any commercial associations that might create or pose a conflict of interest with information presented herein. Such associations include consultancies, stock ownership, or other equity interests, patent licensing arrangements, and payments for conducting or publicizing a study described in the article.
[a] Department of Dermatology, University of Pennsylvania Health System, 3600 Spruce Street, 2 Maloney Building, Philadelphia, PA 19104, USA; [b] Department of Dermatology, Chonnam National University Medical School, 160 Baekseo-Ro, Dong-Gu, Gwangju 61469, Korea (South); [c] Penn Dermatology Oncology Center, University of Pennsylvania Health System, 3400 Civic Center Boulevard, Suite 1-330S, Philadelphia, PA 19104, USA
[1] co-first authors.
* Corresponding author.
E-mail address: christopher.miller@uphs.upenn.edu

Dermatol Clin 39 (2021) 269–280
https://doi.org/10.1016/j.det.2020.12.006

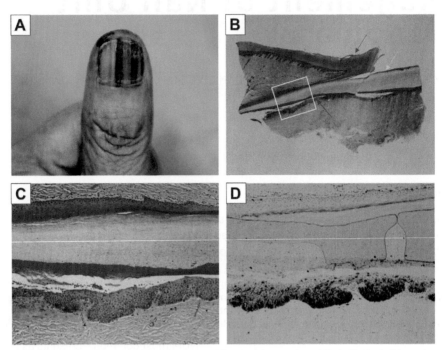

Fig. 1. Biopsy findings of early nail unit melanoma with Hutchinson sign. (*A*) A 62-year-old woman presented with irregular black to brownish longitudinal melanonychia with pigment extending to the hyponychium (Hutchinson nail sign). (*B*) A 6-mm punch biopsy shows the proximal nail fold and cuticle (*blue arrow*), the nail plate (*green arrow*), and nail matrix (*red arrow*) (hematoxylin and eosin [H&E], original magnification ×20). The yellow box indicates the window for higher magnification photomicrographs in C and D. (*C*) Histopathologic findings are subtle, showing only increased pigmentation and melanocytes (H&E, original magnification ×100). (*D*) Melan-A highlights continuous proliferation of melanocytes with prominent dendrites and pagetoid scatter (Melan-A, original magnification ×100).

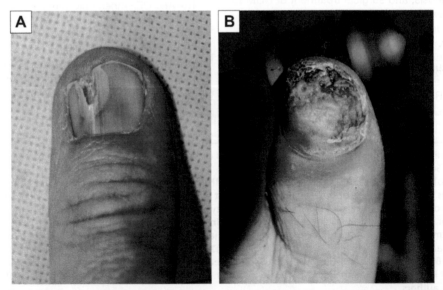

Fig. 2. Amelanotic nail unit melanoma. (*A*) Amelanotic melanoma presenting as onycholysis and splitting of nail plate with faint erythronychia on the thumb of a 36-year-old man with a history of trauma to the nail. (*B*) Amelanotic melanoma presenting as ulcerated red tumor with peripheral yellow and black scale on the left great toenail of a 72-year-old man.

the nail band. "D" stands for the *d*igits most commonly affected (thumb, hallux, or index finger) on the *d*ominant hand. "E" stands for *e*xtension of pigment to the nail folds. "F" stands for *f*amily or personal history of melanoma or dysplastic nevus syndrome.[1,8]

Because the number of ABCDEF criteria often do not differ between NUM and its benign mimickers, history and clinical examination are unreliable to diagnose NUM.[8] Dermoscopy findings showing multiple irregular brown to black lines aid in the clinical diagnosis of early stage NUM (**Fig. 3**),[8,12–14] but benign and malignant lesions also have overlapping dermoscopic features.[8] Biopsy is necessary for definitive diagnosis.[11]

BIOPSY TO DIAGNOSE NAIL UNIT MELANOMA

Like the clinical diagnosis, histopathologic diagnosis of NUM is also difficult.[5] Histologic features of NUM are subtle, and partial biopsies may miss the most prominent diagnostic features. For example, one study reported a median increase in thickness of 1.75 mm of NUM in the excised specimen compared with the initial partial biopsy.[15] Because of the subtle histopathology and risk of sampling error, accurate diagnosis requires a sufficient biopsy specimen and clear communication with an expert dermatopathologist.[14]

Although biopsy of the periungual skin may secure the diagnosis in patients with Hutchinson sign, most NUMs require biopsy from their origin in the nail matrix (see **Fig. 1**).[5] The ideal biopsy technique samples enough of the matrix for an accurate diagnosis while minimizing the risk for nail dystrophy. Proximal matrix biopsies greater than 3 mm wide have the greatest risk for permanent nail dystrophy.

Punch biopsies through the nail plate have an increased risk of sampling error and less control over depth of penetration (**Fig. 4**). After boring through the nail plate, the punch biopsy instrument releases suddenly and often plunges to the periosteum. Like a deep biopsy on the skin, deeper biopsy wounds on the nail matrix increase the risk for scarring and dystrophy.

The matrix shave biopsy is the preferred technique because it allows direct visualization of the matrix, targeted sampling, and controlled depth with less risk of scarring (**Fig. 5**).[16–19] The overlying nail plate is first elevated or removed and the proximal nail fold is retracted for targeted sampling of the grossly visible pathology in the matrix. A 15-blade scalpel is used to score the margins of the biopsy and to shave the nail matrix epithelium with an underlying layer of dermal connective tissue. To aid the pathologist, the specimen is transferred to a paper map of the nail unit and placed directly in formalin.

If the nail plate was fully removed to visualize the matrix, it should also be sent for histologic evaluation, because it may contain atypical melanocytes to support a diagnosis of NUM.[20,21]

If the pigment involves the lateral nail matrix, one could consider a lateral longitudinal excision,[22] but this technique causes permanent narrowing and may cause ipsilateral malalignment of the nail plate.[23]

STAGING OF NAIL UNIT MELANOMA

Like other cutaneous melanomas, NUM is staged according to the American Joint Committee on Cancer TNM (tumor, nodal, metastasis) criteria.[24] However, compared with similar T stages of non-acral melanomas, acral melanomas have higher locoregional recurrence rates and worse survival.[6]

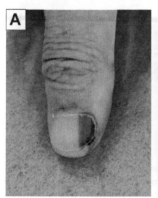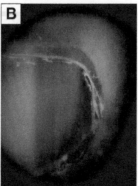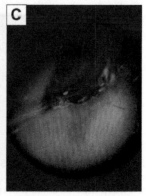

Fig. 3. Dermoscopy of nail unit melanoma. (*A*) A 7-mm-wide longitudinal melanonychia on the right thumbnail in a 56-year-old man. (*B, C*) Dermoscopy shows irregular black to brownish lines and micro-Hutchinson sign.

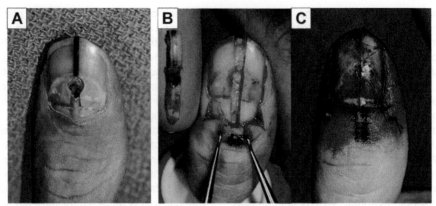

Fig. 4. Sampling error with punch biopsy through the nail plate. (*A*) A 27-year-old Asian man presented after punch biopsy of new-onset longitudinal melanonychia of the thumb. The punch biopsy was interpreted as an atypical intraepidermal melanocytic proliferation of uncertain malignant potential. (*B*) The narrow pigmented streak was excised. (*C*) The wound was closed with bilateral advancement flaps. Pathology confirmed a benign melanocytic proliferation with clear microscopic margins.

In addition, NUM presents unique challenges for accurate tumor staging. Because the normal nail matrix lacks a granular cell layer, accurate measurement of Breslow thickness is difficult. Moreover, the nail unit lacks a clear separation between the papillary and reticular dermis or a distinct fat layer, so determination of accurate Clark levels is also difficult.[5]

For primary melanomas with American Joint Committee on Cancer stage T1b or greater, the National Comprehensive Cancer Network recommends consideration or performance of sentinel lymph node biopsy (SLNB).[25] Several authors recommend SLNB in patients with NUM greater than or equal to 1 mm in depth or between 0.75 and 1.0 mm with ulceration.[15,26–28] SLNB may be particularly important for NUM, because sentinel node metastasis is common.[5] Lieberherr and colleagues[29] reviewed 12 studies of NUM and reported a 23.1% (61/264) rate of positive SLNB. NUM with positive SLNB trends toward worse overall and relapse-free survival.[30] Some

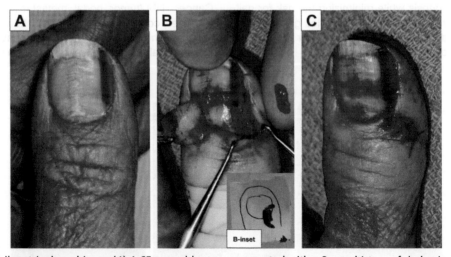

Fig. 5. Nail matrix shave biopsy. (*A*) A 65-year-old woman presented with a 2-year history of darkening longitudinal melanonychia. (*B*) The proximal nail plate was reflected and a matrix shave biopsy was performed (*inset*). The specimen was placed on a nail unit map to maintain precise orientation for the dermatopathologist. Pathology showed a benign melanotic macule. (*C*) The reflected nail plate was replaced and the relaxing incision of the proximal nail fold was repaired with interrupted dissolving sutures.

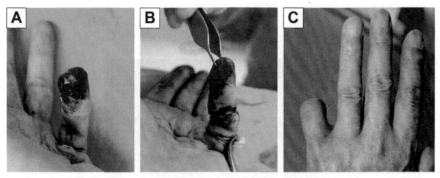

Fig. 6. Proximal digital amputation. (*A*) Black nodule within irregular pigmented patch on the left fifth fingernail in a 66-year-old man. (*B*) Digital amputation at the proximal interphalangeal joint. (*C*) Appearance after reconstruction.

authors have advocated for additional imaging studies, such as PET in patients with thick tumors greater than or equal to 4 mm.[15]

MANAGEMENT OF NAIL UNIT MELANOMA

Surgery of NUM has evolved from proximal amputation to digit-sparing excisions. Surgeons initially favored proximal amputation at the metacarpal or metatarsal joints,[31–33] but this approach results in significant disability. For example, amputation of the thumb at the metacarpophalangeal joint disables the hand by 40%.[4]

As growing evidence showed that proximal amputation did not improve overall or disease-specific survival,[4] surgeons transitioned to more distal amputations.[34,35] Park and colleagues[34] reported on the management of 100 NUM and found no significant difference in survival between tumors treated with metatarsophalangeal joint amputation versus interphalangeal joint amputation and wide local excision (WLE). Distal

amputations have less morbidity. For example, amputation distal to the insertions of the extensor and flexor tendons preserves sensation of the volar skin and function of the distal joint.[4]

Subsequent authors have demonstrated that soft tissue excision with or without removal of the ungual process has outcomes equivalent to amputation.[36] Digit-sparing WLE and Mohs micrographic surgery (MMS) are now common for early-stage NUM.

This section reviews the literature for treatment of NUM with amputation versus digit-sparing surgery.

Digit Amputation

Digit amputation has been the traditional surgery for NUM. In his original description of NUM, Hutchinson[37] advocated for "early amputation," and subsequent literature in NUM recommended amputation at the interphalangeal or more proximal joints.[38] Based on isolated reports of

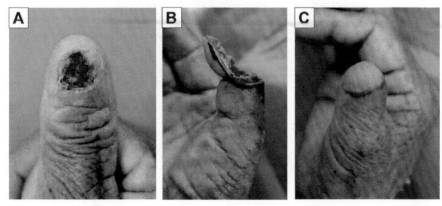

Fig. 7. Digital amputation. (*A*) Black irregular patch on the dystrophic right thumbnail in a 69-year-old woman. (*B*) Digital amputation at the interphalangeal joint. (*C*) Appearance after reconstruction with a volar flap.

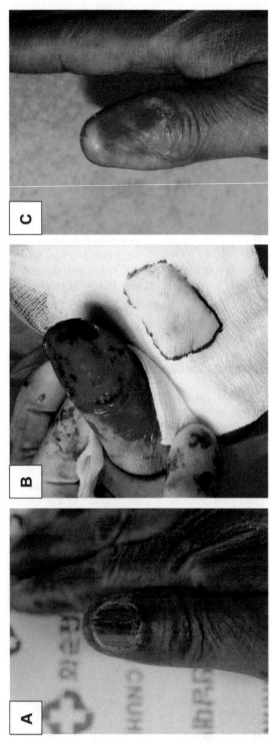

Fig. 8. Wide local excision and skin graft. (*A*) Black to brown longitudinal melanonychia with nail destruction on the right thumbnail in a 50-year-old man. (*B*) The nail unit was removed with wide local excision, and the wound was repaired with a skin graft. (*C*) The patient recovered with full function of the thumb.

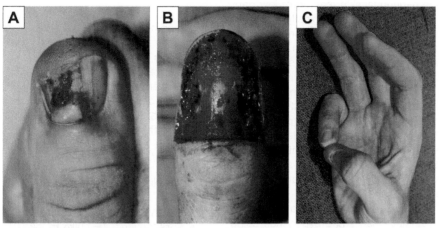

Fig. 9. Nonamputative Mohs micrographic surgery and skin graft. (*A*) Amelanotic melanoma in situ of the thumb. (*B*) Defect after excising the nail unit and confirming clear microscopic margins with Mohs micrographic surgery and frozen section MART-1 immunohistochemical stains. (*C*) The wound was repaired with a skin graft, and the patient has full range of motion 3 months after surgery.

increased recurrence and worse survival after distal amputations, several early studies recommended more aggressive proximal amputations at the carpometacarpal or tarsometatarsal joints.[38–40] However, these studies did not consistently report features, such as tumor thickness, and a significant proportion of the included patients had aggressive tumors with high rates of sentinel lymph node positivity.[38,40]

Proximal joint amputation results in significant functional and cosmetic impairment,[41] and several studies have shown that this morbidity is unnecessary. Nguyen and colleagues[4] retrospectively reviewed 124 cases of NUM and found no

difference in overall survival or melanoma disease-specific survival between proximal and distal digit amputation even after controlling for Breslow thickness and disease burden at the time of diagnosis. Similarly, Chakera and colleagues[42] retrospectively reviewed 103 cases of in situ and invasive NUM of the hand and did not find significant correlation between amputation level and disease-free survival or melanoma-specific survival. Other studies have shown no improvement in outcomes for proximal amputations.[34,35]

Overall, the data from these studies suggest that distal digit amputation (proximal interphalangeal or

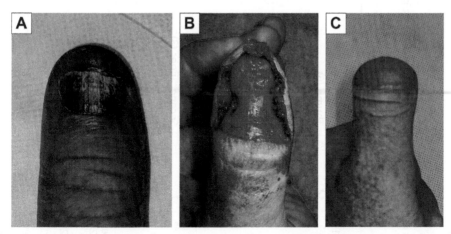

Fig. 10. Functional partial amputation after Mohs micrographic surgery. (*A*) Melanoma in situ of the thumb. (*B*) Defect after excising the nail unit and confirming clear microscopic margins with Mohs micrographic surgery and frozen section MART-1 immunohistochemical stains. The extensor tendon was intact and the patient had full range of motion. (*C*) The patient elected to undergo reconstruction with functional amputation at the waist of distal phalanx and a sensate volar flap. He retained function of the interphalangeal joint.

Table 1
Outcomes after Mohs surgery for acral and nail unit melanoma

Study	N	Tumor Locations (# Cases)	Tumor Characteristics (# Cases)	Stages to Clearance (# Cases)	Immunohistochemical Stains	Recurrence
Banfield et al,[54] 1999	1	Thumb (1)	In situ (1)	4 (1)	HMB-45, S100	No evidence of recurrence at 1 y
Brodland,[55] 2001	14	Thumb (6) Second finger (1) Third finger (3) Fifth finger (1) Great toe (4)	Average depth, 0.98 mm (range, 0–3.3 mm) In situ (4) Clark II (2) Clark III (4) Clark IV (3) Clark V (1)	1 (8) 2 (4) 3–4 (2)	HMB-45 in a subset	No recurrence (6; mean, 6.7 y) Marginal recurrence (3; mean, 5.4 y) Regional metastasis (1; mean, 1.4 y) Death from metastatic disease (2; mean, 9.8 y) Death from other causes (2; mean, 5.3 y)
High et al,[46] 2004	7	Second finger (3) Third finger (1) Fifth finger (1) Great toe (2)	In situ (7)	1 (4) 2 (2) 3 (1)	MART-1 (2)	No recurrence (6; mean, 2 y) Atypical melanocytic hyperplasia in repigmentation (1)
Loosemore et al,[56] 2013	1	Great toe (1)	0.65 mm (1)	2 (1)	MART-1 (1)	No recurrence (3 mo)
Terushkin et al,[45] 2016	62 (40 NUM)	Fingers (33) Toes (29)	In situ (27) Invasive (35; median Breslow depth, 1.06 mm)	Mean 1.7 stages (range, 1–9)	MART-1 (34) HMB-45 (14)	Recurrence rate 12.5% (5/40) for NUM

distal interphalangeal joints on the fingers and toes; interphalangeal joint on the thumb and hallux) results in similar recurrence rates and survival outcomes when compared with proximal digit amputation (**Figs. 6** and **7**).

Digit-Sparing Approaches

More recent studies have advocated for digit-sparing approaches or functional surgery for NUM.[34,36,43–48] In these types of nail procedures, the nail matrix and periungual soft tissues are removed but the bone and joints remain intact (**Figs. 8–10**).[36] Digit-sparing surgery requires careful patient selection and expertise about the anatomy and pathology of the nail unit.

Wide local excision
Moehrle and colleagues[36] performed one of the first studies advocating WLE to treat NUM. The authors retrospectively compared 62 cases of NUM treated with WLE versus digit amputation and showed improved recurrence-free and overall survival in patients who underwent WLE.[36] However, this study was limited by incomplete reporting of tumor depth and higher number of thicker tumors in patients treated with amputation.[36]

The data supporting WLE are strongest for thin NUM.[34,43,44,46–48] Jo and colleagues[43] recently performed a meta-analysis comparing WLE with amputation for in situ and invasive melanoma less than or equal to 0.5 mm of the nail unit. A total of 109 patients from five retrospective studies were included in this meta-analysis.[34,46–49] There were no statistically significant differences in rates of local recurrence, metastasis, or mortality in patients treated with WLE versus amputation.

For more advanced tumors, amputation may be necessary to clear the deep margin.[25] Thicker tumors greater than or equal to 4.0 mm have higher risk of invasion into the periosteum and bone.[44] The data supporting WLE of thick melanomas are less robust, because many retrospective studies defaulted to digital amputation for thicker melanomas.[36,47,50]

A multicenter prospective trial comparing non-amputative digit surgery with historic control subjects treated with amputation is currently ongoing in Japan.[51]

Mohs micrographic surgery
MMS offers the benefit of complete histologic evaluation of the surgical margin and has been used extensively in the treatment of cutaneous melanoma.[52,53] A few reports stress the advantages of MMS to confirm clear NUM with local recurrence rates lower than or comparable with the 0% to 25% rates for WLE (**Table 1**).[43,44,47–49] Banfield

and colleagues[54] first described a single case of in situ NUM treated with fixed-tissue MMS without evidence of recurrence at 1 year. Brodland[55] described 14 cases of NUM treated with MMS. The range of tumor depth was in situ to 3.3 mm. Margin evaluation in a subset of reported cases was aided with HMB-45 immunohistochemical stains. Three cases of marginal recurrence were reported, although these did not affect the overall outcome of these patients. Terushkin and colleagues[45] expanded on the 14 cases reported by Brodland,[55] and described 62 cases of NUM and acral melanoma treated with MMS. Five cases recurred locally after MMS with frozen section hematoxylin and eosin alone or hematoxylin and eosin with HMB-45 immunohistochemical stains.[45] Three of these local recurrences were successfully treated with MMS. None of the 34 cases recurred locally after MMS with melanoma antigen recognized by cytotoxic T cells 1 (MART-1) immunohistochemical stains.[45] These studies support the use of MMS as a digit-sparing modality in the treatment of NUM, especially in tumors less than 2 mm in Breslow thickness.[45]

Metastatic Disease

The introduction of immune checkpoint inhibitors has changed management of metastatic melanoma.[57–59] Few studies have investigated metastatic melanoma of nail unit origin, and metastatic NUM is treated similarly to other metastatic cutaneous melanoma.[25] Lower response to immune checkpoint blockade has been observed in acral lentiginous melanoma (ALM) and NUM, and may be caused by lower number of tumor infiltrating lymphocytes, lower PD-L1 expression, and lower mutational burden in ALM compared with other subtypes of melanoma.[60]

The mutational profile of ALM differs from sun-exposed cutaneous melanomas. *BRAF* mutations are seen in only 15% of ALM compared with up to 50% of sun-exposed cutaneous melanomas.[61] Mutations in *KIT, NRAS, NF1, CDK4,* and *TERT* have also been reported to be enriched in ALM.[62,63] Smaller scale clinical trials have studied inhibitors of these genomic pathways with mixed results.[64,65]

Future directions include focused studies on metastatic NUM; additional targeted, mutation-based approaches; or synergistic approaches with immune checkpoint blockade.

SUMMARY

Knowledge of the clinical presentation, biopsy techniques, and surgery for NUM promotes early detection and effective treatment.

CLINICS CARE POINTS

- Biopsy is necessary to diagnose nail unit melanoma because clinical diagnosis is unreliable.
- The matrix shave is the preferred biopsy technique because it allows direct visualization of the matrix, targeted sampling, and controlled depth.
- Distal amputation has similar recurrence rates and survival outcomes compared to proximal amputation.
- Digit-sparing surgery is preferred for thin melanomas.
- Mohs micrographic surgery has low local recurrence rates for nail unit melanoma.

REFERENCES

1. Levit EK, Kagen MH, Scher RK, et al. The ABC rule for clinical detection of subungual melanoma. J Am Acad Dermatol 2000;42(2 Pt 1):269–74.
2. Banfield CC, Redburn JC, Dawber RP. The incidence and prognosis of nail apparatus melanoma. A retrospective study of 105 patients in four English regions. Br J Dermatol 1998;139(2):276–9.
3. Kato T, Suetake T, Sugiyama Y, et al. Epidemiology and prognosis of subungual melanoma in 34 Japanese patients. Br J Dermatol 1996;134(3):383–7.
4. Nguyen JT, Bakri K, Nguyen EC, et al. Surgical management of subungual melanoma: Mayo Clinic experience of 124 cases. Ann Plast Surg 2013;71(4):346–54.
5. Tan K-B, Moncrieff M, Thompson JF, et al. Subungual melanoma: a study of 124 cases highlighting features of early lesions, potential pitfalls in diagnosis, and guidelines for histologic reporting. Am J Surg Pathol 2007;31(12):1902–12.
6. Gumaste PV, Fleming NH, Silva I, et al. Analysis of recurrence patterns in acral versus nonacral melanoma: should histologic subtype influence treatment guidelines? J Natl Compr Canc Netw 2014;12(12):1706–12.
7. Briggs JC. The role of trauma in the aetiology of malignant melanoma: a review article. Br J Plast Surg 1984;37(4):514–6.
8. Ko D, Oromendia C, Scher R, et al. Retrospective single-center study evaluating clinical and dermoscopic features of longitudinal melanonychia, ABCDEF criteria, and risk of malignancy. J Am Acad Dermatol 2019;80(5):1272–83.
9. Banfield CC, Dawber RP. Nail melanoma: a review of the literature with recommendations to improve patient management. Br J Dermatol 1999;141(4):628–32.
10. Baran R, Kechijian P. Hutchinson's sign: a reappraisal. J Am Acad Dermatol 1996;34(1):87–90.
11. Baran LR, Ruben BS, Kechijian P, et al. Non-melanoma Hutchinson's sign: a reappraisal of this important, remarkable melanoma simulant. J Eur Acad Dermatol Venereol 2018;32(3):495–501.
12. Duarte AF, Correia O, Barros AM, et al. Nail melanoma in situ: clinical, dermoscopic, pathologic clues, and steps for minimally invasive treatment. Dermatol Surg 2015;41(1):59–68.
13. Ohn J, Jo G, Cho Y, et al. Assessment of a predictive scoring model for dermoscopy of subungual melanoma in situ. JAMA Dermatol 2018;154(8):890–6.
14. Starace M, Dika E, Fanti PA, et al. Nail apparatus melanoma: dermoscopic and histopathologic correlations on a series of 23 patients from a single centre. J Eur Acad Dermatol Venereol 2018;32(1):164–73.
15. Reilly DJ, Aksakal G, Gilmour RF, et al. Subungual melanoma: management in the modern era. J Plast Reconstr Aesthet Surg 2017;70(12):1746–52.
16. Zhou Y, Chen W, Liu Z-R, et al. Modified shave surgery combined with nail window technique for the treatment of longitudinal melanonychia: evaluation of the method on a series of 67 cases. J Am Acad Dermatol 2019;81(3):717–22.
17. Haneke E, Baran R. Longitudinal melanonychia. Dermatol Surg 2001;27(6):580–4.
18. Richert B, Theunis A, Norrenberg S, et al. Tangential excision of pigmented nail matrix lesions responsible for longitudinal melanonychia: evaluation of the technique on a series of 30 patients. J Am Acad Dermatol 2013;69(1):96–104.
19. Jellinek N. Nail matrix biopsy of longitudinal melanonychia: diagnostic algorithm including the matrix shave biopsy. J Am Acad Dermatol 2007;56(5):803–10.
20. Boni A, Chu EY, Rubin AI. Routine nail clipping leads to the diagnosis of amelanotic nail unit melanoma in a young construction worker. J Cutan Pathol 2015;42(8):505–9.
21. Gatica-Torres M, Nelson CA, Lipoff JB, et al. Nail clipping with onychomycosis and surprise clue to the diagnosis of nail unit melanoma. J Cutan Pathol 2018;45(11):803–6.
22. Haneke E. Advanced nail surgery. J Cutan Aesthet Surg 2011;4(3):167–75.
23. De Berker DA, Baran R. Acquired malalignment: a complication of lateral longitudinal nail biopsy. Acta Derm Venereol 1998;78(6):468–70.
24. Gershenwald JE, Scolyer RA, Hess KR, et al. Melanoma staging: evidence-based changes in the American Joint Committee on Cancer eighth edition cancer staging manual. CA Cancer J Clin 2017;67(6):472–92.
25. Coit DG, Thompson JA, Albertini MR, et al. Cutaneous Melanoma, Version 2.2019, NCCN Clinical Practice Guidelines in Oncology. J Natl Compr Canc Netw 2019;17(4):367–402.
26. Ito T, Wada M, Nagae K, et al. Acral lentiginous melanoma: who benefits from sentinel lymph node biopsy? J Am Acad Dermatol 2015;72(1):71–7.

27. Pavri SN, Han G, Khan S, et al. Does sentinel lymph node status have prognostic significance in patients with acral lentiginous melanoma? J Surg Oncol 2019;119(8):1060–9.

28. Nunes LF, Mendes GLQ, Koifman RJ. Sentinel lymph node biopsy in patients with acral melanoma: analysis of 201 cases from the Brazilian National Cancer Institute. Dermatol Surg 2019;45(8): 1026–34.

29. Lieberherr S, Cazzaniga S, Haneke E, et al. Melanoma of the nail apparatus: a systematic review and meta-analysis of current challenges and prognosis. J Eur Acad Dermatol Venereol 2019. https://doi.org/10.1111/jdv.16121.

30. Nunes LF, Mendes GLQ, Koifman RJ. Subungual melanoma: a retrospective cohort of 157 cases from Brazilian National Cancer Institute. J Surg Oncol 2018;118(7):1142–9.

31. Patterson RH, Helwig EB. Subungual malignant melanoma: a clinical-pathologic study. Cancer 1980; 46(9):2074–87.

32. Takematsu H, Obata M, Tomita Y, et al. Subungual melanoma. A clinicopathologic study of 16 Japanese cases. Cancer 1985;55(11):2725–31.

33. Daly JM, Berlin R, Urmacher C. Subungual melanoma: a 25-year review of cases. J Surg Oncol 1987;35(2):107–12.

34. Park KG, Blessing K, Kernohan NM. Surgical aspects of subungual malignant melanomas. The Scottish Melanoma Group. Ann Surg 1992;216(6): 692–5.

35. Slingluff CL, Vollmer R, Seigler HF. Acral melanoma: a review of 185 patients with identification of prognostic variables. J Surg Oncol 1990;45(2):91–8.

36. Moehrle M, Metzger S, Schippert W, et al. "Functional" surgery in subungual melanoma. Dermatol Surg 2003;29(4):366–74.

37. Hutchinson J. Melanosis often not black: melanotic whitlow. Br Med J 1886;1(1315):491.

38. Dasgupta T, Brasfield R. Subungual melanoma: 25-year review of cases. Ann Surg 1965;161:545–52.

39. Pack GT, Oropeza R. Subungual melanoma. Surg Gynecol Obstet 1967;124(3):571–82.

40. Papachristou DN, Fortner JG. Melanoma arising under the nail. J Surg Oncol 1982;21(4):219–22.

41. Bhuvaneswar CG, Epstein LA, Stern TA. Reactions to amputation: recognition and treatment. Prim Care Companion J Clin Psychiatry 2007;9(4):303–8.

42. Chakera AH, Quinn MJ, Lo S, et al. Subungual melanoma of the hand. Ann Surg Oncol 2019;26(4): 1035–43.

43. Jo G, Cho SI, Choi S, et al. Functional surgery versus amputation for in situ or minimally invasive nail melanoma: a meta-analysis. J Am Acad Dermatol 2019;81(4):917–22.

44. Nakamura Y, Ohara K, Kishi A, et al. Effects of non-amputative wide local excision on the local control and prognosis of in situ and invasive subungual melanoma. J Dermatol 2015;42(9):861–6.

45. Terushkin V, Brodland DG, Sharon DJ, et al. Digit-sparing Mohs surgery for melanoma. Dermatol Surg 2016;42(1):83–93.

46. High WA, Quirey RA, Guillén DR, et al. Presentation, histopathologic findings, and clinical outcomes in 7 cases of melanoma in situ of the nail unit. Arch Dermatol 2004;140(9):1102–6.

47. Montagner S, Belfort FA, Belda Junior W, et al. Descriptive survival study of nail melanoma patients treated with functional surgery versus distal amputation. J Am Acad Dermatol 2018;79(1):147–9.

48. Goettmann S, Moulonguet I, Zaraa I. In situ nail unit melanoma: epidemiological and clinic-pathologic features with conservative treatment and long-term follow-up. J Eur Acad Dermatol Venereol 2018; 32(12):2300–6.

49. Cohen T, Busam KJ, Patel A, et al. Subungual melanoma: management considerations. Am J Surg 2008;195(2):244–8.

50. Dika E, Patrizi A, Fanti PA, et al. The prognosis of nail apparatus melanoma: 20 years of experience from a single institute. Dermatology (Basel) 2016;232(2): 177–84.

51. Tanaka K, Nakamura Y, Mizutani T, et al. Confirmatory trial of non-amputative digit preservation surgery for subungual melanoma: Japan Clinical Oncology Group study (JCOG1602, J-NAIL study protocol). BMC Cancer 2019;19(1):1002.

52. Ellison PM, Zitelli JA, Brodland DG. Mohs micrographic surgery for melanoma: a prospective multicenter study. J Am Acad Dermatol 2019;81(3):767–74.

53. Etzkorn JR, Sobanko JF, Elenitsas R, et al. Low recurrence rates for in situ and invasive melanomas using Mohs micrographic surgery with melanoma antigen recognized by T cells 1 (MART-1) immunostaining: tissue processing methodology to optimize pathologic staging and margin assessment. J Am Acad Dermatol 2015; 72(5):840–50.

54. Banfield CC, Dawber RP, Walker NP, et al. Mohs micrographic surgery for the treatment of in situ nail apparatus melanoma: a case report. J Am Acad Dermatol 1999;40(1):98–9.

55. Brodland DG. The treatment of nail apparatus melanoma with Mohs micrographic surgery. Dermatol Surg 2001;27(3):269–73.

56. Loosemore MP, Morales-Burgos A, Goldberg LH. Acral lentiginous melanoma of the toe treated using Mohs surgery with sparing of the digit and subsequent reconstruction using split-thickness skin graft. Dermatol Surg 2013;39(1 Pt 1):136–8.

57. Eggermont AMM, Chiarion-Sileni V, Grob J-J, et al. Prolonged survival in stage III melanoma with ipilimumab adjuvant therapy. N Engl J Med 2016; 375(19):1845–55.

58. Robert C, Long GV, Brady B, et al. Nivolumab in previously untreated melanoma without BRAF mutation. N Engl J Med 2015;372(4):320–30.

59. Wolchok JD, Chiarion-Sileni V, Gonzalez R, et al. Overall survival with combined nivolumab and ipilimumab in advanced melanoma. N Engl J Med 2017;377(14):1345–56.

60. Chen YA, Teer JK, Eroglu Z, et al. Translational pathology, genomics and the development of systemic therapies for acral melanoma. Semin Cancer Biol 2019. https://doi.org/10.1016/j.semcancer.2019.10.017.

61. Zhang T, Dutton-Regester K, Brown KM, et al. The genomic landscape of cutaneous melanoma. Pigment Cell Melanoma Res 2016;29(3):266–83.

62. Liang WS, Hendricks W, Kiefer J, et al. Integrated genomic analyses reveal frequent TERT aberrations in acral melanoma. Genome Res 2017;27(4):524–32.

63. Moon KR, Choi YD, Kim JM, et al. Genetic alterations in primary acral melanoma and acral melanocytic nevus in Korea: common mutated genes show distinct cytomorphological features. J Invest Dermatol 2018;138(4):933–45.

64. Kalinsky K, Lee S, Rubin KM, et al. A phase 2 trial of dasatinib in patients with locally advanced or stage IV mucosal, acral, or vulvovaginal melanoma: a trial of the ECOG-ACRIN Cancer Research Group (E2607). Cancer 2017;123(14):2688–97.

65. Kim HK, Lee S, Kim K, et al. Efficacy of BRAF inhibitors in Asian metastatic melanoma patients: potential implications of genomic sequencing in BRAF-mutated melanoma. Transl Oncol 2016;9(6):557–64.

Nail Tumors

Anna Quinn Hare, MD, MS[a], Phoebe Rich, MD[b],*

KEYWORDS

- Onychopapilloma • Superficial acral fibromyxoma • Periungual fibroma/fibrokeratoma
- Pyogenic granuloma • Glomus tumor • Exostosis • Squamous cell carcinoma • Digital myxoid cyst

KEY POINTS

- For the dermatologist assessing a nail tumor, the critical decision is whether to biopsy or monitor the lesion.
- Nail tumor assessment generally follows the basic tenants of skin tumor assessment: lesions with rapid growth, tenderness, and destructiveness warrant further exploration.
- Benign nail tumors are typically slow-growing, slowly evolving, painless (except glomus tumors) lesions.
- In suspected benign lesions, monitoring every 4 to 6 months until lesion stability is certain.
- The definitive treatment is typically excision, but recurrence rate is high for many of these benign lesions.

ONYCHOPAPILLOMA

Onychopapillomas are one of the more common benign nail tumors. Given their painless and relatively static evolution, they are often ignored by patients and likely very underdiagnosed. It remains unknown how or why this distinct clinicopathologic entity develops. Histologically, onychopapillomas exhibit hyperplasia of nail matrix cells in the nail bed epidermis. The origin of this lesion on excision is noted to be in the distal nail matrix, and consequently, the papillomatous hyperplasia follows the undersurface of the nail plate, creating thinning of the nail plate and their resultant, distinct clinical appearance.

Onychopapillomas have a very characteristic appearance, consisting of longitudinal erythronychia, often associated with splinter hemorrhages, a subungual small papilloma, distal V-nicking or V-shaped onycholysis due to thinning of the nail plate,[1] and a tapered interruption of the lunula.[2] The pink-to-red band can be subtle and is often quite thin. Widening of the band over time is not characteristic and suggests alternate diagnosis. An onychopapilloma is a clinical diagnosis, and

after initial early monitoring demonstrates no growth, does not warrant continued monitoring. Atypical signs or symptoms associated, such as widening of the erythronychia, pain, or dystrophy, are more suggestive of squamous cell carcinoma (SCC).[3]

Treatment consists of nail avulsion with careful surgical removal of the lesion longitudinally. Recurrence rate is approximated at 20% for this procedure, greater with transverse excision[4] (**Figs. 1–3**).

Onychomatricomas are rare, benign, fibroepithelial tumors of the nail matrix.[5] These painless, slow-growing tumors are seen most commonly in white adults.[6,7] Origins of these unique tumors are not known. These tumors have characteristic clinical features with some variation, consisting most commonly of transverse overcurvature of the nail plate, yellowing, splinter hemorrhages, and end-on appearance of tubules.[8] Most common dermatoscopic features include free edge thickening and pitting, splinter hemorrhages, and parallel lesion edges.[9]

The tumor of Onychomatricoma (OMO) consists of a fibrous lesion located at the distal matrix, and

[a] Oregon Dermatology and Research Center, 2565 Lovejoy Street, Suite 200, Portland, OR 97210, USA;
[b] Dermatology OHSU, Oregon Dermatology and Research Center, 2565 Northwest Lovejoy Street, Portland, OR, USA
* Corresponding author.
E-mail address: prich419@gmail.com

Dermatol Clin 39 (2021) 281–292
https://doi.org/10.1016/j.det.2020.12.007

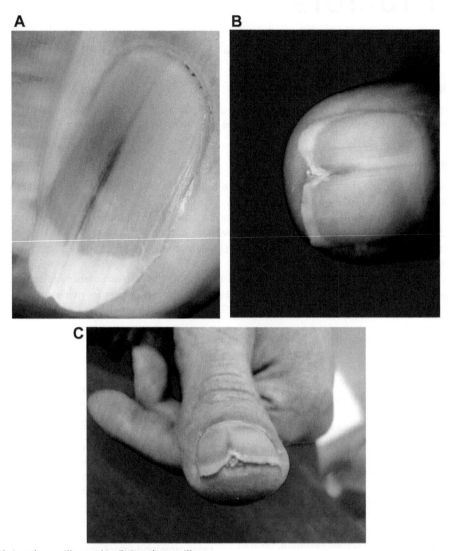

Fig. 1. (*A*) Onychopapilloma. (*B, C*) Onychopapilloma.

the stroma typically exhibits fingerlike projections of fibrous tissue extending out along and within the nail plate.[10] As the nail plate grows around these projections, holes are left once the plate grows past the tumor. The resultant nail is thickened with appreciation of a honeycomb appearance of tubules when viewed end-on. These tubules can be colonized by dermatophyte, which

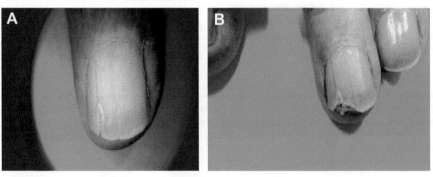

Fig. 2. (*A, B*) Onychopapilloma before and after clipping.

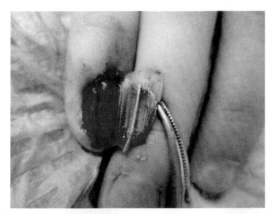

Fig. 3. Onychopapilloma visualization upon avulsion of the nail plate.

complicates the diagnosis and often leads to early misdiagnosis.[11]

The only treatment for these lesions is excision, and if they are not bothersome to the patient, they may be left alone. They may recur if excised. An onychomatricoma, which has been likened to a seborrheic keratosis of the nail histologically, presents identically to an onychomatricoma in the authors' experience (**Fig. 4**).

SUPERFICIAL ACRAL FIBROMYXOMA

Superficial acral fibromyxoma is a relatively common acral tumor that was first described in 2001.

It affects predominantly middle-aged people and is twice as common in men than women. It is a benign, slow-growing tumor with about 50% affecting a periungual and subungual location. Clinically, the tumor appears as a pink or white nontender subungual mass; however, in up to 40% of cases, there may be pain.[12,13] The tumor may grow to up to 5 cm, at which point there is usually anatomic distortion of the nail unit and occasionally bony erosions.[14] The diagnosis is made by biopsy, which characteristically shows a myxofibromatous tumor composed of spindle-shaped fibroblast-like cells that are immunoreactive to CD34.[15]

Surgical excision of the entire lesion is the treatment of choice for acral fibromyxoma; however, the recurrence rate has been reported to be about 25% within an average of 27 months and is more likely to occur in larger tumors[16] (**Figs. 5–7**).

PERIUNGUAL FIBROMA/FIBROKERATOMA

Acquired digital fibrokeratoma is a firm skin-colored nodule that usually has a fibrokeratotic tip. These benign periungual tumors often emanate from the ventral aspect of the proximal portion of the proximal nail fold or less likely from the matrix or nail bed. It may act as a space-occupying lesion pressing on the nail matrix, resulting in a longitudinal depression in the nail plate distal to the lesion.[17] Patients with tuberous sclerosis have multiple periungual fibromas called

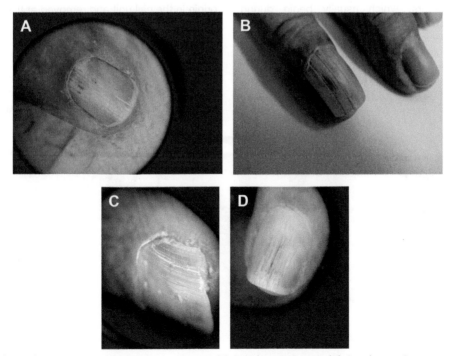

Fig. 4. (*A*) Onychomatricoma. (*B*) Onychomatricoma. (*C*) Onychomatricoma. (*D*) Onychomatricoma.

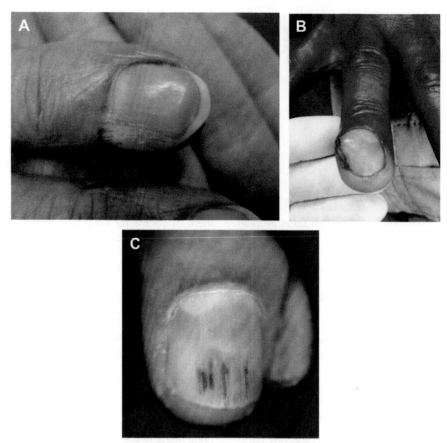

Fig. 5. (*A*) Fibromyxoma. (*B*) Fibromyxoma. (*C*) Fibromyxoma.

Koenon tumors, which usually begin during adolescence and can increase in number with aging. There are no histopathologic differences between acquired fibromas/fibrokeratomas and the Koenen tumors seen in tuberous sclerosis.[18]

Surgical excision is the treatment of choice. The lesion must be dissected back to its most proximal origin in the nail unit and removed at that location to prevent recurrence (**Fig. 8**).

PYOGENIC GRANULOMA

Pyogenic granuloma (PG) is a benign reactive vascular neoplasm that occurs frequently in the periungual and subungual area. PG can be caused

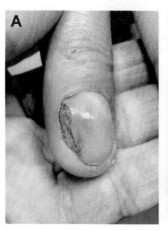
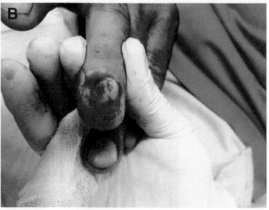

Fig. 6. (*A*, *B*) Fibromyxoma visualization after nail plate avulsion.

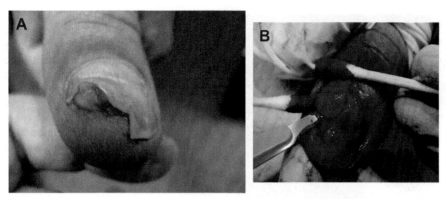

Fig. 7. (*A*, *B*) Fibromyxoma excision.

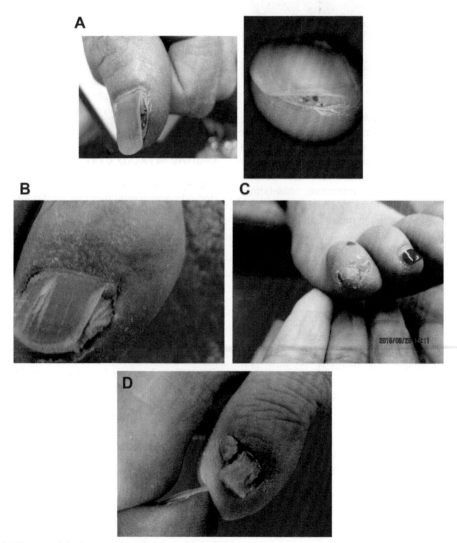

Fig. 8. (*A*) Fibroma. (*B*) Fibroma. (*C*) Fibroma. (*D*) Fibroma.

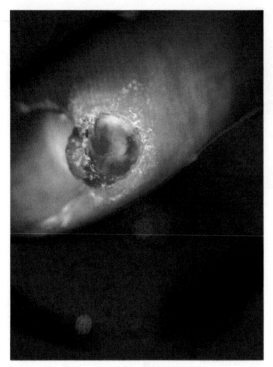

Fig. 9. Pyogenic granuloma.

by or related to several different clinical conditions, the most common of which is periungual injury or local trauma. It can follow acute nail fold or bed injury or sometimes can be associated with other nail issues, such as ingrown nail, torn cuticle, aggressive manipulation manicure, nail-biting, and picking.[17] There have been reports of PG associated with reflex sympathetic dystrophy, casts for fractures, suggest an underlying traumatic event that includes nerve damage may be associated with PG formation.[19]

PG may drug induced. The drugs responsible for PG in a dermatology office are retinoids, specifically acitretin and etretinate, as well as topical retinoids like tazarotene and tretinoin. Some antineoplastic chemotherapy drugs in cancer chemotherapy are associated with the development of PG, notably EGF inhibitors, taxanes, and 5-fluorouracil. Often the PG associated with drugs occur on multiple on fingers and toenails.[20]

Treatment of PG involves removing or treating the underlying trauma or stopping the offending drug. When local conservative measures are not helpful, surgical removal with curettage and electrocautery may be indicated (**Fig. 9**).

GLOMUS TUMOR

Glomus tumors arise from glomus bodies, which are specialized arterial-venous anastomoses responsible for temperature regulation. Glomus tumors commonly occur on the hands and feet, where glomus bodies are the most prevalent.[21] Glomus tumors account for around 2% of hand tumors. They occur in middle age and more frequently in women than men.[21]

Glomus tumors typically present with highly localized pain on pressure in the precise location of the tumor, which is describes as a positive Love sign. Hildreth sign, which restricts blood flow using an inflatable blood pressure cuff, is positive if it relieves the pain of pressure on the glomus tumor.[22]

Most glomus tumors result in pain on pressure and sensitivity to cold, findings which are highly specific to glomus tumors. However, up to 20% of glomus tumors are asymptomatic.

Clinical features are a blue or red subungual macule seen through the nail plate. Occasionally, a glomus tumor presents as longitudinal erythronychia, presumably because the tumor impinges on the distal matrix and results in thinning of the nail plate distally. An MRI with contrast will localize the tumor if clinical findings are ambiguous.[23] Bone erosion from the pressure of a growing glomus tumor occurs in about 50% of cases and can be demonstrated on a plane film of the digit (**Fig. 10**).

DIGITAL MYXOID CYST

Digital myxoid cysts (also called myxoid pseudocysts and digital mucous cysts) are common, benign, slow-growing nodules that occur over a joint of the distal finger or toe. These space-occupying, slow-growing lesions can affect nail plate growth, causing dystrophy and mimicking other space-occupying tumors. This lesion consists of a pseudocyst (no true cyst lining) caused by outpouching of synovial fluid from the distal interphalangeal joint of the finger. The connection between the pseudocyst and the joint space typically contains one-way valves that allows the joint fluid to flow into the cyst but prevents retrograde flow back to the joint space.[24] Clinically, the pseudocyst occupies space either above the nail matrix, creating a longitudinal groove in the nail plate, or below the nail matrix, creating longitudinal thinning. If located superficially, there is often a skin-colored nodule noted at the proximal nail fold, and there may be separation of the cuticle from the nail plate. These cysts are most commonly associated with finger joint arthritis,[25] and the cyst size can fluctuate depending on the degree of joint inflammation, which can create a wavelike pattern in the longitudinal groove corresponding to the size of the

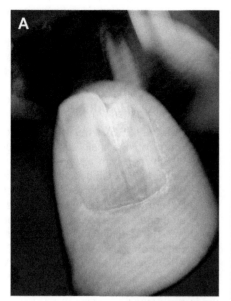

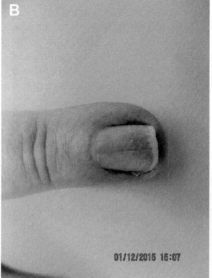

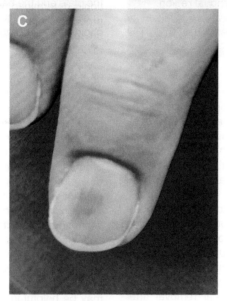

Fig. 10. (*A*) Glomus tumor. (*B*) Glomus tumor. (*C*) Glomus tumor.

cyst and resultant degree of nail matrix pressure.

These benign lesions can be drained with an 18-gauge needle, expelling myxoid contents with a jellylike consistency for definitive diagnosis. Although the most effective definitive treatment is surgery with removal of the pseudocyst and ligation of the valve,[26] sometimes drainage and injection of steroid or a sclerosis agent (polidocanol and sodium tetradecyl sulfate are reported) followed by continued pressure on the lesion can result in resolution of the cyst.[27–29] If not painful, it is acceptable to leave them

untreated after definitive diagnosis has been made (**Figs. 11–15**).

EXOSTOSIS

Exostosis is a benign nail tumor of osteochondral origin that occurs as an outgrowth of the underlying bone of the distal pharynx. The cause is unknown, but most investigators think that trauma to the digit plays a role in its onset. Any digit can be involved, but more than 7% occur on the great toe.[30,31] Subungual exostosis is most common in adolescents and young adults and occurs in men

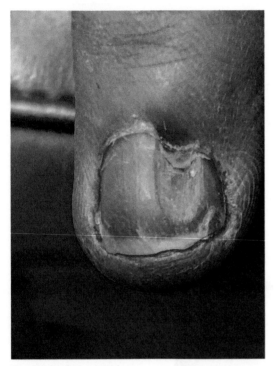

Fig. 11. Digital myxoid cyst.

and women equally. They are slow-growing tumors and have minimal symptoms initially, but as the lesion enlarges, it causes nail plate dystrophy and lifting, which result in pressure and increasing pain. The appearance through the nail plate is often a white area with surrounding telangiectasias on dermoscopy, and more advanced lesions have a hard surface with a collarette of hyperkeratosis. Subungual exostosis can mimic other nail conditions, including fibroma, verruca, enchondroma (benign tumor of cartilage), paronychia, onycholysis, and SCC of the nail unit. Diagnosis is confirmed with a radiograph, which should be performed before attempted biopsy.[32]

Treatment is complete surgical removal after exposure of the subungual lesion under sterile

conditions. A bone rongeur is used to transect the lesion at the base, and the nail bed is carefully repaired. Alternatively, the nail bed can be left to heal by secondary intention. Recurrence is possible with incomplete excision[17] (**Figs. 16** and **17**).

SQUAMOUS CELL CARCINOMA

Bowen disease (SSC) is the most common malignant tumor of the nail unit. It occurs most frequently in men with an average age of 50 to 70 years. Up to 75% OF periungual SCC are associated with human papillomavirus,[33] especially the high-risk serotypes 16,18,35,56. Other risk factors are trauma and exposure to high levels of ionizing radiation. The effect of chronic infection and inflammation on the development of SCC of the nail has been speculated, although direct causality has not been established.[34]

As with most nail disease, the clinical presentation is determined by the location of the pathologic process within the nail unit. The most common presentation occurs on the proximal, lateral nail folds and hyponychium and is characterized by erythematous, verrucous papules and plaques, nodules, or onycholysis and oozing.[35,36] When nail matrix is involved, there may be longitudinal erythronychia, melanonychia, and usually nail plate destruction.[37] Nail bed SCC may present with onycholysis and oozing as well as red papules and nodules in the nail bed.[38] SCC of the nail unit is progressive and invasive, and there is often a delay in diagnosis of many years. Lesions often present with pain. Because the variations of SCC of the nail unit can mimic many common benign nail disorders, such as paronychia, verruca, onychomycosis, PG, and infectious onycholysis, it behooves the clinician to have a high index of suspicion and to biopsy any nail lesion that does not respond to therapy. Dermoscopy of the nail may be helpful in cases of subungual squamous cell.

A

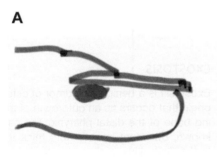

B

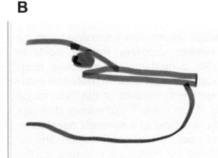

Fig. 12. (*A, B*) How a digital myxoid cyst causes nail dystrophy (*below matrix:* bulge in nail plate; *above matrix:* groove in nail plate).

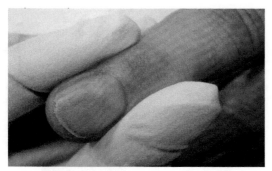

Fig. 13. Digital myxoid cyst located under nail matrix.

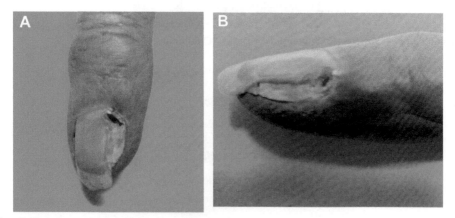

Fig. 14. (*A*, *B*) Digital myxoid cyst located on top of nail matrix.

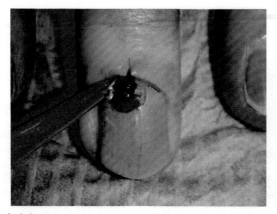

Fig. 15. Digital myxoid cyst draining.

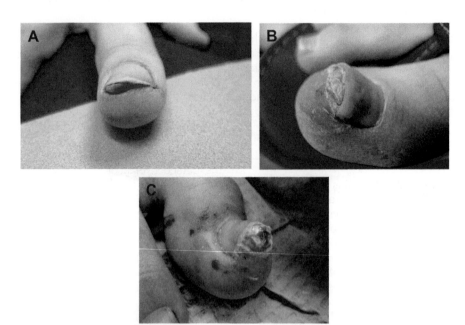

Fig. 16. (*A*) Subungual exostosis. (*B*) Subungual exostosis. (*C*) Subungual exostosis.

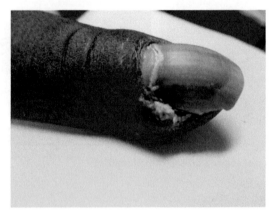

Fig. 17. SCC verrucous subtype.

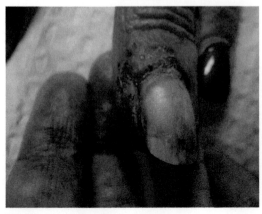

Fig. 18. SCC paronychial subtype.

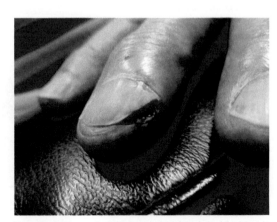

Fig. 19. SCC onycholytic/oozing subtype.

The treatment of choice is surgery with Moh's micrographic surgery or surgical excision with margin control.[39] For invasive lesions, full nail unit excision can be performed. Nonsurgical treatments have been reported to be effective, including photodynamic therapy and 5-fluorouracil topically, but these treatments are less reliable and not appropriate for sequestered areas of the nail unit. Radiograph of the digit is indicated in invasive tumors because bone invasion is an indication for digit disarticulation,[40] but it is not clear that radiograph on in situ lesions is necessary and would change the outcome (see **Fig. 17**; **Figs. 18** and **19**).

DISCLOSURE

The authors have nothing to disclose.

REFERENCES

1. de Berker DAR, Perrin C, Baran R. Localized longitudinal erythronychia: diagnostic significance and physical explanation. Arch Dermatol 2004;140(10): 1253–7.
2. Tosti A, Schneider SL, Ramirez-Quizon MN, et al. Clinical, dermoscopic, and pathologic features of onychopapilloma: a review of 47 cases. J Am Acad Dermatol 2016;74(Issue 3):521–6.
3. Baran R, Perrin C. Longitudinal erythronychia with distal subungual keratosis: onychopapilloma of the nail bed and Bowen's disease. Br J Dermatol 2000;143(1):132–5.
4. Delvaux C, Richert B, Lecerf P, et al. Onychopapillomas: a 68-case series to determine best surgical procedure and histologic sectioning. J Eur Acad Dermatol Venereol 2018;32:2025–30.
5. Perrin C. Tumors of the nail unit. A review. Part II: acquired localized longitudinal pachyonychia and masked nail tumors. Am J Dermatopathol 2013; 35(7):693–709.
6. Piraccini BM, Antonucci A, Rech G, et al. Onychomatricoma: first description in a child. Pediatr Dermatol 2007;24(1):46–8.
7. Tosti A, Piraccini BM, Calderoni O, et al. Onychomatricoma: report of three cases, including the first recognized in a colored man. Eur J Dermatol 2000; 10(8):604–6.
8. Haneke E, Fränken J. Onychomatricoma. Dermatol Surg 1995;21(11):984–7.
9. Lesort C, Debarbieux S, Duru G, et al. Dermoscopic features of onychomatricoma: a study of 34 cases. Dermatology 2015;231(2):177–83.
10. Perrin C, Baran R, Balaguer T, et al. Onychomatricoma: new clinical and histological features. A review of 19 tumors. Am J Dermatopathol 2010; 32(1):1–8.
11. Rushing CJ, Ivankiv R, Bullock NM, et al. Onychomatricoma: a rare and potentially underreported tumor of the nail matrix. J Foot Ankle Surg 2017; 56(5):1095–8.
12. Al-Daraji WI, Miettinen M. Superficial acral fibromyxoma: a clinicopathological analysis of 32 tumors including 4 in the heel. J Cutan Pathol 2008;35: 1020–6.
13. Andre J, Theunis A, Richert B, et al. Superficial acral fibromyxoma: clinical and pathological features. Am J Dermatopathol 2004;26:472–4.
14. Quaba O, Evans A, Al-Nafussi AA, et al. Superficial acral fibromyxoma. Br J Plast Surg 2005;58:561–4.
15. Ashby-Richardson H, Rogers GS, Stadecker MJ. Superficial acral fibromyxoma: an overview. Arch Pathol Lab Med 2011;135:1064–6.
16. Hollmann TJ, Bovee JV, Fletcher CD. Digital fibromyxoma (superficial acral fibromyxoma): a detailed characterization of 124 cases. Am J Surg Pathol 2012;36:789–98.
17. Richert B, Lecerf P, Caucanas M, et al. Nail tumors. Clin Dermatol 2013;31:602–17.
18. Kint A, Baran R. Histopathologic study of Koenen tumors. Are they different from acquired digital fibrokeratoma? J Am Acad Dermatol 1988;18(2 Pt 1): 369–72.
19. Tosti A, Baran R, Peluso AM, et al. Reflex sympathetic dystrophy with prominent involvement of the nail apparatus. J Am Acad Dermatol 1993;29(5 Pt 2):865–8.
20. Piraccini BM, Bellavista S, Misciali C, et al. Periungual and subungual pyogenic granuloma. Br J Dermatol 2010;163:941–53.
21. Mravic M, LaChaud G, Nguyen A, et al. Clinical and histopathological diagnosis of glomus tumor: an institutional experience of 138 cases. Int J Surg Pathol 2015;23:181–8.
22. Baran R, Richert B. Common nail tumors. Dermatol Clin 2006;24:297–311.
23. Ham KW, Yun IS, Tark KC, et al. Glomus tumors: symptom variation and MRI imaging for diagnosis. Arch Plast Surg 2013;40(No. 4):392–6.
24. Budoff JE. Mucous cysts. J Hand Surg 2010;35A: 828–30.
25. Lin YC, Wu YH, Scher RK. Nail changes and association of osteoarthritis in digital myxoid cyst. Dermatol Surg 2008;34(3):364–9.
26. Johnson SM, Treon K, Thomas S, et al. A reliable surgical treatment for digital mucous cysts. J Hand Surg Eur 2014;39(8):856–60.
27. Esson GA, Holme SA. Treatment of 63 subjects with digital mucous cysts with percutaneous sclerotherapy using polidocanol. Dermatol Surg 2016;42(1): 59–62.
28. Park SE, Park EJ, Kim SS, et al. Treatment of digital mucous cysts with intralesional sodium tetradecyl sulfate injection. Dermatol Surg 2014;40(11):1249–54.

29. Jabbour S, Kechichian E, Haber R, et al. Management of digital mucous cysts: a systematic review and treatment algorithm. Int J Dermatol 2017;56(7): 701–8.
30. Russell JD, Nance K, Nunley JR, et al. Subungual exostosis. Cutis 2016;97:128–9.
31. Starnes A, Crosby K, Rowe DJ, et al. Subungual exostosis: a simple surgical technique. Dermatol Surg 2012;38:258–60.
32. Lee SK, Jung MS, Lee YH, et al. Two distinctive subungual pathologies: subungual exostosis and subungual osteochondroma. Foot Ankle Int 2007;28: 595–601.
33. Riddel C, Rashid R, Thomas V. Ungual and periungual human papillomavirus-associated squamous cell carcinoma: a review. J Am Acad Dermatol 2011;64:1147–53.
34. Grigorov Y, Philipov S, Patterson J, et al. Subungual squamous cell carcinoma associated with long standing onychomycosis: aggressive surgical approach with a favourable outcome. Open Access Maced J Med Sci 2017;5(4):480–2.

35. Lecerf P, Ricaeart B, Theunis A, et al. A retrospective study of squamous cell carcinoma of the nail unit diagnosed in a Belgian general hospital over a 15-year period. J Am Acad Dermatol 2013;69(2): 253–61.
36. Starace M, Alessandrini A, Dika E, et al. Squamous cell carcinoma of the nail unit. Dermatol Pract Concept 2018;8(3):238–44.
37. Jellinek NJ, Lipner SR. Longitudinal erythronychia: retrospective single-center study evaluating differential diagnosis and the likelihood of malignancy. Dermatol Surg 2016;42(3):310–9.
38. Haneke E. Important malignant and new nail tumors. J Dtsch Dermatol Ges 2017;15(4):367–86.
39. Deberker DA, Dahl MG, Malcolm AJ, et al. Micrographic surgery for subungual squamous cell carcinoma. Br J Plast Surg 1996;49(6):114–9.
40. Starace M, Allessandrini A, Piraccini B. Squamous Cell Carcinoma of the Nail Unit Dermatology Practical & Conceptual 8(3):238-244.

Dermoscopy of the Nail Unit

Michela Starace, MD, PhD*, Aurora Alessandrini, MD, Bianca Maria Piraccini, MD, PhD

KEYWORDS

- Nail dermoscopy • Onychoscopy • Onycholysis • Pitting • Capillary alterations • Melanonychia

KEY POINTS

- Nowadays onychoscopy should be used routinely in presence of nail alterations, and sometimes it is diagnostic.
- With onychoscopy, many nail signs can be magnified and combined together with clinical examination to reach the diagnosis.
- Initial dry observation can be followed by application of an interface medium gel.
- Onychoscopy has a great impact during daily practice where it is possible to use for differential diagnosis.
- The clinical sign where onychoscopy is helpful in differential diagnosis is onycholysis, pitting, nail pigmentation, and capillary alterations.

INTRODUCTION

Nail dermoscopy is helpful in analyzing nail disease with an enhanced visualization of the clinical aspects of nail diseases and to follow the prognosis and result of the therapy, especially with the possibility to observe the new nail formation.[1]

As in skin diseases, dermoscopy was initially used in the management of nail melanocytic lesions, but in the last few years, its utility has expanded to general nail diseases and is used routinely in daily practice. Knowledge of the technique as applied to nail diseases, as well as knowledge of the normal aspect of the nail with dermoscopy to better identify the pathologic aspects is very important. Another important presupposition before using dermoscopy on the nail is the pathogenesis of the nail diseases in order to know on which part of the nail to focus.

With dermoscopy (onychoscopy), many nail signs can be magnified and combined together with clinical examination to reach the diagnosis.

First aspect, the nail is visible as a whole only with 10x magnification using a hand-held dermoscope, but with a videodermoscope it is possible to have a magnification range from 20x to 70x, with which observation can be improved by moving the lens back and forth and transversally.

Second aspect, the dermoscope may be used dry or with ultrasound gel. Initial dry observation can be followed by application of an interface medium gel. The patient undergoing the examination must initially be seated comfortably with the hand or foot to be examined placed on a flat surface, because the whole procedure may take 15 to 20 minutes.

The suspected disease leads the choice of the method to use. In case of nail plate alteration, the dry method is the option to choose, to not cover surface abnormalities, but, on the other hand, in cases of color alterations the use of ultrasound gel is recommended because it increases visibility and permits staying on the nail plate and filling any concavities (**Fig. 1**). The unique anatomy of the nail apparatus makes nail dermoscopy technically more difficult to perform than on skin and not as easily interpreted, due to the convexity and hardness of the nail plate, which make it difficult to obtain complete contact of the lens to the surface.

Dermatology, Department of Experimental, Diagnostic and Specialty Medicine, University of Bologna, Via Massarenti 1, Bologna 40138, Italy
* Corresponding author.
E-mail address: Michela.starace2@unibo.it

Dermatol Clin 39 (2021) 293–304
https://doi.org/10.1016/j.det.2020.12.008

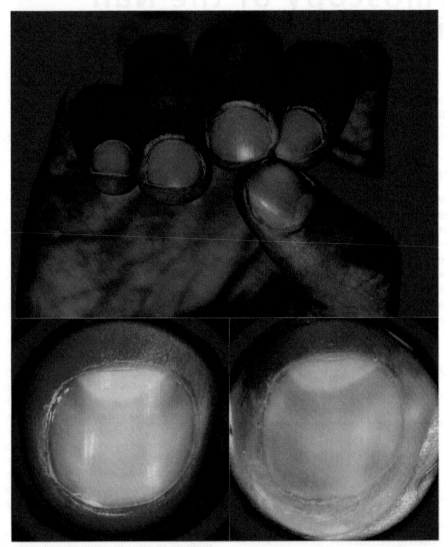

Fig. 1. Normal nail, with dry dermoscopy (on the left) and dermoscopy with gel (on the right).

Moderate knowledge of nail anatomy and the different nail diseases are necessary to use the dermoscope on the nails. The normal nail plate at 10x magnification appears pale pink in color, and its surface is smooth and shiny. It is adherent to the nail bed and with a free edge of regular thickness. The normal proximal nail fold at 10x magnification appears pale pink in color, and its epithelium has a smooth surface. The cuticle is easily visible as a transparent transverse band that seals the plate to the epithelium of the fold. The nail bed is visible deep due to the increased transparency of the plate and appears pale pink in color. The hyponychium and distal pulp can be observed putting the lens under the nail plate free margin: the epithelium shows the digital creases. The use of dermoscopy can be performed to all visible parts of the nail unit, but in conjunction with intraoperative methods observation of the nail matrix, the only nonvisible part to the naked eye, is possible.

Where onychoscopy is really useful? Onychoscopy has a great impact during daily practice where it is possible to use for differential diagnosis. The clinical sign where onychoscopy is helpful in differential diagnosis is onycholysis, pitting, nail pigmentation, and capillary alterations.

Onycholysis

Onycholysis describes the detachment of the nail plate from the nail bed, and it can be the result of different causes, such as traumatic event, nail psoriasis, onychomycosis, and presence of subungual mass.

All of these conditions determine a specific type of onycholysis, and onychoscopy can be very useful for the diagnosis.

Traumatic onycholysis

Traumatic onycholysis generally involves the toenails, especially in adults with anatomic abnormalities of the feet, such as hallux rigid. The detachment of the nail plate due to trauma appears frequently bilateral and symmetric. The line of detachment of the plate from the bed is linear, regular and smooth, and surrounded by a normally pale pink-bed, without hyperkeratosis[2] (**Fig. 2**). The subungual space is usually whitish to yellow, and frequent black drops or lines corresponding to hemorrhages due to traumas can be observed.

Distal subungual onychomycosis

In distal subungual onychomycosis (DSO), there are 4 important dermoscopic pattern to consider:

a. jagged edge of the proximal margin of the onycholytic area, with sharp structures (spikes) directed toward the proximal fold (**Fig. 3**);
b. white-yellow longitudinal striae in the onycholytic nail plate;
c. an overall appearance of the affected nail plate in parallel bands of different colors, resembling aurora borealis and in fact named *Aurora borealis pattern*[2] (**Fig. 4**); and
d. "ruin appearance" of the subungual hyperkeratosis due to the accumulation of dermal debris of fungal invasion, better visible with frontal dermoscopy.[3]

In particular, onycholysis is yellow-whitish in color due to the colony's formation and corresponds to longitudinal striae pattern. The detachment runs along the nail bed horny layer, which is thicker in the longitudinal furrows between the dermal creases: this explains the ragged border of the

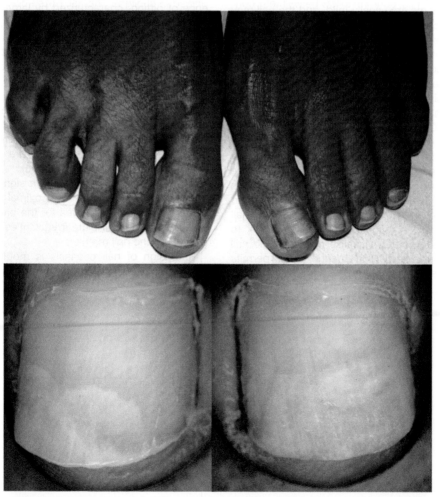

Fig. 2. Toenail traumatic onycholysis: it is bilateral and symmetric, and the line of detachment is linear, regular, and smooth, without hyperkeratosis.

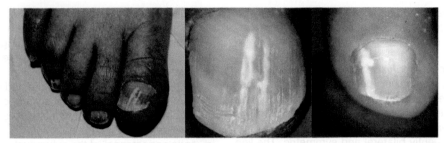

Fig. 3. In DSO, a jagged edge of the proximal margin of the onycholytic area and sharp structures (spikes) directed toward the proximal fold are typical.

onycholysis and the frequent striped shape of the DSO due to dermatophytes.

Diagnosis is made by mycology, but the dermoscopy observation of the onycholysis can aid the dermatologist in differential diagnosis, together with the other listed patterns.

Nail psoriasis

Nail symptoms are usually mild, and the nail may be the sole localization of the disease. Involvement of the nails has no relationship with type of psoriasis or duration or extent of disease. Fingernails are more affected than toenails. Nail psoriasis can involve the matrix or the bed, and the signs differ accordingly but an extremely wide spectrum of symptoms may be present, which vary in severity and type. Dermoscopy can be helpful for the diagnosis of psoriasis when the clinical features are not typical.

Dry dermoscopy is suggested to better visualize the alteration of the surface of the nail plate, which are typical when the nail matrix is involved, and dermoscopy with ultrasound gel in cases of nail bed psoriasis. A magnification power of 40x to 70x is used to better visualize nail plate and nail bed abnormalities. High magnification permits detecting subclinical signs that can be very helpful

for a definitive diagnosis of nail psoriasis in doubtful cases. The typical clinical signs of nail matrix psoriasis are irregular pitting and nail plate abnormalities such as crumbling or trachyonychia. Nail bed psoriasis usually produces salmon patches, onycholysis, and subungual hyperkeratosis.

Dry onychoscopy of nail plate abnormalities, due to matrix damage one can observe the presence of pitting, characterized by large and deep pits, that are typically irregular in shape, size, and distribution, and often full of scales. Diffuse scales may be present especially in the onset of a new nail, and they are helpful for the prognosis of the disease. Dermoscopy of pitting is very helpful to distinguish other diseases appearing with pitting, especially in cases where the pitting is the only sign of nail psoriasis. The other most important disease that can be presented only with pitting is alopecia areata, where the pits are regular in shape, size, and distribution (**Fig. 5**).

Crumbling of the nail plate is a sign of severe psoriasis: dermoscopy of the proximal part of the nail plate, where it emerges for the proximal nail fold, shows the nail plate irregularities produced directly by the nail matrix.

Rare sign of nail psoriasis is mottled lunula, where the lunula may be irregularly red as a sign

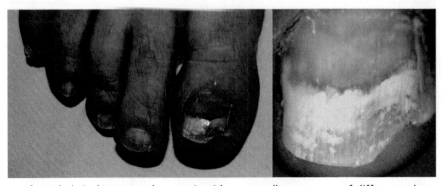

Fig. 4. A case of onycholysis due to onychomycosis with an overall appearance of different colors, resembling aurora borealis.

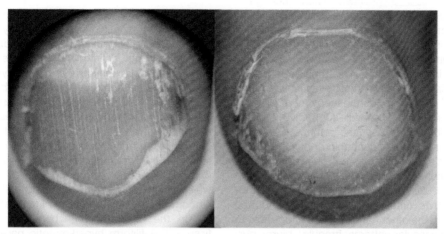

Fig. 5. Nail psoriasis pitting (on the *left*) is typically deep and irregular in shape, size, and distribution, whereas alopecia areata pitting (on the *right*) is very regular.

of inflammation.[4] In this case, it is better to use dermoscopy with gel.

Onychoscopy of nail abnormalities to nail bed alterations shows onycholysis with erythematous border, salmon oil spot, whereas nonspecific signs are splinter hemorrhages and subungual hyperkeratosis, better observed with gel (**Fig. 6**). Dermoscopy of the nail bed is very helpful in patients with fingernail onycholysis, allowing visualization of the erythematous border surrounding the distal edge of the detachment.

A bright orange-yellow border surrounding the distal edge of the detachment surrounded by a slightly dented margin is the most typical aspect, and it is impossible to be observed with naked-eye. It is important to differentiate diagnosis from other diseases appearing with onycholysis such as onychomycosis and traumatic onycholysis.

Less typical sign of nail psoriasis is the presence of several splinter hemorrhages. They appear as thin, longitudinal lines running in the direction of the nail growth. They are due to capillary trauma and reflect the aspect of nail bed capillaries; for this reason it is possible to find them in a lot of other diseases with fragility. By onychoscopy the salmon patches are irregular in shape and size, with a color from red to orange.[5]

Dermoscopy of the hyponychium is helpful in observation of an accumulation of scales under the nail plate to distinguish onychomycosis, where the scales are usually yellow or black in cases of the pigmented variant, and the margin of the detatched part is fringed, whereas in nail psoriasis the scales are white. The absence of scales with the presence of onycholysis is typical of traumatic onycholysis where the margin of onycholytic part is linear. Dermoscopy at hyponychium is very helpful to confirm the diagnosis of psoriasis in patients with simple onycholysis or mild nail bed hyperkeratosis. It may be used as well, showing irregularly distributed, dilated, tortuous, elongated, and capillaries.[6] Capillary density is positively correlated with the disease severity and response to treatment. Capillaries are better visualized at 40x magnifications, but also with handheld dermatoscope they appear as regular red dots[7] and may also be visible on the proximal nail fold in very marked inflamed diseases. Nail fold dermoscopy is useful to evaluate the severity of psoriasis, as it reflects the degree of

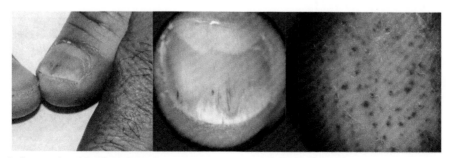

Fig. 6. Typical case of nail bed psoriasis.

microvascular changes,[8] as well as both quantitative and morphologic abnormalities are presented in the capillaries of proximal nail fold.

Some investigators stated that dermoscopy is the most important tool for diagnosis in a patient with psoriasis especially in cases of isolated onycholysis.[9] Moreover, dermoscopy of the hyponychium may be a useful supportive tool for differentiating early psoriatic arthritis (PsA) sine psoriasis from early rheumatoid arthritis (RA). Differential diagnosis of these 2 diseases may be quite difficult, as both may be present with symmetric articular involvement. In the PsA, dermoscopy shows diffusely distributed, red, dotted vessels. On the other hand, in RA it is possible to observe 3 vascular patterns: irregular, blurry, purple vessels or avascular appearance or sparse, dotted, purple vessels.[10]

A rare variant of nail psoriasis is pustular psoriasis (Hallopeau acrodermatitis), where dermoscopy can be useful to better observe when the alterations are localized in nail bed, especially in subacute phase: scaling, dilated vessels, hemorrhages, small pustules, not visible with the naked eye, and sometimes the possible melanic pigmentation due to melanocyte activation.[11]

Subungual mass

Onycholysis due to the presence of subungual masses can affect any digit, and it usually has an irregular aspect with bulgy distal margin and a slightly dented border. The color is white, pink, or different based on the mass, and the presence of subungual mass cause other specific alterations.

Onychopapilloma occurs most commonly on the thumb, in fingernails much more frequently than toenails. It presents itself as a longitudinal band and is often associated or composed entirely of splinter hemorrhages. With clipping the onycholysis of the distal nail plate the free margin of the band is occupied by hyponychial hyperkeratosis[12] (**Fig. 7**). The colors of the band may differ, such as red, white, or brown. For this reason, the presentation of onychopapilloma may vary. Recently all the possible aspects of onychopapilloma—longitudinal leukonychia; longitudinal melanonychia; long splinter hemorrhages without erythronychia, leukonychia, or melanonychia; and short splinter hemorrhages without erythronychia, leukonychia, or melanonychia with subungual mass and distal fissuring—have been described.[13]

Generally, an onychopapilloma induces nail plate thinning and red discoloration involving the length of the nail plate. These different aspects can be seen with dermoscopy, which reveals a well-defined longitudinal red band with splinter hemorrhages, starting from the lunula and reaching to the distal margin where they cause a fissure ± a filiform hyperkeratotic papule under the hyponychium. These aspects are diagnostic with dermoscopy, performed with gel. Splinter hemorrhages are usually present in the distal part of the band, whereas the filiform mass is evident at the margin of the distal nail plate. Larger onychopapillomas can induce onycholysis and an evident subungual mass that make differential diagnosis difficult versus onychomatricoma, but the observation of the distal part of the nail plate is diagnostic with dermoscopy, highlighting the honeycomb aspect of the onychomatricoma.

Onychomatricoma is a benign tumor originating in the nail matrix. It typically affects the fingernails, usually one digit, but it is possible to find multiple onychomatricomas, especially in young people. Clinical examination shows plate thickening, hypercurvature, and whitish yellow color. To the naked eye, the nail plate appears with white-yellow longitudinal ridging and splinter hemorrhages, more concentrated distally. It is important to have a frontal view of the nail to better observe the characteristic aspect of the nail plate that shows multiple holes in its thickened free margin (**Fig. 8**). These honeycomb holes correspond to longitudinal hollows that contain the digitations of the tumor that perforate within the nail plate.

These clinical aspects are reflected with dermoscopy. The typical dermoscopic findings

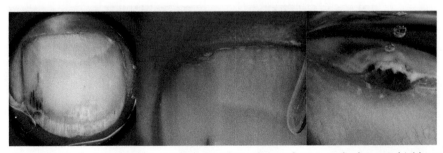

Fig. 7. Onychopapilloma characterized by onycholysis, splinter hemorrhages, and a hyponychial hyperkeratosis.

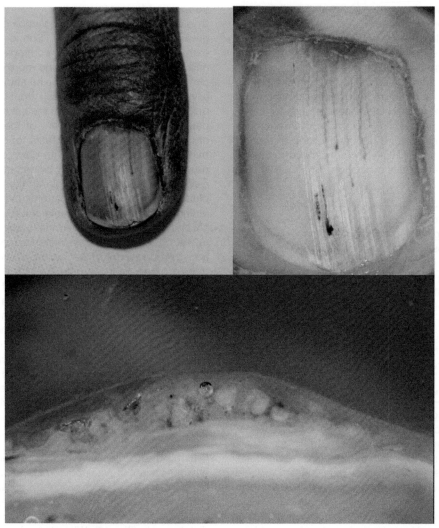

Fig. 8. Onychomatricoma showing plate thickening, splinter hemorrhages, and honeycomb aspect at the free margin.

include the following: yellowish discoloration with longitudinal striae due to the tunnels of the digitations of the tumor that detach the nail plate from the nail bed due to the presence of the tumor within the nail, also called xanthonychia; nail plate thickening and transverse overcurvature due to the presence of the tumor that cause increased difficulties to perform the technique; and splinter hemorrhages appear as a black thin and short striae because of pinpoint bleeding of nail capillaries with successive incorporation of the blood in the ventral nail plate due to trauma, especially in thickened nails.

In cases of onychomatricoma it is always recommended to perform frontal dermoscopy, so it is necessary to apply the dermoscope at the distal margin of the nail plate to have a frontal view of the thickened nail plate. This position is very important

and diagnostic of onychomatricoma. The typical dermoscopic aspect of the onychomatricoma in the frontal view is the honeycomb pattern that corresponds to the tunnels excavated from the tumor within the nail plate. This pattern is represented by white longitudinal grooves corresponding to the holes oriented around antero-oblique connective tissue axes.[14]

With onychomatricoma, dermoscopy is helpful to gain an enhanced visualization of the typical patterns that help the diagnosis and help in differential diagnosis with other benign lesions such as warts, onychopapilloma, or more recently onychomycosis[15] or malignant lesions such as squamous cell carcinoma. It can also be used as a preoperative method, to select the right margin of the excision of the tumor and avoid the relapses after surgery.

A recent paper summarized all the clinical and dermoscopic aspects of onychomatricoma through a large series of patients. And if the clinical criteria are not exclusive of onychomatricoma, some dermoscopic parameters are clearly and frequently observed. These findings are parallel white lines and a sharp lateral demarcation of the lesion with parallel lesion lateral edges, which are considered "specific" enough for onychomatricoma, whereas dark dots and pitting of the free edge of the nail plate are considered indicators for the preoperative evaluation.[16]

Pitting

Pits are small depression of the nail plate surface. Depending on the size and distribution, pitting may be diagnostic for a specific disease. Dermoscopy of pitting is very helpful to distinguish diseases appearing with pitting, especially in cases where pitting is the only sign. Pitting is commonly seen in nail psoriasis and in nails of patients with alopecia areata. The pits of psoriasis are large, deep, and irregular in shape, size, and distribution, whereas the pits of alopecia areata are regular in shape, size, and distribution.

Nail Pigmentation

Onychoscopy is very useful to differentiate exogenous nail pigmentation from melanonychia. Generally, melanic pigmentation is brown-black and within the nail plate and the aspect is a longitudinal band, whereas exogenous pigmentation includes different substances that adhere to the nail plate and does not usually have a longitudinal appearance. Common causes of nonmelanic pigmentation are subungual hematoma, fungal melanonychia, or Pseudomonas infection.

Subungual hematoma

One of the best uses of onychoscopy is to distinguish blood from melanin.[17] Subungual blood extrusion due to trauma is very common in the toenails, where it is rarely acute and more commonly chronic. The round shape of the hematoma is usually easy enough to distinguish from a band of melanic nail pigmentation with the naked eye; the patient usually becomes aware of the presence of a brown-black nail pigmentation of one toenail that lasts for a long time. With dermoscopy, we observe the round shape of hematoma, associated with a homogeneous color in the red-brown pigmentation, with globular pattern, and peripheral fading of the color with multiple blood globules or splinter hemorrhages around the hematoma.

The color of hematoma depends on the time from the occurrence of the trauma: a recent hematoma is deep under the plate and red-purple to black in color, with irregular margins but generally round at the proximal edge and with a streaked and filamentous distal end.[7] A new term is coined as *"pseudopods"* to refer to the distal end of a nail hemorrhage.[18] In cases of older lesions, dermoscopy observes a lesion more superficial on the ventral nail plate that are roundish, red-brown in color, often surrounded by small globules of paler color or dots of coagulated blood with fading around the center of the lesion (**Fig. 9**).

Fungal melanonychia

In fungal melanonychia, due to colonization of melanoides variant of *Trichophyton rubrum* or *Scytalidium dimidiatum* dermoscopy shows black pigmentation of the nail due to the presence of black scales under the nail plate evident from the distal margin (**Fig. 10**). When there is a black nail pigmentation the role of dermoscopy is crucial.

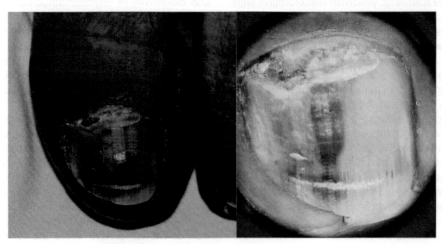

Fig. 9. Subungual hematoma of the toenail with onycholysis.

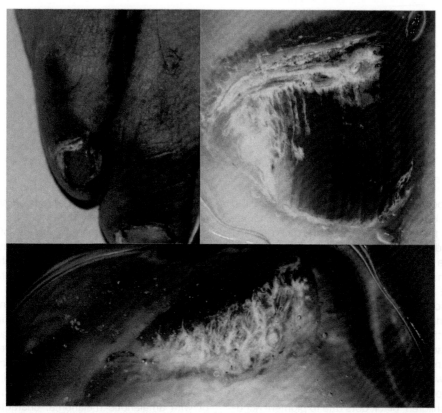

Fig. 10. Fungal melanonychia: black pigmentation of the nail due to the presence of black scales under the nail plate evident from the distal margin.

In fact, dermoscopy is very helpful in distinguishing if the pigmentation is due to melanocytic or nonmelanocytic lesions.[19]

Pseudomonas aeruginosa infection

Pseudomonas aeruginosa is a bacterial infection, type Gram negative, which can colonize the nail with a typical green or black discoloration usually with onycholysis. Known as chloronychia or green nail syndrome, for the presence of greenish-yellow, greenish-brown, greenish-black discoloration, it affects healthy people whose hands are constantly exposed to water, soaps, and detergents or are subject to mechanical trauma, especially in the elderly, inducing proximal chronic nontender paronychia and distolateral onycholysis. The pigmentation is due to the colonization of a bacterium that product a pigment named pyocyanin.[20,21] The color of pigmentation may vary from pale green to very dark green to black nail pigmentation to the naked eye, and for this reason it is important to exclude it from melanic pigmentation, especially when this coloration appears as a longitudinal arrangement along the lateral side of the nail plate.[22] The great adherence of the color to the nail plate is due to the

production of an irregular nail plate surface, so in this case dermoscopy can be very helpful and it is better visualized with dry dermoscopy. Onychoscopy helps in identifying the source of the pigmentation. In cases where nail coloration is above the nail plate, friable, and irregular, dermoscopy shows a bright green color that fades to yellow. In case of onycholysis, dermoscopy permits observing the border of the subungual pigmentation where the color typically fades into pale green at the margin of the detachment **(Fig. 11)**.

Melanonychia

As mentioned, the term melanonychia describes a black-brown pigmentation of the nail due to the presence of melanin within the nail plate. Usually it appears as a longitudinal band that starts from the proximal margin extending to the distal margin of the nail, following the growth of the nail, or involves all the nail plate (total melanonychia). The presence of melanonychia can be due to melanocytic activation or melanocytic proliferation due to benign or malignant causes, and onychoscopy is essential for the first evaluation of the pigmentation.[23]

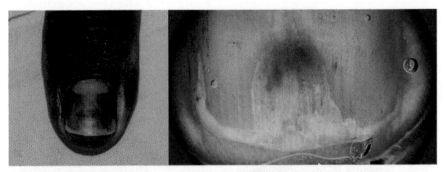

Fig. 11. *Pseudomonas aeruginosa* colonization with its typical color.

The aspect of the band can be very different: the color can be more or less pronounced and homogeneous, the borders can be well defined or less sharp, and the width can range from a few millimeters to the entire nail plate. The corresponding nail plate can show some changes or be normal. Finally, a brown black periungual pigmentation (Hutchinson sign) may be present, and this sign is very important for the diagnosis of malignant pigmentation (**Fig. 12**).

Dermoscopic patterns that suggest a nevus are the presence of a brown background with longitudinal brown to black regular and parallel lines with regular spacing and thickness and more importantly in children, black dots due to pigment accumulation in the nail plate. These dots appear black in color, with a regular size and shape (less than 0.1 mm), irregularly distributed along the lines, and sometimes form a shallow pit at the periphery or they are within the pigmented lines often interrupting the lines. In most young patients, the dots will disappear over time, together with fading of melanonychia.

These dots are a sign of a regression of a nevus and not a warning sign of a melanoma[24]: in fact, dermoscopic parameters used in adults are not valid for children.[25]

Dermoscopic patterns that may suggest a melanoma in children are a rapid evolution of brown background with longitudinal, brown to black lines with irregular color, spacing, and thickness and ending abruptly. However, these features can also be seen in longitudinal melanonychia in children and for this reason they are not specific in youth.[26]

Dermoscopic features that suggest nail melanoma in adults include a brown to black background of the band with longitudinal lines irregular in their thickness, spacing, color, or parallelism[27] (**Fig. 13**). This rule has its exceptions, as lines that are irregular in width or color can be observed also in benign lesions.[11]

A study identifies 3 important dermoscopic patterns that could help the physician in the differential diagnosis between benign and malignant nail pigmentation: the width of the band that involves more than two-thirds of the nail plate in melanoma, the presence of gray to black color, and the presence of nail dystrophy that increases 3 times the risk of detecting a nail melanoma.[28]

Onychoscopy of the hyponychium and periungual tissues permits discovering the micro-Hutchinson sign, a periungual pigmentation seen with dermoscope but not with naked eye that corresponds to the initial radial growth if melanoma into adjacent tissue. The micro-Hutchinson sign could be associated with a band of melanonychia or with amelanotic melanoma, characterized by the lack of melanin pigment. The clinical features of this type of melanoma are the absence of the nail plate, a nail dystrophy with nail bed hyperkeratosis, or ulceration.

Onychoscopy reliability in diagnosis of melanoma is particularly true in the presence of micro-Hutchinson sign, even if the gold standard for a definitive diagnosis of nail pigmentation is histopathology.[29]

A recent study[30] created an algorithm to apply in case of suspected nail melanoma. In the presence of periungual tissue pigmentation a malignant diagnosis is highly suggestive. The most frequent aspect of nail apparatus melanoma is an irregular

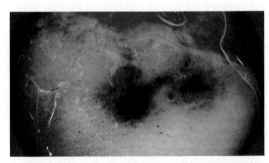

Fig. 12. A brown black periungual pigmentation (Hutchinson sign) in a patient with nail melanoma.

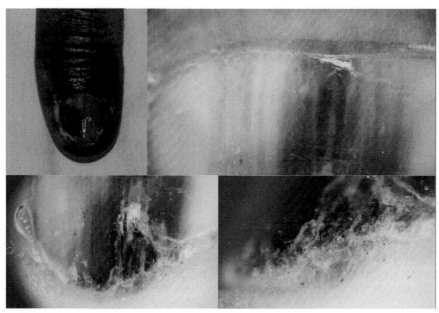

Fig. 13. Nail melanoma: brown to black background of the band with longitudinal lines irregular in their thickness, spacing, color, or parallelism.

line pattern with brown to black background. Nail plate changes, which indicate nail matrix damage, also suggest a malignancy. In cases of a nail bed nodule with ulceration, its association with Hutchinson sign is diagnostic for invasive nail melanoma. The use of a dermatoscope may detect micro-Hutchinson sign and the irregular vascular structures with atypical vessels. All cases should indeed be biopsied.

Capillaries Alterations

Connective diseases

Nail fold onychoscopy is a valid technique used to study patients with connective tissue diseases.[31] Dermoscopy observation of nail fold capillaries is usually done in the fourth or the third fingers, avoiding the thumb whose skin has a lower transparency.

In systemic sclerosis, there are 3 different patterns: early (limited number of giant capillaries, rare microhemorrhages), active (numerous giant capillaries, frequent microhemorrhages, moderate reduction of capillary density), and late (marked loss of capillaries with evident extensive avascular areas and ramified or bushy neoangiogenesis).[32] In dermatomyositis, the capillaroscopic pattern can be observed, characterized by giant capillaries, microhemorrhages, and complete change of the microvascular architecture. The most typical alteration is the tortuous and arborescent aspect of the capillaries.[33]

SUMMARY

All nail diseases can be observed with onychoscopy, but in a few conditions this technique is not only used to magnify the symptoms but also to make the diagnosis. In particular, different types of onycholysis are determined by different causes, and a better visualization of the onycholytic border can be very useful. In case of nail pigmentation, onychoscopy is essential to distinguish type and nature of the pigmentation itself and can be the only step to make in case of benign melanonychia. Moreover, its reliability in diagnosis of melanoma is particularly true in presence of micro-Hutchinson sign. In our opinion, nowadays onychoscopy should be used routinely in presence of nail alterations, and sometimes it is diagnostic.

DISCLOSURE

The authors have nothing to disclose.

REFERENCES

1. Piraccini BM, Alessandrini A, Starace M. Onychoscopy: dermoscopy of the nails. Dermatol Clin 2018;36(4):431–8.
2. Piraccini BM, Balestri R, Starace M, et al. Nail digital dermoscopy (Onychoscopy) in the diagnosis of onychomycosis. J Eur Acad Dermatol Venereol 2013; 27(4):509–13.

3. De Crignis G, Valgas N, Rezende P, et al. Dermato-scopy of onychomycosis. Int J Dermatol 2014;53(2): e97–9.

4. Shelley WB. The spotted lunula. A neglected nail sign associated with alopecia areata. J Am Acad Dermatol 1980;2(5):385–7.

5. de Farias D, Tosti A, Di Chiacchio N, et al. Dermo-scopy of nail psoriasis. An Bras Dermatol 2010; 85(1):101–3.

6. Iorizzo M, Dahdah m, Vincenzi C, et al. Videodermo-scopy of the hyponychium in nail bed psoriasis. J Am Acad Dermatol 2008;58(4):714–5.

7. Lencastre A, Lamas A, Sà D, et al. Onychoscopy. Clin Dermatol 2013;31(5):587–93.

8. Ohtsuka T, Yamakage A, Miyachi Y. Statistical defini-tion of nail fold capillary pattern in patients with pso-riasis. Int J Dermatol 1994;33(11):779–82.

9. Tosti A, Piraccini BM, de Farias D. Nial diseases. Dermatoscopy in clinical practice: beyond pig-mented lesions. London: Informa healthcare Ltd; 2010.

10. Errichetti E, Zabotti A, Stinco G, et al. Dermoscopy of nail fold and elbow in the differential diagnosis of early psoriatic arthritis sine psoriasis and early rheumatoid arthritis. J Dermatol 2016;43:1217–20.

11. Piraccini BM, Dika E, Fanti PA. Nail disorders: prac-tical tips for diagnosis and treatment. Dermatol Clin 2015;33:185–95.

12. Perrin C. Tumors of the nail unit. A review. Part I ac-quired localized longitudinal melanonychia and er-ythronychia. Am J Dermatopathol 2013;35:621–36.

13. Tosti A, Schneider SL, Ramirez-Quizon Mn, et al. Cli-cal, dermoscopic and pathologic features of ony-chopapilloma: a review of 47 cases. J Am Acad Dermatol 2016;74(3):521–6.

14. Joo HJ, Kim Mr, Cho BK, et al. Onychomatricoma: a rare tumor of nail matrix. Ann Drmatol 2016;28(2): 237–41.

15. Kallis P, Tosti A. Onychomycosis and Onychomatri-coma. Skin Appendage Disord 2016;1(4):209–12.

16. Lesort C, Debarbieux S, Duru G, et al. Dermoscopic features of onychomatricoma: a study of 34 cases. Dermatology 2015;231:177–83.

17. Ronger S, Touzet S, Ligeron C, et al. Dermoscopic examination of nail pigmentation. Arch Dermatol 2002;138:1327–33.

18. Haas N, Henz BM. Pitfall in pigmentation: pseudo-pods in the nail plate. Dermatol Surg 2002;28(10): 966–7.

19. Elewski BE, Rich P, Tosti A, et al. Onychomycosis: an overview. J Drugs Dermatol 2013;12(7):s96–103.

20. Maes M, Richert B, de la Brassinne M. Green nail syndrome or chloro-nychia. Rev Med Liege 2002; 57:233–5.

21. Chiriac A, Brzezinski P, Foia L, et al. Chloronychia: green nail syndrome caused by Pseudomons aeru-ginosa in elderly persons. Clin Interv Aging 2015; 14(10):265–7.

22. Leung LK, harding J. A chemical mixer with dark-green nails. BMJ Case Rep 2015;3:2015.

23. Starace M, Alessandrini A, Brandi N, et al. Use of nail dermoscopy in the management of melanony-chia: review. Dermatol Pract Concept 2019;9(1): 38–43.

24. Kikuchi I, Inoue S, Sakaguchi E, et al. Regressing nevoid nail melanosis in childhood. Dermatology 1993;186:88–93.

25. Chu DH, Rubin AI. Diagnosis and management of nail disorders in children. Pedriatr Clin 2014;61: 293–308.

26. Iorizzo M, Tosti A, Di Chiacchio N, et al. Nail mela-noma in children: differential diagnosis and man-agement. Dermatol Surg 2008;34:974–97.

27. Thomas L, Dalle S. Dermoscopy provides useful in-formation for the management of melanonychia striata. Dermatol Ther 2007;20:3–10.

28. Benati E, Ribero S, Longo C, et al. Clinical and der-moscopic clues to differenziate pigmented nail bands: an international dermoscopy society study. J Eur Acad Dermatol Venereol 2017;31(4):732–6.

29. Ruben BS. Pigmented lesions of the nail unit: clinical and histopathology features. Semin Cutan Med Surg 2010;29:148–58.

30. Starace M, Dika E, Fanti PA, et al. Nail apparatus melanoma: dermoscopic and histopathologic corre-lations on a series of 23 patients from a single centre. J Eur Acad Dermatol Venereol 2017;32(1): 164–73.

31. Hasegawa M. Dermoscopy findings of nail fold cap-illaries in connective tissue disease. J Dermatol 2011;38(1):66–70.

32. Pizzorni C, Sulli A, Smith V, et al. Capillaroscopy in 2016: new perspective in systemic sclerosis. Acta Rheumatol Port 2016;41:8–14.

33. Shenavandeh S, Nezhad MZ. Association of nail fold capillary changes with disease activity, clinical and laboratory findings in patients with dermatomyositis. Med J Islam Repub Iran 2015;29:233.

Nail Surgery
Six Essential Techniques

Julia O. Baltz, MD[a,b], Nathaniel J. Jellinek, MD[a,b,c],*

KEYWORDS

- Nail • Nail surgery • Matrix • Bed • Nail melanoma • Matrix shave • En bloc excision

KEY POINTS

- Adequate anesthesia is of utmost importance in nail surgery.
- Punch biopsy of the nail unit is a relatively simple procedure with high diagnostic accuracy in the evaluation of melanonychia and inflammatory nail diseases.
- The tangential matrix excision is optimal for histologic examination of melanonychia and erythronychia. The lateral longitudinal biopsy is especially useful in the diagnosis of inflammatory disease.
- Nail wedge biopsy provides robust sampling of a suspected nail bed neoplasm.
- En bloc excision for treatment of nail melanoma in situ is emerging as the standard of care as a digit-sparing alternative to distal amputation.

INTRODUCTION

Successful nail surgery requires an understanding of specific disease processes and anatomy of the nail unit, and fluency with only a few key techniques. This article focuses on 6 high-yield procedures, facility with which will allow the clinician to approach most of the clinical scenarios requiring surgical intervention (**Table 1** provides indications of each procedure). Mastery of these techniques will create a logical jumping-off point to other, unrelated but overlapping surgeries occasionally required on the nail unit (treatment of exostosis, digital myxoid cysts, ingrown nail surgery, and so forth). In all cases, the patient must be aware of the unique risks of each surgery. These risks have been summarized in **Table 2**.

DISTAL DIGITAL NERVE BLOCK

Historically, digital and nail unit anesthesia has been achieved with traditional digital blocks or local infiltrative blocks (**Fig. 1**).[1] Single-injection techniques (transthecal or subcutaneous) have also been advocated[2]; however, the distal digital block is the most useful in the authors' practice. Anecdotally, it appears that patients experience less postoperative paresthesias with this method. Complete and rapid anesthesia using a relatively painless technique is paramount for successful nail surgery and is an absolute prerequisite for performing any of the following procedures.

Innervation of the fingernail unit is supplied by the ulnar, radial, and median nerves, the branches of which run longitudinally as dorsal and volar branches along the lateral aspects of each digit, trifurcating just beyond the distal interphalangeal joints (DIPJ) to supply the nail bed, distal tip, and pulp.[3,4] The targets of the distal digital block are these paired digital nerves.[1] Importantly, the long fingernails (second to fourth) are innervated exclusively by the volar branches, whereas the thumb and fifth fingernail receive dual innervation from the volar and dorsal branches.[5]

Prior presentation: None.

[a] Dermatology Professionals, Inc, 1672 South County Trail, Suite 101, East Greenwich, RI 02818, USA; [b] Department of Dermatology, University of Massachusetts Medical School, 281 Lincoln Street, Worcester, MA 01605, USA; [c] Department of Dermatology, The Warren Alpert Medical School at Brown University, 593 Eddy Street, Providence, RI 02903, USA

* Corresponding author. Dermatology Professionals, Inc, 1672 South County Trail, Suite 101, East Greenwich, RI 02818.

E-mail address: winenut15@yahoo.com

Dermatol Clin 39 (2021) 305–318
https://doi.org/10.1016/j.det.2020.12.015

Table 1
Indications and nail procedures

	First Line	Second Line
Melanonychia	Matrix shave	Matrix punch
Erythronychia[a]	Longitudinal matrix/bed tangential excision	Longitudinal full-thickness biopsy
Inflammatory nail disease	Lateral longitudinal excision	Punch biopsy of involved tissue
Nail bed tumor	Nail bed wedge biopsy	Punch biopsy of nail bed
Nail melanoma in situ[b]	En bloc excision of all nail tissues or Mohs surgery	Distal digital amputation

[a] For epithelial lesions. Submatrix lesions (eg, glomus tumors) are approached in a different manner.
[b] Primary goal is extirpation with clear margins.

The 3 most commonly used anesthetics in cutaneous surgery include lidocaine (with or without epinephrine), bupivacaine, and ropivacaine. Lidocaine has the most rapid onset of action but the shortest duration of effect, whereas bupivacaine is the opposite. Ropivacaine and bupivacaine have similar duration of efficacy; however, ropivacaine has a quicker onset and inherent vasoconstrictive properties.[6] The use of lidocaine with epinephrine has historically been frowned upon in digital surgery because of a theoretic risk of ischemia and subsequent necrosis; however, in the absence of contraindications, the literature supports its use safely in digital blocks.[7,8] Nevertheless, ropivacaine appears to be the ideal choice for digital anesthesia because of its mild vasoconstrictive properties, its long duration of effect postprocedurally, and its relative lack of adverse effects.[9] Buffering to physiologic pH can decrease pain with injection and is most commonly done with lidocaine. Buffering of ropivacaine should be done cautiously, if at all, as buffered ropivacaine has been shown to precipitate out of solution, thereby decreasing bioavailability and anesthetic effect.[10,11]

In order to facilitate relatively painless anesthesia, the authors advocate the use of multiple distractive techniques. The patient should be positioned in such a way that the clinician has access to the digit of interest and the patient is comfortable and supine. The importance of the environment of the procedure cannot be underestimated. The authors find that music and lively conversation with the patient ("talkesthesia") are the first steps in decreasing

Table 2
Risks of nail surgery (to include during informed consent)

Nail Bed Wedge Biopsy or Nail Bed Punch Biopsy	Matrix Shave	Matrix Punch	Lateral Longitudinal Excision	En Bloc Excision of all Nail Tissues
Paresthesias	Paresthesias	Paresthesias	Paresthesias	Paresthesias
Cold sensitivity	Cold sensitivity	Cold sensitivity	Cold sensitivity	Cold sensitivity
Onycholysis	Erythronychia	Erythronychia	Nail plate narrowing ~10%	Incomplete excision
	Split nail	Split nail	Lateral malalignment (toward side of excision)	Tumor upstaging
	Recurrent pigment	Recurrent pigment	Spicule	Recurrence
			Cyst	Spicule
				Cyst
				Mallet deformity

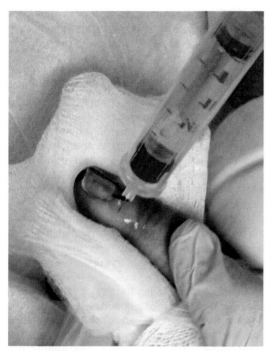

Fig. 1. Distal digital block. The anesthesia is injected into the dorsal proximal nail fold skin. The needle is then inserted nearly perpendicular to the skin and anesthetic injected toward the volar digit until it passes the midsagittal line. This process is performed bilaterally for complete distal digital anesthesia.

the pain and fear responses heightened in those patients about to undergo a nail procedure.[12] In order to decrease discomfort of injection, the gate theory of pain can be exploited. By creating sensory noise proximal to the injection point, the afferent pathways that transmit pain to the spinal cord are narrowed or closed, leading to decreased sensation of painful stimuli.[13] The clinician and his or her assistant can use multiple modalities to capitalize on this, including a massager, refrigerant spray, or pinching or tapping the skin proximal to the surgical site.[14]

The primary injection points are a few millimeters distal to the DIPJ on both the ulnar and the radial side of each finger (or medial and lateral on the toe). These injection points directly target the main sensory supply to the nail apparatus, ideally before the distal trifurcation. The needle should be inserted perpendicular to the digit and advanced extraordinarily slowly while injecting anterograde. Blanching beyond the midsagittal line of the digit indicates anesthesia to the level of the volar branch of the nerve and will include dorsal branch innervation. In order to target nerve endings that may not have been directly anesthetized by the lateral injections, one should inject

superficially starting at the initial injection point and marching across the proximal nail fold. By injecting through an area previously anesthetized, one can limit the discomfort of additional needle insertions. Typically, 1 to 3 mL overall are necessary based on the size of the digit.[1] A delay of onset can range from 1 to 10 minutes; therefore, it is recommended to test the patient for areas of pain before beginning the procedure. The benefits of this are 2-fold. First, additional anesthetic can be applied before beginning the procedure, and second, showing the patient that they are indeed numb can help the procedure to go more smoothly. That said, it is prudent to have additional anesthesia easily accessible should there be any breakthrough pain.

Use of this procedure with 0.5 or 1% ropivacaine will provide anesthesia that lasts for well over an hour, often several hours.[6] Pain can be further minimized when combined with postoperative immobilization and elevation.

PUNCH BIOPSY

The punch biopsy is a perfect introductory, yet high-yield, procedure that can be applied to the nail unit (**Fig. 2**). Punches are generally affordable, sharp, single-use devices that come in a range of sizes, although 3 to 4 mm is appropriate for most nail surgeries. As opposed to more involved nail procedures, in a punch biopsy, a tourniquet is not usually required, and application of lateral digital pressure or simply use of ropivacaine (or lidocaine with epinephrine) will provide adequate hemostasis during the operation. In addition, nail plate avulsion (either partial or complete) is not required, so recovery is faster with less postoperative paronychia and pain.[15]

There are 2 categories of disease in which the punch is useful: inflammatory (or occasionally infectious) and neoplastic. In the former, when the clinical diagnosis is ambiguous and/or noninvasive studies have been inconclusive, more direct tissue sampling is often the next diagnostic step. The clinician must assess whether there is bed or matrix disease and direct the biopsy specifically to the area affected. Not unusually, both matrix and bed are involved in inflammatory nail disease, and sampling both is appropriate. In the authors' practice, however, a slender lateral longitudinal excision of the involved nail tends to be higher yield than 1 or 2 punch biopsies and is the preferred procedure; more thorough explanation is provided in later discussion.

For punch biopsies, nail plate avulsion is unnecessary: the biopsy should be performed directly through the intact nail plate and carried deep to

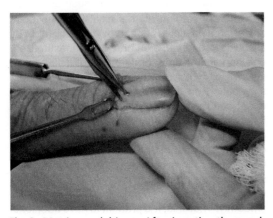

Fig. 2. Matrix punch biopsy. After inserting the punch until bone is reached, the plate may or may not separate from the underlying matrix when removed. Gradle scissors are inserted perpendicular to the surface and used to extract the minute punch specimen without crush.

the underlying bone. The clinician should identify areas of nail matrix that show disease activity, although being aware that creating a full-thickness wound in the proximal matrix (even with a 3-mm punch) may result in a permanently split nail. The nail bed location is more straightforward to identify clinically, and of significantly less risk of creating a permanent dystrophy; in nearly all cases, nail bed punch biopsies heal without enduring sequelae.[16]

The procedure is uncomplicated. The punch is applied directly to the plate and twisted with downward pressure until the bone is reached. The punch instrument should be withdrawn slowly and delicately. Doing so may prevent detachment of the nail plate and underlying tissue.

Fine tissue cutting scissors (Gradle) are used to remove the punch specimen from the nail apparatus, with minute nibbling at the bony base until the tissue sample is elevated and can be placed in formalin. Ideally, the specimen is removed with both plate and bed (or plate and matrix) as 1 block. When the plate separates and is retained in the punch instrument, this should be removed and placed in a separate formalin jar for processing.[17]

For neoplastic disease diagnosis, the punch is also useful. In most instances, the punch biopsy is incisional rather than excisional and tumor remnants remain. Despite this, the diagnostic yield tends to be quite high. In melanonychia, the punch must be targeted at the origin of pigment in the matrix. Traditional teaching has advocated making 2 tangential incisions in the proximal nail fold in order to reflect the proximal nail fold and visualize the entire matrix through the nail plate before the punch biopsy, necessitating subsequent nail fold

repair. The authors have found that, in many instances, using an elevator or spatula to simply push the proximal nail fold further proximally can expose nearly all of the matrix, allowing for adequate identification of the pigment origin, thereby decreasing rates of postoperative paronychia associated with nail fold reflection while still yielding a biopsy of the appropriate site.

Full-thickness punch wounds are not sutured, and chemical hemostatic agents or electrosurgery is unnecessary. Hemostasis is obtained with pressure. Subsequent morbidity is low. The residual intact nail plate acts as a splint, and the wound is inherently immobilized. The punch defect will grow out longitudinally. For distal matrix defects, the resulting nail may be entirely normal, although a degree of longitudinal erythronychia is commonly seen, and the preoperative consent should reflect this.

There are advantages to using a punch over a shave in the setting of longitudinal melanonychia despite the incisional nature of the procedure and the fact that it creates a full-thickness (albeit small) defect. The morbidity is less without nail fold reflection and (partial) plate avulsion. The predictable resultant chronic paronychia from nail fold reflection and nail plate avulsion is usually avoided.[18] Scars, when resulting from distal matrix injury (most adult melanonychia), are usually minimal and in the spectrum of erythronychia rather than split nails. Punch scars do not result in dorsal pterygium, as the nail plate is not avulsed. In toenail surgery, whereby the friction/microtrauma postoperatively tends to exacerbate inflammation with partial plate avulsion (a prerequisite for tangential biopsy), the punch is particularly well tolerated.

Despite this, the authors prefer to use tangential techniques (shave) for most cases of melanonychia biopsy and erythronychia biopsy. As discussed later, these tend to be excisional rather than incisional, leave behind a partial-thickness wound that not only reepithelializes faster than full-thickness ones, but heals without contraction and with very little scarring, even in the setting of large extirpation.

SHAVE BIOPSY (TANGENTIAL EXCISION)

The tangential matrix shave is an excisional biopsy technique most appropriate in cases of longitudinal melanonychia and erythronychia and most frequently used to diagnose nail unit neoplasms. This technically demanding procedure has many advantages. This biopsy is a partial-thickness biopsy; ideally the specimen should be less than 1 mm thick.[19] Partial-thickness wounds of the bed and matrix granulate rapidly and scar only minimally, if at all.[20] If margins are appropriately planned, one can excise the lesion completely. In the case of a benign melanocytic process, complete removal with biopsy can prevent future clinical confusion in the case of recurrent pigment. If a neoplasm is diagnosed that requires total or partial removal of the nail unit, the lack of full-thickness scarring allows for an easier subsequent procedure. Despite the paucity of tissue depth, in the authors' practice, these tangential excisions have without exception provided adequate tissue for histologic diagnosis.[21]

FOR MELANONYCHIA

The first step in a matrix shave is exposure of the matrix. Before anesthesia, the origin of the lesion should be estimated based on clinical examination, including the use of onychoscopy (**Fig. 3**).[22] In the case of lighter pigmented lesions, mapping of the lesion preoperatively is paramount, as findings can be much more subtle after digital anesthesia, a bloodless field, and nail fold and plate reflection. In most cases, a partial proximal plate avulsion provides adequate exposure without necessitating complete removal of the nail plate.

Occasionally, a lateral plate curl is preferable for truly laterally oriented pigmented bands.[23]

After adequate anesthesia is attained, the appendage has been appropriately sterilized, and a bloodless field has been established, one should use a nail elevator; the authors prefer a pediatric nail elevator/spatula in order to free the nail plate from the cuticle. To increase access to the proximal matrix, 2 tangential incisions are made in the proximal nail fold in order to retract the proximal nail fold as a trapezoidal flap. When incising the proximal nail fold, it is wise to insert the elevator under the proximal nail fold in the path of the blade in order to prevent inadvertent damage to the underlying matrix. Alternatively, the scalpel can be inserted with the sharp side up and incised through the proximal nail fold from the plate to the skin, eliminating the risk of matrix injury.[24] A partial nail plate avulsion is performed in standard fashion, most commonly a partial proximal or alternatively a lateral plate curl. Total plate avulsions are discouraged.[23]

Once the matrix is exposed, the area of interest should be confirmed with an assistant to limit confusion if histology is not consistent with the preoperative clinical impression. The visualized lesion is scored with 1- to 2-mm margins in a

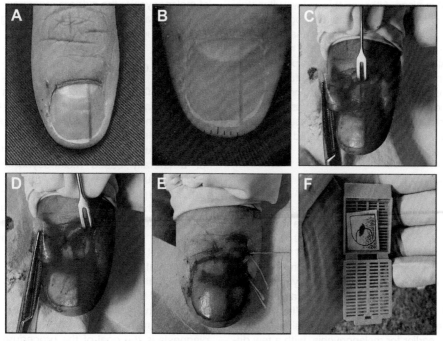

Fig. 3. Matrix shave biopsy. (*A*) Slender band of longitudinal melanonychia. (*B*) Dermoscopy shows a brown background with slightly irregular brown lines. (*C*) A partial proximal plate avulsion is performed with reflection of the proximal nail fold. The pigmented lesion is appreciated grossly as a longitudinally oriented band of pigment in the matrix. (*D*) The pigmented lesion has been excised tangentially as a rectangular specimen. Onychodermis is visualized at the depth of the defect. (*E*) The nail plate and nail fold are returned to anatomic position and sutured. (*F*) The specimen is uncurled and placed flat on a nail map in a cassette and then placed in formalin.

rectangular fashion. The blade is then inserted tangentially, and the specimen is freed from underlying tissue using slow sweeping and stabbing motions. Forceps or a cotton-tipped applicator can be used to gently stabilize the specimen during removal, taking care not to curl or crush the specimen.

Once completely removed, the specimen should be placed on a paper nail map in a cassette before placing in formalin. The nail map allows the pathologist to accurately orient the specimen and prevents specimen curling. It is important to stipulate that the specimen be sectioned longitudinally.

The nail bed and matrix should be inspected for residual pigment or masses. If significant pigment is noted on the ventral nail plate overlying the matrix, this can be removed (by curettage or scraping with a no. 15 blade) to prevent reimplantation of melanocytes and ambiguity in the case of recurrent pigment at the site of a biopsy-proven benign lesion. Alternatively, when the surgeon is concerned about the possibility of leaving any melanocytes, this small section of plate can be sent for pathologic processing and a faux nail inserted in its place to prevent postoperative dorsal pterygium.[25] For most matrix shave biopsies in the setting of longitudinal melanonychia, however, removing and sending the nail plate are unnecessary, and it can be left in place. Although this nail will ultimately elevate and fall off, it serves as a biologic dressing over and splint for the matrix during healing. Suture is used to reapproximate the proximal nail fold and set the nail plate back in the anatomic position. The authors prefer a rapidly absorbable suture, such as rapidly absorbable Polyglactin 910. The tourniquet is removed, and digital reperfusion must be appreciated and documented. A sterile pressure dressing is applied, and the patient is instructed on postoperative analgesia.

FOR ERYTHRONYCHIA

Erythronychia is usually the result of a process in the distal matrix: neoplastic, pressure related, inflammatory, scarring, or idiopathic, that leads to ventral plate groove in which the nail bed swells, leading to the clinically apparent red line observed through the plate. Given that erythronychia can be a sign of malignancy, biopsy is warranted in the setting of a new or changing lesion (**Fig. 4**).[26]

The procedural process is similar to that described earlier for melanonychia, with a few differences based on clinical findings. As with all nail procedures, total anesthesia is required, and a bloodless field is imperative. The lesion should be mapped preoperatively, as erythronychia can disappear completely with anesthesia.

Nail plate avulsion is tailored to the size and location of the area of interest. In the case of larger ill-defined lesions, total plate avulsion is often necessary, while a trap door, hemi-trap door, strip avulsion, or lateral curl can be used from slim well-defined lesions.[23] Once the bed and matrix are exposed, one should identify the lesion based on preoperative markings on surrounding skin, and identify any submatrical process, if present. When a process is appreciated under the bed and matrix, a full-thickness excision is recommended. However, in the case of localized submatrical glomus tumors, for instance, dissection of the lesion from beneath the matrix is both diagnostic and curative.[27]

In most instances, however, the band of erythronychia represents an onychopapilloma versus squamous cell carcinoma in situ (as epithelial processes) and can be excised tangentially.[28] As previously described, 2- to 3-mm margins are incised around the area of interest, and the specimen is delicately removed as detailed earlier as a tangential excision. The margins must include the distal matrix, the entire bed (in a longitudinal specimen), and often the hyperkeratotic papule at the hyponychium. The nail plate can nearly always be reapproximated, as melanocyte implantation is not a concern.

As with tangential specimens excised in cases of melanonychia, the authors recommend placing the tissue flat on a nail map and marking it specifically for longitudinal sectioning.

LATERAL LONGITUDINAL EXCISION

When an inflammatory process such as psoriasis or lichen planus is suspected, a lateral longitudinal excision provides a full-thickness specimen that samples each segment of the nail unit (**Fig. 5**).[29] Although one could use this technique for a laterally based melanocytic lesion, the resultant full-thickness scar complicates any further surgical treatment. When performed correctly, the affected nail will be narrowed by approximately 10%. If a larger specimen is taken, one can induce lateral malalignment of the nail unit with respect to the distal phalanx.[30] If the lateral horn of the matrix is not removed in full, the patient will develop a cyst or spicule. Because of these potentially troubling outcomes, the chosen digit is ideally on the patient's nondominant hand; however, a histopathologic diagnosis is the goal of the procedure, and this should not be compromised in the service of cosmesis.

Before the procedure, a surgical marking pen should be used to outline a slender fusiform sample that includes the proximal nail fold (and

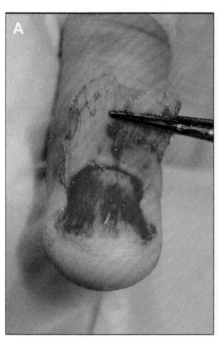 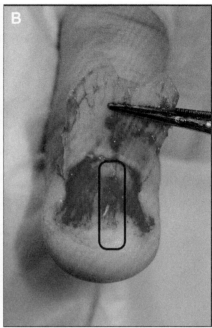

Fig. 4. Matrix and bed tangential excision for longitudinal erythronychia. (*A*) A trap door avulsion is performed demonstrating the longitudinal disease process extending from the distal matrix to the distal bed. (*B*) The black marking shows the margins for tangential excision. Like the matrix shave biopsy, the specimen is less than 1 mm in thickness; the resultant wounds are left to heal by second intention and usually are covered by the partially avulsed nail plate.

underlying matrix), lateral nail plate (and underlying bed), lateral nail fold (only if involved in the clinical presentation), hyponychium, and distal tip skin (see **Fig. 5**A). Including the entirety of the lateral matrix horn is imperative to prevent spicule formation as previously discussed. Of note, the lateral matrix horn of the great toe extends far more laterally and proximally than that on the fingers.[29]

The first incision is made at the proximal nail fold and extending onto the nail plate. When advancing the blade through the nail plate, it is important to rock the blade over the dorsal phalanx to prevent an inadvertent full-thickness incision through the distal pulp, which can lead to injury to the clinician and complicate the procedure. Once this incision is extended to the distal tip skin, a full-thickness incision is made, and the fusiform excision is completed with a uniform deep plane of dissection over bone, tendon, and joint, with special care to include the entire lateral matrix horn. The lateral nail fold is included if involved clinically; otherwise, the incision is made in the lateral sulcus. Fine tissue cutting scissors (Gradle or tenotomy) are inserted at the distal edge of the sample with tips down, and the specimen is removed at the level of the dorsal phalanx for the entirety of the procedure. This tissue is also placed on a nail map as noted above, with instructions for longitudinal (and not bread loaf) sectioning.

The surgical site is inspected for residual matrix proximally; any suspected tissue is excised, and the defect may be curetted. The proximal nail fold and digital tip skin are reapproximated with rapidly absorbable suture, after which the lateral nail fold is sutured to the lateral nail plate. As the nail plate dulls the suture needle, it is prudent to place these sutures last. As always, the tourniquet is removed, reperfusion is appreciated and documented, and a sterile pressure dressing applied.

NAIL BED WEDGE BIOPSY

Nail bed wedge biopsies are useful for a small but specific presentation: nail bed tumors. These tumors are often but not necessarily warty, although the differential diagnosis may include nail bed wart, squamous cell carcinoma, melanoma (more commonly primary to the nail bed presenting as amelanotic), as well as a variety of benign soft tissue tumors, such as lipomas and superficial acral fibromyxomas (**Fig. 6**).[31] Usually patients present with nail bed tumefaction and resultant overlying onycholysis or nail plate loss. A radiograph to rule out underlying exostosis is recommended.[32] With a negative radiograph and nail bed tumor, a nail bed wedge biopsy is indicated and almost always preferable to using a single (or even double)

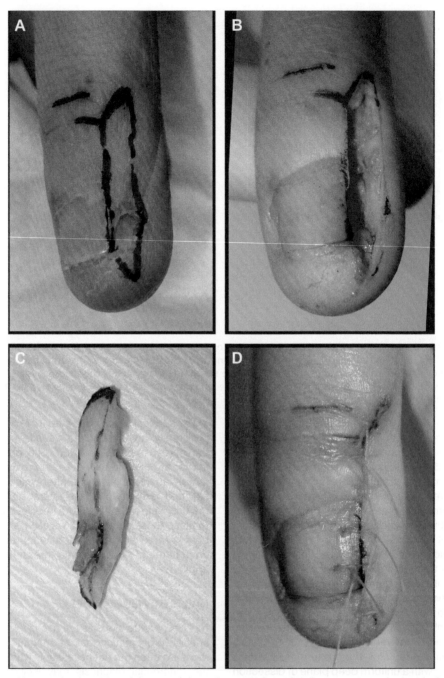

Fig. 5. Lateral longitudinal excision. (*A*) Scarred, hyperkeratotic lateral nail process is marked with the margins for a lateral longitudinal excision, with care to include the proximal lateral matrix horn and extending through the lateral nail sulcus. (*B*) The excision is completed with a dissection plane above bone. Proximally, the defect should demonstrate no evidence of residual matrix tissue, which could cause postoperative spicules or cysts. (*C*) The specimen is marked for longitudinal (as opposed to bread loaf) sectioning. (*D*) The defect is sutured with 5-0 Polyglactin 910 rapidly absorbable suture.

punch biopsy. The diagnostic yield is higher; recovery is only slightly longer, and patients are only marginally at higher risk of permanent dystrophy. The chance for accurate diagnosis and cure is significantly greater.

In the setting of warty nail bed tumors, the wedge is particularly important. The differential diagnosis is usually wart versus squamous cell carcinoma (in which up to 90% of cases demonstrate the associated high-risk human

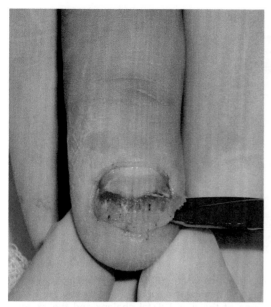

Fig. 6. Nail bed wedge biopsy. After the tumor is scored and the incision extended to the underlying bone, Gradle scissors are used to complete the wedge excision above bone.

papillomavirus). It is not uncommon for smaller and/or more superficial biopsies to show features of verruca and not carcinoma, even in the presence of underlying cancer; the most diagnostic elements of these human papillomavirus–related carcinomas tend to be deep and may collide with benign verruca.[33] Only a wedge biopsy with serial section histopathologic processing makes this diagnosis reliably.

This procedure is truly simple, largely because of the phenomenal wound-healing properties of the nail bed; reconstruction is nil, and the wound heals by second intention. The goal of this procedure is to remove the nail bed tumor in its entirety, not with wide margins as in a wide local excision, but with narrow (0.5–1 mm) margins in order to provide the pathologist with adequate tissue sampling (including any shoulder) with which to make a diagnosis as well as to minimize recurrence in many benign diagnoses.

A tourniquet is placed. The nail bed tumor is scored with a scalpel blade, following the often well-defined margin at the periphery of the tumor; this is then extended deep to the underlying bone. The growth is excised just above the dorsal phalanx with scissors as a tissue wedge specimen. The base of the wound will be periosteum and bone. The tourniquet is removed, and hemostasis is obtained with pressure. Only rarely is electrosurgery necessary; pressure is adequate, and electrosurgery necrosis and char will discourage and delay optimal wound healing by granulation.

Patients must be reassured that second intention healing is preferred and that the defect does not require primary repair, local tissue rearrangement, or skin grafting. Essential aspects of wound care include keeping a greasy dressing and education about sterile wound care. Antibiotics are optional, with variables including degree of bone exposure, patient hygiene and motivation, and ability/accessibility for clinical follow-up.

Healing is predictable and efficient, although the size of the wound as well as the innate genetic, vascular, and nutritional attributes of the patient will affect the speed of healing. Most fingernail defects 1 cm or smaller will completely reepithelialize in 4 to 6 weeks, with larger defects taking 6 to 8 weeks. Toenail wounds are always slower to heal.[34] It is helpful to have a photograph of the defect; this will demonstrate to patients the progress they are making and the miraculous ability for the nail unit to reform itself after wedge biopsy.

EN BLOC EXCISION OF ALL NAIL TISSUES

Historically, all nail melanomas, including in situ melanomas, were treated with some form of disarticulation. Over time, the more radical limb removals were replaced with digital amputation, and then more distal digital amputation (**Figs. 7 and 8**).[35] Only recently has the practice of digit-sparing surgery (termed "functional" or "conservative" excision, wide local excision, or en bloc excision of all nail tissues) been advocated widely (thanks to an expanding group of data) and adopted by a wider range of surgeons.[36,37]

Nail melanomas occur most frequently on the thumb and great toe.[38] The morbidity of even distal amputation of these digits is significant.[39] Excision with clear margins is the most critical factor in melanoma survival and the most basic tenet for surgical treatment. That said, the medical community must balance the morbidity and resultant quality of life of amputation versus more conservative wide local excision, while maintaining the strictest adherence to obtaining clear oncologic margins. The data suggest, and the authors espouse, that en bloc surgery of all nail tissues is the treatment of choice for nail melanoma in situ. Mohs surgery with immunostains is used by some and can be considered an effective form of digit-sparing/conservative surgery as well.[40] Its discussion is not included herein.

This procedure is perhaps the most complicated and involved of all nail surgeries. It features manipulation of and around all the nail subunits, including meticulous excision above the dorsal

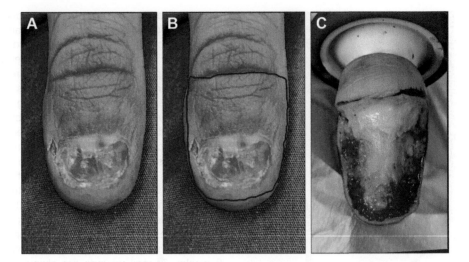

Fig. 7. En bloc excision of all nail tissues. (*A*) Recurrent nail melanoma in situ. (*B*) Margins are marked in black, from the DIPJ crease to the midsagittal lines bilaterally, extending beyond the hyponychium by at least 3- to 4-mm margins. (*C*) Postoperative defect showing exposed bone of the dorsal distal phalanx and the extensor tendon inserting into bone. This will be resurfaced immediately with a full-thickness skin graft.

phalanx and extensor tendon to the (distal) interphalangeal joint, often reconstruction with a full-thickness skin graft, and much more complicated recovery than any of the prior procedures. It is not a surgery for novices; however, it represents an elegant alternative to the more barbaric disarticulation procedures. Loss of the thumb, for example, results in 40% loss of hand function.[41] Conversely, quality of life of those having undergone en bloc excision of all nail tissues is unchanged from preoperative quality of life, including physical and psychological measures.[42]

Detailed preoperative examination guides the extent of surgery; at the very least, 9 mm is excised around the clinical margins of the melanoma in situ.[43] In some instances, this allows a "hemi-en bloc excision" that can leave a third or more of the nail plate and still achieve excision with adequate margins. Leaving remnant plate allows for the plate to serve as counterpressure to the sensate pulp and facilitates pincer action with the finger. Leaving too small a fragment of plate, however, will result in an irritating spicule that constantly catches on clothing, causing pain and persistent annoyance. Determining surgical margins and purposely leaving remnant matrix is an important judgment call that is made individually on a case-by-case basis.

The surgeon must assess for any periungual melanoma in situ, either proximally, laterally, or distally. Dermoscopy can be quite helpful in this analysis. Occasionally, subtle periungual pigment is present (representing a true Hutchinson sign) and must be included before margins are drawn.[44]

When there is significant periungual pigment, excision with appropriate margins may unfortunately result in digit degloving; this carries with it several unique risks and complicates the benefits provided by conservative excision.[45] Because this clinical scenario represents the exception rather than the rule, further discussion is left out of this article; multidisciplinary consultation and possibly management should be initiated in such cases.

The authors routinely reconstruct the excision defects with a full-thickness skin graft and harvest this graft before the wide local excision to minimizes tourniquet time. For smaller defects on the fingers, the ulnar (acral skin) hand site is used, and for larger defects, the upper inner arm is the preferred donor site. The graft is harvested in standard fashion, defatted, and placed in saline. The graft donor site is reconstructed. All attention is then paid to the nail unit for en bloc excision.

The following procedural steps represent an evolution from those previously published by one of the authors (N.J.J.) and reflect his current practice in 2020.

A tourniquet is placed. In most cases, the entire nail apparatus is excised (minus the hemi-en bloc cases discussed earlier). The margins are scored, from the DIPJ crease bilaterally to the midsagittal line, extended distally on either side of the digit to several millimeters (as little as 2 to 3, as many as 7 to 8, depending on the suspicion of periungual spread of tumor) distal to the hyponychium. These parameters create a nearly rectangular-shaped excision when viewed from above. The subsequent excision must elevate this tissue off of the

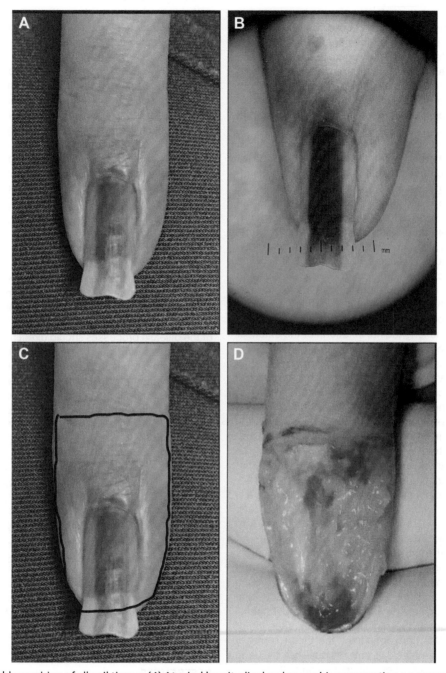

Fig. 8. En bloc excision of all nail tissues. (*A*) Atypical longitudinal melanonychia representing a nevus with severe atypia. (*B*) Dermoscopy shows a brown background and irregular brown lines. (*C*) Margins marked in black, from the DIPJ crease to the midsagittal lines bilaterally, extending beyond the hyponychium by at least 3- to 4-mm margins. (*D*) Postoperative defect showing exposed bone of the dorsal distal phalanx and the extensor tendon inserting into bone. This will be resurfaced immediately with a full-thickness skin graft.

dorsal phalanx, the extensor tendon, and DIPJ, excising all nail tissues in toto.

The authors start the excision distally. The scalpel blade is inserted on either side of the ungual process of the distal phalanx and advanced until the bone is reached. Then, the blade is moved millimeter by millimeter until the dorsal surface is appreciated by loss of resistance, a delicate and blind process accomplished by feel. At this point, the blade can be used to sharply dissect over the ungual process from either side, creating a distal plane of dissection above the bone. Unlike the looser periosteal attachments more proximally on the distal phalanx, the ungual process is tenaciously adherent via tight collagen attachments from the periosteum to the ventral nail plate and cannot be dissected easily. Sharp and precise cutting in this location is the only way to establish the correct plane for excision.

Once the distal third of the nail apparatus is elevated sharply, forceps or skin hooks can retract the leading edge of the nail unit. With bright surgical lighting, the waist of the distal phalanx is appreciated, and the blade again is used to cut in this deep plane, moving distally to proximally, to maintain a uniform dissection above bone. Frequently, the periosteum is removed, and resultant dry bone observed. This is ok. At this point, the dissection shifts from the scalpel blade to fine tissue cutting scissors (either Gradle or tenotomy). With "tips down," the dissection is carried further proximally using minute "nibbling" of the tips until the longitudinal striations of the extensor tendon are appreciated.

The remaining dissection is carried out proximal to distal and lateral to midline. The proximal nail fold skin can be tumesced with local anesthesia, and starting at the DIPJ crease, a clean dissection plane is appreciated from the joint over the tendon distally to its insertion into the distal phalanx. Similarly, a lateral approach from the joint over the tendon can be initiated and dissected. These dissections are carried proximally over the tendon until the two planes come together. This procedure is performed with delicate tissue-cutting scissors. The entire nail apparatus is then excised in toto as 1 block. The radial and ulnar (or medial and lateral on the toe) margins are inked for orientation. The specimen is placed on a nail map[46] and marked for serial longitudinal sectioning. Such steps are critical to maintain orientation and assess margins. The authors have found it helpful to photograph the digit immediately after tumor removal; this can document the clean plane of dissection and lack of any residual nail tissue in the event of perceived transection on pathology.[47]

The skin graft is placed over the defect and sutured in standard fashion. The authors prefer to use rapidly absorbable polyglactin 910 (5-0 on a P3 needle), running locked sutures, basting sutures throughout, and a xeroform bolster dressing sutured over the graft. (The purpose of this bolster is to prevent shearing and provide pressure for and protection of the graft.)[48] Electrosurgery and chemical hemostatic agents are unnecessary. The tourniquet is removed, and a pressure dressing is applied, with care to wrap top to bottom and side to side to avoid creating a dressing tourniquet. Tourniquet time is documented, as is the rapid reperfusion of the surgical site. Antibiotics are prescribed.

A splint for the digit will lower risks of development of mallet deformity; this is maintained for 3 weeks after surgery.[49] Subsequent hand therapy (either home or instituted formally) will be needed to reachieve full range of motion. A sling (for finger surgeries) or orthopedic open-toed boot with crutches (for toe surgeries) is also recommended for surgical site immobilization. The graft is examined with bolster removal at 1 week. Wound care is standard until fully healed.

LIMITATIONS

There are several specific presentations of nail disease that were not covered in this review: ingrown nails, exostoses, myxoid cysts, painful nail tumors (ie, glomus tumor), and about which a robust literature exists. In each of these instances, knowledge of the disease processes should direct the differential diagnosis and guide the clinician toward the appropriate procedure. Nevertheless, knowledge of the 6 procedures highlighted herein is an invaluable base from which to explore and expand into these more specific surgical techniques.

CLINICS CARE POINTS

- Multiple techniques can be utilized to achieve anesthesia in nail surgery, however employing a technique that prioritizes patient comfort is of the utmost importance.
- Diagnostic nail procedures are often very different from therapeutic nail procedures, and surgical procedure should be chosen based upon clinical intent.

CONFLICTS OF INTEREST, FUNDING SOURCES

None.

REFERENCES

1. Jellinek NJ, Vélez NF. Nail surgery: best way to obtain effective anesthesia. Dermatol Clin 2015; 33(2):265–71.
2. Huang L. Comparison of transthecal digit block and single injection volar subcutaneous digit block. Wounds 2011;23(4):93–6.
3. de Berker DA, André J, Baran R. Nail biology and nail science. Int J Cosmet Sci 2007;29(4):241–75.
4. Haneke E. Anatomy of the nail unit and the nail biopsy. Semin Cutan Med Surg 2015;34(2):95–100.

5. Dankmeijer J, Waltman JM. Sur l'innervation de la face dorsale des doigts humains. Acta Anat 1950; 10:377–84.

6. Park KK, Sharon VR. A review of local anesthetics: minimizing risk and side effects in cutaneous surgery. Dermatol Surg 2017;43(2):173–87.

7. Harness NG. Digital block anesthesia. J Hand Surg Am 2009;34(1):142–5.

8. Ilicki J. Safety of epinephrine in digital nerve blocks: a literature review. J Emerg Med 2015;49(5): 799–809.

9. Haneke E. Nail surgery. Clin Dermatol 2013;31(5): 516–25.

10. Vent A, Surber C, Graf Johansen NT, et al. Buffered lidocaine 1%, epinephrine 1:100,000 with sodium bicarbonate (hydrogen carbonate) in a 3:1 ratio is less painful than a 9:1 ratio: a double-blind, randomized, placebo-controlled, crossover trial. J Am Acad Dermatol 2020;S0190-9622(20):30066–9.

11. Fulling PD, Peterfreund RA. Alkalinization and precipitation characteristics of 0.2% ropivacaine. Reg Anesth Pain Med 2000;25(5):518–21.

12. Molleman J, Tielemans JF, Braam MJI, et al. Distraction as a simple and effective method to reduce pain during local anesthesia: a randomized controlled trial. J Plast Reconstr Aesthet Surg 2019;72(12): 1979–85.

13. Ueki S, Yamagami Y, Makimoto K. Effectiveness of vibratory stimulation on needle-related procedural pain in children: a systematic review. JBI Database System Rev Implement Rep 2019;17(7):1428–63.

14. Strazar AR, Leynes PG, Lalonde DH. Minimizing the pain of local anesthesia injection. Plast Reconstr Surg 2013;132(3):675–84.

15. Jellinek NJ. Nail surgery: practical tips and treatment options. Dermatol Ther 2007;20(1):68–74.

16. Rich P. Nail biopsy: indications and methods. Dermatol Surg 2001;27(3):229–34.

17. Jellinek N. Nail matrix biopsy of longitudinal melanonychia: diagnostic algorithm including the matrix shave biopsy. J Am Acad Dermatol 2007;56(5): 803–10.

18. Jellinek NJ, Vélez NF. Dermatologic manifestations of the lower extremity: nail surgery. Clin Podiatr Med Surg 2016;33(3):319–36.

19. Di Chiacchio N, Loureiro WR, Michalany NS, et al. Tangential biopsy thickness versus lesion depth in longitudinal melanonychia: a pilot study. Dermatol Res Pract 2012;2012:353864.

20. Richert B, Theunis A, Norrenberg S, et al. Tangential excision of pigmented nail matrix lesions responsible for longitudinal melanonychia: evaluation of the technique on a series of 30 patients. J Am Acad Dermatol 2013;69(1):96–104.

21. Jellinek NJ, Vélez NF, Knackstedt TJ. Recovery after matrix shave biopsy. Dermatol Surg 2016;42(10): 1227–9.

22. Piraccini BM, Alessandrini A, Starace M. Onychoscopy: dermoscopy of the nails. Dermatol Clin 2018;36(4):431–8.

23. Collins SC, Cordova K, Jellinek NJ. Alternatives to complete nail plate avulsion. J Am Acad Dermatol 2008;59(4):619–26.

24. Di Chiacchio N, Fonseca Noriega L, Borges Figueira de Mello CD, et al. Do not hurt the nail matrix: safe technique for proximal nail fold incision. Skin Appendage Disord 2018;4(4):347–8.

25. Jellinek NJ, Cressey BD. Nail splint to prevent pterygium after nail surgery. Dermatol Surg 2019; 45(12):1733–5.

26. Jellinek NJ. Longitudinal erythronychia: suggestions for evaluation and management. J Am Acad Dermatol 2011;64(1):167.e1-11.

27. Baltz JO, Jellinek NJ. Commentary on transungual excision of glomus tumors. Dermatol Surg 2020; 46(1):113–5.

28. Jellinek NJ, Lipner SR. Longitudinal erythronychia: retrospective single-center study evaluating differential diagnosis and the likelihood of malignancy. Dermatol Surg 2016;42(3):310–9.

29. Jellinek NJ, Rubin AI. Lateral longitudinal excision of the nail unit. Dermatol Surg 2011;37(12):1781–5.

30. De Berker DA, Baran R. Acquired malalignment: a complication of lateral longitudinal nail biopsy. Acta Derm Venereol 1998;78(6):468–70.

31. Haneke E. Important malignant and new nail tumors. J Dtsch Dermatol Ges 2017;15(4):367–86.

32. Nowillo KS, Simpson RL. Subungual exostosis of the finger with nail plate induction. Hand (N Y) 2010; 5(2):203–5.

33. Tang N, Maloney ME, Clark AH, et al. A retrospective study of nail squamous cell carcinoma at 2 institutions. Dermatol Surg 2016;42(Suppl 1):S8–17.

34. Bosley R, Leithauser L, Turner M, et al. The efficacy of second-intention healing in the management of defects on the dorsal surface of the hands and fingers after Mohs micrographic surgery. Dermatol Surg 2012;38(4):647–53.

35. Dika E, Patrizi A, Fanti PA, et al. The prognosis of nail apparatus melanoma: 20 years of experience from a single institute. Dermatology 2016;232(2):177–84.

36. Montagner S, Belfort FA, Belda Junior W, et al. Descriptive survival study of nail melanoma patients treated with functional surgery versus distal amputation. J Am Acad Dermatol 2018;79(1):147–9.

37. Jo G, Cho SI, Choi S, et al. Functional surgery versus amputation for in situ or minimally invasive nail melanoma: a meta-analysis. J Am Acad Dermatol 2019;81(4):917–22.

38. Mannava KA, Mannava S, Koman LA, et al. Longitudinal melanonychia: detection and management of nail melanoma. Hand Surg 2013;18(1):133–9.

39. Hattori Y, Doi K, Ikeda K, et al. A retrospective study of functional outcomes after successful replantation

versus amputation closure for single fingertip amputations. J Hand Surg 2006;31:811–8.

40. Brodland DG. The treatment of nail apparatus melanoma with Mohs micrographic surgery. Dermatol Surg 2001;27(3):269–73.

41. Rondinelli R. Guides to the evaluation of permanent impairment. Chicago (IL): American Medical Association; 2007.

42. Knackstedt TJ, Baltz JO, Wilmer EN, et al. Assessing patient outcomes after digit-sparing en bloc surgery of nail apparatus melanoma in situ using two validated surveys. J Am Acad Dermatol 2019;82(3): 746–7.

43. Kunishige JH, Doan L, Brodland DG, et al. Comparison of surgical margins for lentigo maligna versus melanoma in situ. J Am Acad Dermatol 2019;81(1): 204–12.

44. Koga H, Saida T, Uhara H. Key point in dermoscopic differentiation between early nail apparatus melanoma and benign longitudinal melanonychia. J Dermatol 2011;38(1):45–52.

45. Proietto G, Giaculli E, De Biasio F, et al. Conservative surgical treatment of a thin acral lentiginous melanoma of the thumb with no recurrences: a case report. Dermatol Ther 2013;26(3):260–2.

46. Available at: https://www.cta-lab.com/pdfs/CTALab_Nail_Cutouts.pdf. Accessed February 1, 2021.

47. Jellinek NJ, Bauer JH. En bloc excision of the nail. Dermatol Surg 2010;36(9):1445–50.

48. Lazar A, Abimelec P, Dumontier C. Full thickness skin graft for nail unit reconstruction. J Hand Surg Br 2005;30(2):194–8.

49. Cressey BD, Clark A, Jellinek NJ. Mallet finger as a complication of dermatologic surgery: diagnosis, treatment, and prevention. Dermatol Surg 2019; 45(7):997–9.

Pathology of the Nail Unit

Beth S. Ruben, MD

KEYWORDS

- Nail unit pathology • Nail disease • Psoriasis • Onychomycosis • Nail unit inflammatory disease
- Nail unit neoplasms • Melanonychia

KEY POINTS

- Clinical findings in inflammatory diseases such as psoriasis stem from specific alterations in different compartments of the nail unit epithelium.
- Nail clippings can be used to diagnosis psoriasis, onychomycosis, *Pseudomonas*, and sometimes neoplasms such as onychomatricoma, as well as other conditions.
- Without submission of the nail plate, it may be impossible to render a pathologic diagnosis of onychopapilloma.
- Nail nevi in children may demonstrate concerning clinical, dermatoscopic, and histologic features, but melanoma in this setting is exceedingly rare.
- An important pitfall in the interpretation of nail unit melanoma is low cellularity areas, especially in partial samples, which can mimic a lentigo. Attention to other features such as cytologic atypia is important in this setting.

INTRODUCTION

Nail unit pathologic assessment represents an important component of the diagnosis of nail disease. The hard nature of the nail plate can make procuring and processing these specimens an impediment to optimal diagnosis, however.[1,2] In this section, the histopathology of common and uncommon or emerging entities in the nail unit, which have been covered clinically elsewhere in this issue, are presented, with attention to the clinicopathologic correlates, best practices to demonstrate the relevant histopathologic features, and pitfalls in diagnosis.

INFLAMMATORY NAIL DISEASE
Psoriasis

The clinical hallmarks of psoriasis depend on the area of the nail unit involved, and there are recognizable histologic correlates that can be observed in nail unit biopsies, and also, often in nail clippings. For example, nail pitting and nail crumbling, which can be observed on the surface of the nail, are the result of proximal and dorsal matrix involvement.[3,4] The proximal matrix and dorsal matrix epithelium are responsible for the formation of the surface of the nail plate. In psoriasis, parakeratosis is produced in those compartments, and ends up on the surface defects of the plate. As the nail plate exits from under the proximal nail fold, these foci of parakeratosis are shed, resulting in small surface (pits), or larger ones (crumbling). Such findings can occasionally be observed in nail clippings (**Fig. 1**). The distal matrix forms the bulk of the lower portions of the nail plate. When this is affected in psoriasis, retained nuclei or parakeratosis are found in the lower nail plate. This finding corresponds with leukonychia clinically. The nail bed epithelium is responsible for a minor contribution to the formation of the lower most nail plate, but is responsible for the remaining characteristic clinical findings of psoriasis that occur in the subungual space. These findings include oil spots, onycholysis, subungual hyperkeratosis, pustules, and splinter hemorrhages. Histologically, the nail bed epithelium is usually hyperplastic. Whereas in cutaneous psoriasis hypogranulosis is common, in nail unit psoriasis, paradoxical hypergranulosis may be observed. Oil spots represent serum and

Palo Alto Medical Foundation Medical Group, Dermatology, 795 El Camino Real, Clark Building, 2nd Floor, Palo Alto, CA 94301, USA
E-mail addresses: bsruben@alumni.stanford.edu; RubenBS@sutterhealth.org

Dermatol Clin 39 (2021) 319–336
https://doi.org/10.1016/j.det.2020.12.009

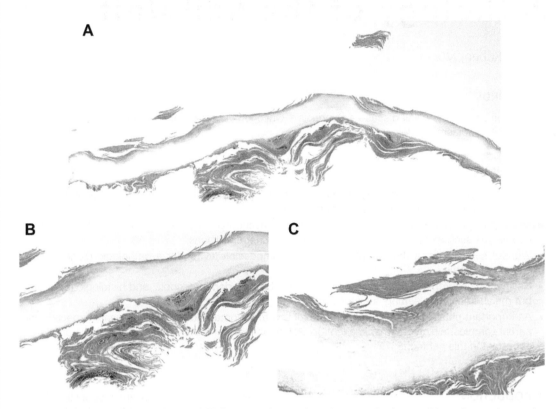

Fig. 1. Psoriasis. Nail clippings. (*A*) An undulating surface with nail pits, and subungual hyperkeratosis, parakeratosis. and neutrophils (hematoxylin-eosin, original magnification ×20x). (*B*) Closer view of subungual material, arising from nail bed involvement and nail pits, arising from proximal/dorsal matrical involvement (hematoxylin-eosin, original magnification ×40x). (*C*) Nail pits are formed when parakeratosis on the nail plate surface shells out as the nail plate exits from under the proximal nail fold (hematoxylin-eosin, original magnification ×20x).

neutrophils accumulating alongside parakeratosis in the subungual space. As this process intensifies, onycholysis can occur, because the nail plate can become separated from the nail bed. Subungual hyperkeratosis, often observed most distally in the nail unit, is due to the subungual accumulation of hyperkeratosis and parakeratosis with neutrophils owing to the abnormal cornification in psoriasis (**Fig. 2**). Pustular psoriasis of the nail unit occurs when neutrophilic pustules form within the epithelium, which are often associated with onycholysis. As in cutaneous psoriasis, dilated tortuous blood vessels can be found in the superficial nail unit dermis. When minor trauma occurs, hemorrhage accumulates in the longitudinal ridges of the undersurface of the nail plate, causing splinter hemorrhages clinically. In longstanding lesions, marked epithelial hyperplasia may occur, and the other diagnostic findings may be limited to hyperkeratosis laced with occasional neutrophils. Especially when the nail bed is exposed, diagnostic findings may be lacking altogether.[5] Nail clippings in nail bed psoriasis usually demonstrate subungual hyperkeratosis and parakeratosis with neutrophils, as detailed elsewhere in this article. The latter are almost never observed in patients with normal nails, but can actually even be found in the normal-appearing nails in patients with psoriasis.[6]

Lichen Planus

Characteristic clinical findings in lichen planus may vary.[7] There is often longitudinal ridging, thinning, and splitting (onychorrhexis), atrophy, hyperkeratosis, and in severe cases, progression to nail loss. When the inflammatory infiltrate has destroyed the nail matrix, pterygium may occur as the proximal nail fold fuses with the nail bed epithelium. Without the formation of a nail plate, these structures blend together. Histologically, the findings in nail unit lichen planus are similar to those elsewhere. There is a band-like

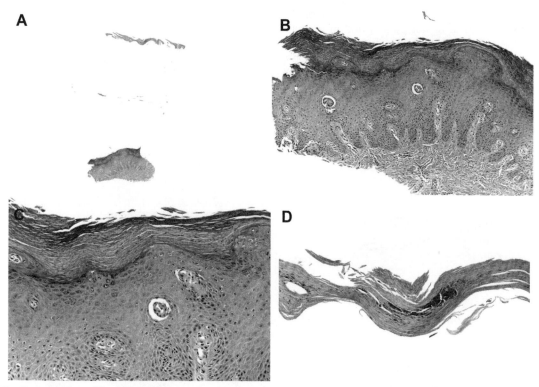

Fig. 2. Psoriasis. Nail bed biopsy. (*A*) Low power view of punch biopsy with some detached cornified material (hematoxylin-eosin, original magnification ×20x). (*B*) Punch biopsy with epithelial hyperplasia of nail bed, hyperkeratosis, and prominent dermal blood vessels (hematoxylin-eosin, original magnification ×40x). (*C*) Closer view of nail bed also showing hypergranulosis instead of hypogranulosis found at cutaneous sites, parakeratosis laced with neutrophils, and dilated dermal blood vessels (hematoxylin-eosin, original magnification ×100x). (*D*) Detached cornified material with parakeratosis and neutrophils (hematoxylin-eosin, original magnification ×100x).

lymphohistiocytic infiltrate, sometimes with occasional eosinophils or plasma cells, which variably obscures the junctional zone of the epithelium, which is irregular, where there may be necrotic keratinocytes. These changes can occur anywhere in the nail unit, from the proximal nail fold to the hyponychium. A longitudinal biopsy is often very helpful in capturing the inflammatory infiltrate, which can vary along the length of the nail unit. Hypergranulosis, a finding that is not observed in the nail matrix or bed normally,[8] may be observed in involved areas, as well as hyperkeratosis. As the process continues and the matrical epithelium is compromised, there may be breaking up of the nail plate (onychorrhexis), as well as thinning of the plate. The nail unit epithelium may also be thickened or thinned (**Fig. 3**). In late lesions, there may be a sparse infiltrate, superficial dermal fibrosis, and sometimes only scattered necrotic keratinocytes, indicative of the prior lichenoid reaction. In such cases, there may be pronounced

hypergranulosis and hyperkeratosis, and the normal nail plate may be inconspicuous. In pterygium, the normal architecture in the vicinity of the proximal nail fold can be altered, as the nail fold blends with the nail bed. In advanced cases, complete nail loss can occur, with no remaining normal architectural features of the nail unit.

Lichen Striatus

Lichen striatus, when it affects the nail unit, often does so secondarily. Reported cases are rare[9,10] and, as expected, occur more commonly in children, as does lichen striatus. Skin lesions are usually found in the surrounding acral skin, and possibly even more proximally on the affected extremity, as linear papules in a blaschkoid distribution. The nail changes are identical to those in lichen planus, both clinically and histologically. In fact, if the nail unit is sampled for diagnosis, it may not be possible to distinguish between these entities. Therefore, in this setting, it may be more

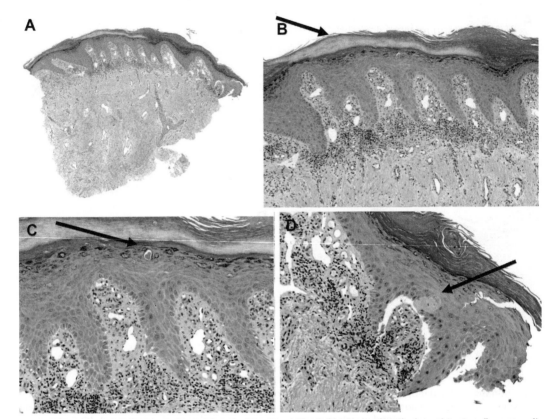

Fig. 3. Lichen planus. (*A*) Later lesion with a patchy band-like infiltrate and nail plate thinning (hematoxylin-eosin, original magnification ×40x). (*B*) Nail bed epithelial hyperplasia, hypergranulosis, and hyperkeratosis, with a thin nail plate (hematoxylin-eosin, original magnification ×100x) Arrow, nail plate. (*C*) Angular/sawtooth nail ridges, and scattered necrotic keratinocytes (hematoxylin-eosin, original magnification ×200x) Arrow, necrotic keratinocyte within hypergranulosis). (*D*) Interface changes with necrotic keratinocytes, and a mostly lymphocytic infiltrate (hematoxylin-eosin, original magnification ×200x) Arrow, necrotic keratinocytes and nearby lymphocytic infiltrate.

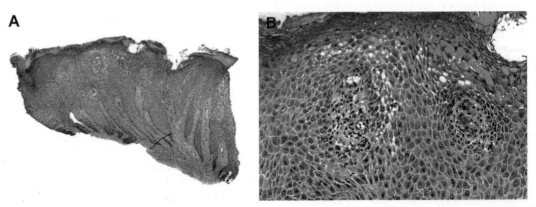

Fig. 4. Eczematous dermatitis (allergic contact dermatitis). Nail bed biopsy. (*A, B*) Epithelial hyperplasia of nail bed with spongiosis and serum ([A] hematoxylin-eosin, original magnification ×400x; [B] hematoxylin-eosin, original magnification ×200x).

helpful to biopsy a cutaneous lesion. This biopsy may demonstrate more distinctive features of lichen striatus, especially, a deeper perieccrine or perifollicular infiltrate, in addition to a variably psoriasiform, lichenoid, and/or spongiotic reaction more superficially.

Eczematous Dermatitis

Eczematous dermatitis may also involve the nail unit secondarily. However, an increasing number of cases are primary, owing to the application of various nail cosmetics. Gel manicures are a particular emerging culprit[11] for allergic contact dermatitis and may cause a variety of clinical manifestations, including nail dystrophy and onycholysis. Histologically, the nail unit epithelium is altered by spongiosis and there is a variable infiltrate, which may include eosinophils. Serum accumulation can occur, along with parakeratosis under the nail plate (**Fig. 4**). Similar findings can be seen in onychomycosis; therefore, it is

important to complete Periodic acid-Schiff staining in such cases.

Trachyonychia

Trachyonychia is not a condition sui generis, but may be the clinical manifestation of several different inflammatory conditions that can affect the nail unit, including psoriasis, lichen planus, eczematous dermatitis, and alopecia areata.[12] It is more common in children. Affected nails usually demonstrate pronounced surface changes, including ridging, fissures, striations, pitting, and hyperkeratosis. They may seem to be roughened to opalescent or shiny. Koilonychia may also occur.[13] Any number of nails may be involved, although the other name used for this condition is "20 nail dystrophy." Histologically, the features may vary, depending on the underlying condition. Alopecia areata may present with spongiosis nonspecifically. Because it is a self-limited condition, especially in children, biopsies of trachyonychia are infrequent.

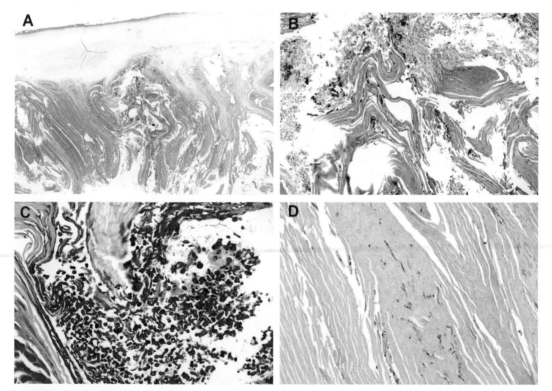

Fig. 5. Onychomycosis. Dermatophytoma. (*A, B*) A loculated collection of fungi/mold under the nail plate, with yellow discoloration of the nail plate owing to *Pseudomonas* ([A] hematoxylin-eosin, original magnification ×40x; [B] hematoxylin-eosin, original magnification ×100x). (*C*) Periodic acid-Schiff staining highlighting irregular hyphae and spores, suggesting a nondermatophyte may be present (Periodic-Schiff, 200x). (*D*) In other areas of the nail plate, more characteristic dermatophytic hyphae can be found (Periodic-Schiff, 100x).

ONYCHOMYCOSIS

This common infection of the nail unit may be caused by dermatophytic fungi, molds, and/or *Candida*.[14–16] The diagnosis can be made in nail clippings, but it is often unsuspected in a range of nail dystrophies, and may be picked up in other types of nail unit sampling. Periodic acid-Schiff or Grocott methenamine silver staining of nail clippings are more sensitive methods for detection than culture. Superficial, intraungual, and/or subungual spaces may be involved. In dermatophytoma, a loculated area of organisms, which may also include bacteria, occurs under the nail plate (**Fig. 5**). This pattern of infection, often presenting as a discolored nail streak, may resist therapy and should therefore be mentioned specifically in pathology reports.[17] Dematiaceous fungi and molds may give rise to pigmented oncyhomycosis, which can mimic melanonychia clinically. Such organisms do contain melanin in their cell walls, accounting for their pigmentation. *Candida* species present as yeast forms, with occasional budding and pseudohyphae (**Fig. 6**). Dermatophytic hyphae are small and characteristically septate. They tend to respect the boundaries of onychocytes in the nail plate. Molds, however, are often larger, may be pigmented, and spores may be seen. Tortuous hyphae, and so-called perforating hyphae, which can be found perpendicular to onychocytes, may be observed. Associated changes in the nail plate include subungual hyperkeratosis and parakeratosis, often with neutrophils, which may simulate the findings in nail clippings in psoriasis. Likewise, nail unit biopsies can present similar findings, with variable epithelial hyperplasia, hypergranulosis, and parakeratosis with neutrophils. Concurrent infections may occur, especially *Pseudomonas*, giving the nail a lemon-yellow hue in histologic sections, owing to fluorescein pigment that has diffused from the bacterium, which is not itself usually identifiable histologically. This process gives the nail a greenish color clinically (see **Figs. 5** and **6**).

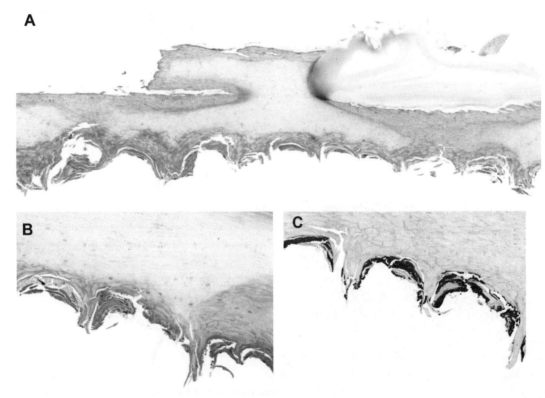

Fig. 6. Onychomycosis. *Candida*. (A) Nail plate with lemon yellow discoloration owing to *Pseudomonas*, and subungual *Candida* (hematoxylin-eosin, original magnification ×100x). (*B, C*) Many subungual yeast, some budding, are evident, in routine and Periodic acid-Schiff–stained sections ([B] hematoxylin-eosin, original magnification ×20x; [C] Periodic-Schiff, 20x).

NEOPLASMS OF THE NAIL UNIT
Epithelial Neoplasms

Benign
Onychomatricoma This distinctive benign nail matrix proliferation was first reported in 1992 by Drs. Baran and Kint.[18] Since then, more than 200 cases have been reported, with some larger series.[19–21] Clinically, it presents with a nodular portion under the proximal nail fold, with a thickened nail plate, also demonstrating transverse overcurvature. It tends to be yellowish, but can be pigmented. Splinter hemorrhages are also a common finding. When looking at the thickened nail plate from its distal end, one may see cavities within it, and these cavities are evident proximally when the nail plate is avulsed. Histologically, the nodular proximal portion corresponds to the fibroepithelial portion of tumor in the matrix, with reduplicated matrix epithelium, covering a fibrocellular stroma, containing bland spindle cells of varying density, with a collagenous to myxoid stroma. The stromal cells usually label with CD34 immunostain,[22] as do many spindle cell proliferations in this area. There is a pleomorphic variant,[23] which display occasional larger and sometimes multinucleate cells, without biologic significance. Some of these cases had been reported as subungual pleomorphic fibromas. Without seeing the associated nail plate, some cases of onychomatricoma can be misdiagnosed as subungual angiofibroma or superficial fibromyxoma, which are also CD34+. Pigmented onychomatricoma results when the matrix epithelium contains melanin pigment, possibly owing to melanocytic activation. The nail plate interdigitates with the fibroepithelial portion in a finger and glove configuration. Characteristic large loculations of serum, and foci of hemorrhage, can be observed in the nail plate (**Fig. 7**). Nail clippings can be used for diagnosis, and will demonstrate these

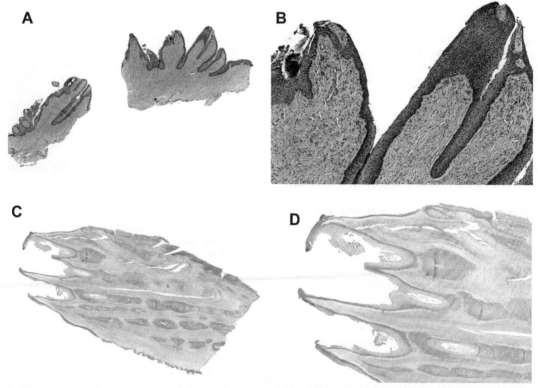

Fig. 7. Onychomatricoma, pigmented. (*A, B*) The proximal fibroepithelial portion displays a fibrocellular stroma, and is covered by reduplicated matrix epithelium. In this case, it demonstrates some pigmentation, as did the clinical lesion, a rare variant ([A] hematoxylin-eosin, original magnification ×20x; [B] hematoxylin-eosin, original magnification ×40x). (*C, D*) The thickened nail plate interdigitates proximally with the fibroepithelial portion in vivo. It contains superficial matrix epithelium. The nail plate is thickened and contains loculated serum and hemorrhage ([A]hematoxylin-eosin, original magnification ×20x; [B] hematoxylin-eosin, original magnification ×40x).

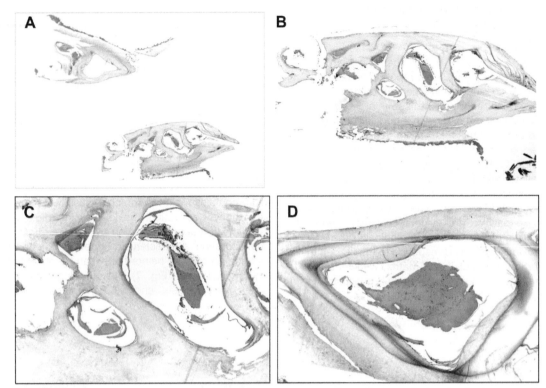

Fig. 8. Onychomatricoma. Nail clippings. (*A–D*) When sectioned transversely, the nail plate in clippings contains typical loculated serum and hemorrhage and on occasion, some matrix epithelium from the digitations formed more proximally ([A] hematoxylin-eosin, original magnification ×20x; [B] hematoxylin-eosin, original magnification ×40x; [C] hematoxylin-eosin, original magnification ×100x; [D] hematoxylin-eosin, original magnification ×100x).

findings; occasionally, the digitate epithelium can be captured more distally as well[19,24,25] (**Fig. 8**).

Onychopapilloma A benign and relatively common proliferation in the nail unit, onychopapilloma presents as longitudinal erythronychia of varying widths, usually originating from the distal matrix and lunula. More distally, splinter hemorrhages can often be found overlying the nail bed. Under the free edge of the nail plate, a nail spicule, composed of keratotic material, is also usually present.[26] Pigmented variants have also been described, usually owing to melanocytic activation in the matrix.[27] Onychomycosis has also been observed coincidentally in occasional reported lesions. Histologically, although distinctive clinically, a proper diagnosis depends on the nature of the specimen. If the overlying nail plate has been avulsed, and then not submitted, it may be difficult to identify diagnostic features in the remaining nail bed. Significant portions of the epithelium are often removed with the nail plate, a common

occurrence.[28] In an ideal setting, one can find so-called matrical metaplasia in the nail bed. This entity consists of a nucleated zone over the nail bed epithelium, similar to what can be observed in the nail matrix keratogenous zone under normal conditions. More distally, the epithelium may be papillated and hypergranulosis may be evident, simulating a verruca. There is associated parakeratosis and hyperkeratosis most distally, forming the subungual nail spicule. Hemorrhage can be seen in the cornified material overlying the nail bed and within the area of the spicule (**Fig. 9**). When pigmentation is present, melanin granules may be found in the nail bed epithelium, as well as in the keratotic material overlying it.

Onychocytic matricoma Although the first series of 5 cases was reported in 2012,[29] other cases reported under various headings, such as subungual seborrheic keratosis, represent the same entity.[30,31] Clinically, they may present with so-called pachymelanonychia, that is, a thickened

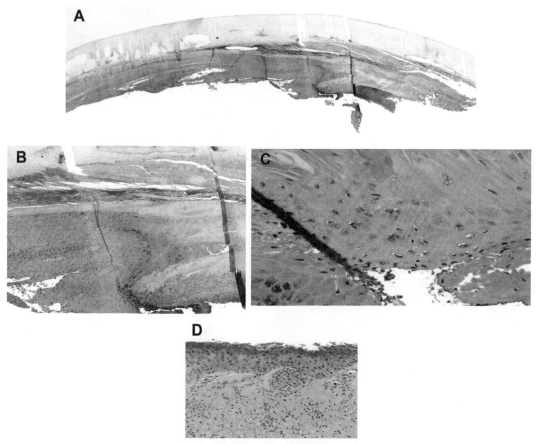

Fig. 9. Onychopapilloma. (*A*) A longitudinal excision is the best way to observe the diagnostic features of this entity, sampling the matrix, bed, and hyponychial area (hematoxylin-eosin, original magnification ×20x). (*B*) Distally, the nail bed epithelium is papillated and demonstrates subungual hyper- and parakeratosis, forming a distal keratotic nail spicule. Hemorrhage is often visible in the subungual space including distally. These changes may simulate a verruca (hematoxylin-eosin, original magnification ×40x). (*C*) In the distal nail bed, slightly enlarged and often multinucleate keratinocytes may be found (hematoxylin-eosin, original magnification ×200x). (*D*) In a different case, after nail plate avulsion, it is fortunate that a portion of the nail bed demonstrating matrical metaplasia could be found. This consists of an area of nail bed that resembles the keratogenous zone of the matrix (hematoxylin-eosin, original magnification ×100x).

and pigmented nail plate. Hypopigmented variants, with a thickened but yellowish nail plate, have also been reported, and these occurrences may simulate onychomatricoma clinically. Histologically, 3 patterns were described in the series of 5 cases, including acanthotic, keratogenous, and papillated. However, the author's experience with a number of similar cases is that the acanthotic and papillated patterns often occur together, and that observation of those features depending on the plane of section visualized for diagnosis. More proximal portions of this benign proliferation usually demonstrate an acanthotic, seborrheic keratosis-like pattern, and more distal portions are papillated, often closely simulating a verruca (**Fig. 10**). The acanthotic pattern may be mistaken for squamous cell carcinoma in situ, but does not demonstrate cytologic atypia. The keratogenous pattern presents as a thickening of the keratogenous zone. Melanin pigment may be present, and scattered melanocytes are present among keratinocytes.

Subungual epidermoid inclusions This benign finding may not be an epithelial neoplasm per se, but its importance lies in being a pitfall in diagnosis, because it can be mistaken for squamous cell carcinoma or onycholemmal carcinoma. These inclusions probably result from implantation of nail bed epithelium in the nail dermis, often as

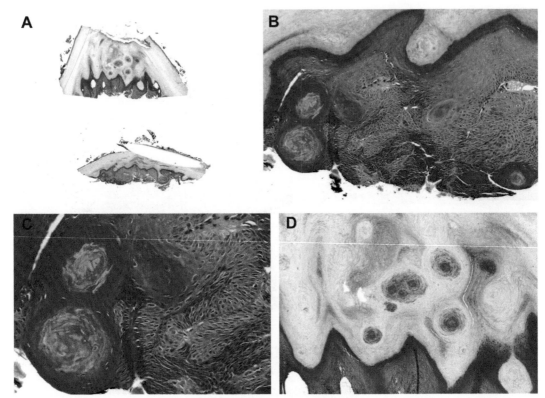

Fig. 10. Onychocytic matricoma. (*A*) This example is transversely sectioned, showing the proximal acanthotic portion of nail matrix with incipient formation of prekeratogenous zones in whorls, below, and the distal papillated nail bed, with the thickened nail plate, above (hematoxylin-eosin, original magnification ×40x). (*B*) The matrical zone is acanthotic and may be pigmented, although not in this case (hematoxylin-eosin, original magnification ×100x). (*C*) A closer view of the prekeratogenous zones with incipient nail plate formation (hematoxylin-eosin, original magnification ×20x). (*D*) The nail plate also contains a whorled pattern based on the contour of the underlying matrix (hematoxylin-eosin, original magnification ×100x).

the result of trauma. They may be found incidentally in a wide variety of other nail conditions, both inflammatory and neoplastic. When a distinctive clinical presentation has been described, it usually consists of a shortened and dystrophic nail plate and nail bed hyperkeratosis.[32–35] Histologically, small aggregates, some cystic and/or elongated, of the nail bed epithelium are found in the nail bed dermis (**Fig. 11**). Some may calcify.

Malignant

Squamous cell carcinoma

Although squamous cell carcinoma represents the most common epithelial malignancy of the nail unit, the incidence is relatively infrequent overall. There is often a link to oncogenic human papilloma virus subtypes. Both in situ and invasive carcinoma often present with a nail dystrophy, mimicking inflammatory nail disease, or even paronychia, and can thus elude diagnosis. Of course, any

monodactylic process should be suspected of being neoplastic until ruled out. Nodular tumors are more likely to be invasive. Histologically, they present similarly to those as other cutaneous sites. Squamous cell carcinoma in situ may be digitate and have other features suggesting a human papilloma virus effect (**Fig. 12**). On occasion, pigmentation may occur and, in this case, longitudinal melanonychia may be the presenting sign.[36]

Keratoacanthoma and subungual tumors of incontinentia pigmenti

Subungual keratoacanthoma, unlike at cutaneous sites, does not display a tendency to involute, and is often painful. Osteolysis may occur. The appearance is similar to a conventional squamous cell carcinoma. A subungual keratotic mass or spicule may form under the nail plate. Histologically, a crateriform to cystic proliferation of keratinocytes, with central hyperkeratosis is typical, and it may impinge on underlying bone. Unusual

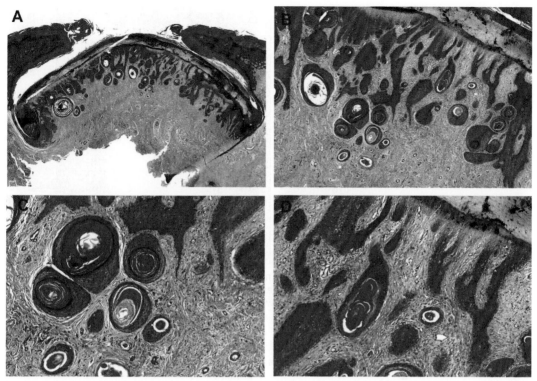

Fig. 11. Subungual epidermoid inclusions. (*A–C*) The nail bed, sectioned transversely, displays many downgrowths of the epithelium, some solid and some more cystic ([A] hematoxylin-eosin, original magnification ×20x; [B] hematoxylin-eosin, original magnification ×40x; [C] hematoxylin-eosin, original magnification ×100x). (*D*) Some of these inclusions resemble ducts (hematoxylin-eosin, original magnification ×100x).

features that distinguish from keratoacanthoma at other sites include multiple dyskeratotic keratinocytes within the epithelium, and calcified keratinocytes and corneocytes[37] (**Fig. 13**). The painful subungual tumors of incontinentia pigmenti[38,39] show identical histologic features.

Melanocytic proliferations

The clinical features of the common entities associated with melanonychia have been covered elsewhere in this article, and so are addressed in more limited fashion here. It is important to note that excellent technical preparation of nail unit sections is especially important when evaluating pigmented lesions of the nail unit. Although there is not enough space for a full discussion of the latter, these references in this area may be of use.[1,2]

Melanocytic activation (hypermelanosis)

Melanocytic activation usually presents with a solitary or with multiple pigmented bands. They tend to be lightly pigmented bands, usually tan or gray. When solitary, they are usually narrow. Melanocytic activation can be found secondarily in many other nail

conditions, including onychomycosis and with various nail neoplasms, as a secondary event, owing to the stimulation of melanin production. Histologically, there is a normal density of single often inconspicuous melanocytes in the matrix (in the range of 4–9 per millimeter across the matrix epithelium[40]), but an increase in melanin. Sometimes, the pigmentation is so sparse that a Fontana stain may be needed to identify it, and may also show occasional thin melanocytic dendrites. Immunostaining, using preferably a nuclear melanocytic marker, such as SOX-10 or MiTF will be needed to assess melanocytic density.[41] Occasionally, such stains fail in the matrix, and Melan-A would be the most reliable stain in this setting. It can overemphasize melanocytic density, however, being a cytoplasmic marker. S100 protein has been shown to be unreliable in this setting, because it may fail to label matrical melanocytes.

Lentigo

Nail unit lentigo usually darker band, brown or sometimes even black, of variable width, although generally narrow. Histologically, there is an increase in single melanocytes, without nests. There

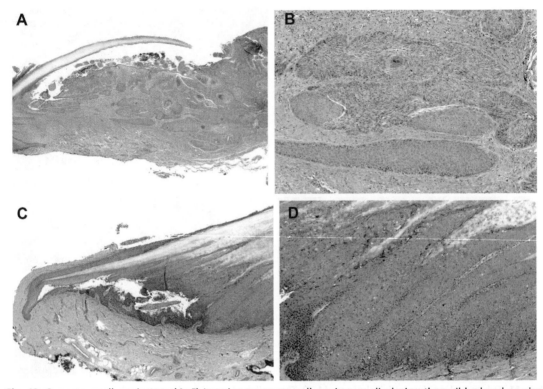

Fig. 12. Squamous cell carcinoma. (*A, B*) Invasive squamous cell carcinoma, displacing the nail bed and causing interruption in the nail plate ([A] hematoxylin-eosin, original magnification ×20x; [B] hematoxylin-eosin, original magnification ×100x). (*C, D*) Squamous cell carcinoma in situ, showing a thickened and digitate epithelium with confluent atypical keratinocytes. Some viropathic changes are present superficially, suggesting oncogenic human papilloma virus effect ([C] hematoxylin-eosin, original magnification ×40x; [D] hematoxylin-eosin, original magnification ×100x).

is usually more intense melanin pigmentation of the nail matrix. Often, melanocytes in this setting will be more conspicuous, although not always, and may be dendritic. Therefore, immunostaining is again useful to identify them (**Fig. 14**). The range of density reported in 1 series is roughly 10 to 31 per mm across the matrix.[40] Melanocytic nuclei are small, and this can be highlighted in a SOX-10 immunostain. An important pitfall is that melanoma in situ may contain relatively lower density areas of single melanocytes. Therefore, attention to any atypical cytologic features, and correlation with clinical findings is crucial in this setting.

Nevus

Nail unit nevi may present in a similar clinical fashion to a lentigo. However, especially in children, they may be broad, and may also involve the periungual skin. Histologically, single melanocytes and nests may be found, and they may be arranged somewhat irregularly, but are generally confined to the lower epithelium. Any significant

suprabasilar scatter in the nail matrix or the finding of melanocytes in the nail plate should raise some concern. Extension onto the nail bed, or eponychial epithelium (ventral nail fold) may indicate poor circumscription, and should also raise concern. However, again, such findings are not unusual in children.[42,43] Most nail unit nevi are junctional, and discrete nests are reassuring (see **Fig. 14**). Compound nevi are relatively rare. On occasion, junctional nevi in the matrix may be accompanied by compound features in periungual skin. Melanocytes are generally cytologically bland, with small nuclei. Pigmented epithelioid melanocytes can be observed with more abundant dusty cytoplasmic melanin. Spitz nevus-like epithelioid and spindled cytologic features may also occur. Heavily melanized nevi are challenging to evaluate, because the background epithelium may be nearly black in some cases, complicating the assessment of the density and distribution of the melanocytes. In this case, immunostaining with a red chromogen is especially crucial. It is

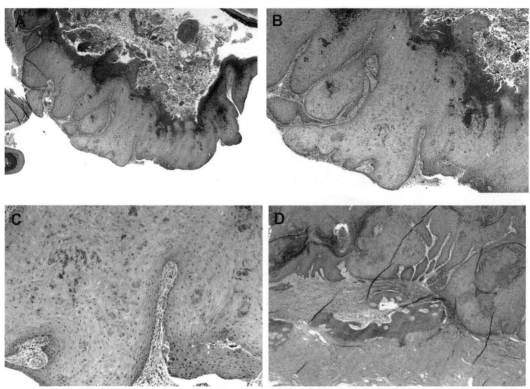

Fig. 13. Keratoacanthoma and subungual tumors of incontinentia pigmenti. (*A–C*) Typical crateriform to cystic contour with lobules of eosinophilic keratinocytes, and many dyskeratotic keratinocytes, which are distinctive in the subungual variant ([A] hematoxylin-eosin, original magnification ×20x; [B] hematoxylin-eosin, original magnification×40x; [C] hematoxylin-eosin, original magnification ×100x). (*D*) Osteolysis is common, including in this example of a subungual tumor or incontinentia pigmenti, which shares other features of keratoacanthoma (hematoxylin-eosin, original magnification ×40x).

paramount to keep in mind that reports of nail unit melanoma in children are exceedingly rare, so as not to overinterpret unusual histologic findings.

Melanoma

Nail unit melanoma and generally presents as a broader, irregularly pigmented band, with irregular lines within it. As it extends from its usual origin in the nail matrix, it may involve the periungual skin, including the proximal nail fold, as well as the nail bed, hyponychium, and lateral nail folds (Hutchinson sign). Amelanotic melanoma usually arises from the nail bed, where melanocytes do not generally produce melanin pigment. This entity may present with nail destruction, features similar to pyogenic granuloma, or it may mimic other nail tumors, such as squamous cell carcinoma. Histologically, early nail unit melanoma in situ may be very difficult to distinguish from a lentigo. However, the density of single melanocytes is generally greater, in 1 series in the range of 39 to 136 (mean, 58.9)[40] It is worth

noting that the high end of density reported in this series in lentigo and the low end of melanoma in situ are very close, and low cellularity areas of melanoma captured in partial biopsies can create a diagnostic pitfall. Therefore, it is important to rely on other diagnostic clues as well, such as cytologic atypia (melanocytes with large hyperchromatic nuclei),[41,44] anisodendrocytosis (melanocytic dendrites of varying thickness), poor circumscription, and suprabasilar scatter of melanocytes, including melanocytes within the nail plate on occasion. An avulsed nail plate and its attached epithelium should be scrutinized for such clues as well.[45] As for other melanocytic lesions at this site, immunostaining is often critical in examining melanocytic density and other features such as circumscription (**Fig. 15**). SOX-10, Melan-A, MiTF, and HMB45 stains tend to work in the nail matrix, but S100 protein may be negative.[46] MiTF staining creates a pitfall, because it stains the nuclei of keratinocytes in the superficial nail matrix.[41] Melanoma in situ

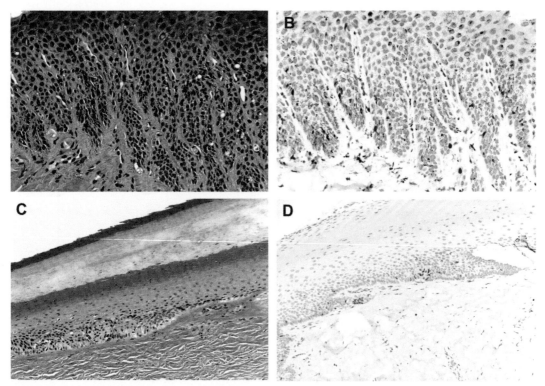

Fig. 14. Nail unit lentigo and nevus. (*A*) Lentigo: Pigmentation of the matrix epithelium is accompanied by an increase in single melanocytes which may be difficult to identify in routine sections (hematoxylin-eosin, original magnification ×200x). (*B*) SOX-10 immunostain with red chromogen is helpful in quantifying melanocytes (SOX-10, 100x). (*C*) Nevus: Longitudinal excision with a mostly nested proliferation of melanocytes, in a child (hematoxylin-eosin, original magnification ×100x). (*D*) SOX-10 immunostain helps to delineate nests and occasional single melanocytes along the junctional zone (SOX-10, 100x).

involving the periungual skin may be of low density and sometimes is cytologically relatively bland (see **Fig. 17**). The Hutchinson sign may sometimes consist only of melanin pigmentation.[47] Newer immunostains such as p16 have yet to show promise diagnostically in this area in smaller studies.[48] Regression at this site may create a lichen planus-like inflammatory pattern that can present another diagnostic pitfall. Invasive nail unit melanoma is usually less difficult to diagnose, with a dermal component of atypical cells, some in mitosis. Desmoplastic and myxoid variants may occur as well (**Figs. 16** and **17**). Molecular techniques have not been extensively studied in lesions here, but the author and other investigators[49] have had some experience using fluorescence in situ hybridization analysis, which is useful in lower cellularity lesions. Other techniques such as comparative genomic hybridization can also be used, but require a greater volume of DNA. Whole exome sequencing has suggested some differences between nail unit melanoma and acral melanoma.[50]

SUMMARY

In this article, we have explored the histologic features of a range of inflammatory, infectious, and neoplastic conditions, both common and uncommon. Understanding the pathology of these disorders enhances clinical acumen and may affect choice of biopsy procedures and treatment measures, with the outcome of better clinical care for patients with nail disease.

CLINICS CARE POINTS

- Nail clippings can be a less invasive method to make a diagnosis of nail disease, from onychomycosis to onychomatricoma.
- Melanonychia in children can display concerning clinical and histopathologic findings. However, melanoma of the nail unit in children is exceptionally rare and therefore there should be a high level of skepticism when such a diagnosis is made.
- Sampling of low cellularity areas of nail unit melanoma is a diagnostic pitfall especially in

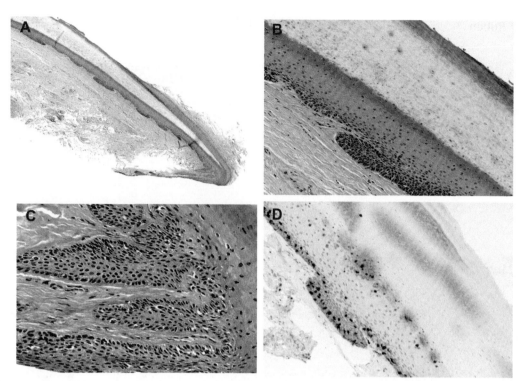

Fig. 15. Melanoma in situ. (*A–C*) A low cellularity example of melanoma in situ, but with atypical melanocytes containing hyperchromatic nuclei in irregular array within matrical epithelium and also in the nail plate ([A] hematoxylin-eosin, original magnification ×20x) ([B] hematoxylin-eosin, original magnification ×100x; [C] hematoxylin-eosin, original magnification ×400x). (*D*) MiTF immunostain highlights the irregular density and distribution of melanocytes, including within nail plate. A pitfall is that this stain also labels the smaller nuclei of keratinocytes in the superficial keratogenous zone which in this image are admixed with slightly darker-staining melanocytes (MiTF, 100x).

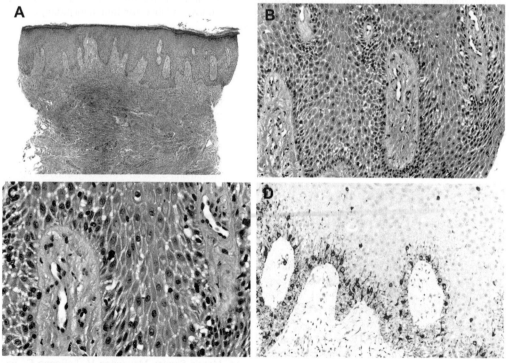

Fig. 16. Hutchinson sign in invasive melanoma. (*A–C*) This was the initial biopsy of the tumor pictured in **Fig. 17**, taken from the proximal nail fold area. This illustrates the possible pitfall in biopsies of the Hutchinson sign (periungual pigmentation), which can be hypocellular, and in this case, also obscured by spongiosis ([A] hematoxylin-eosin, original magnification ×40x; [B] hematoxylin-eosin, original magnification ×100x; [C] hematoxylin-eosin, original magnification ×200x). (*D*) Melan-A immunostain was helpful in confirming that many melanocytes are actually present and in pagetoid array (Original magnification ×100x).

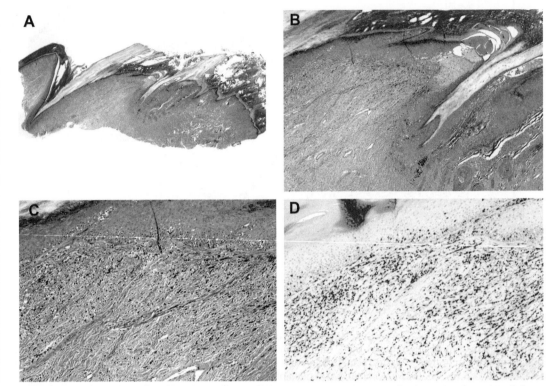

Fig. 17. Melanoma, invasive. (*A–C*) This invasive melanoma sampled in a longitudinal excision, has caused disruption of the nail plate. It involves the matrix and nail bed, and the nail dermis in a spindled/desmoplastic pattern ([A] hematoxylin-eosin, original magnification ×20x; [B] hematoxylin-eosin, original magnification ×40x; [C] hematoxylin-eosin, original magnification ×100x). (*D*) SOX-10 immunostain labels the tumor, including the desmoplastic invasive component (Original magnification ×100x).

adults. If the clinician is highly suspicious of melanoma clinically, and the pathology report seems benign, it may be useful to discuss with the dermatopathologist.

DISCLOSURE

The author has nothing to disclose.

REFERENCES

1. Wlodek C, Lecerf P, Andre J, et al. An international survey about nail histology processing techniques. J Cutan Pathol 2017;44(9):749–56.
2. Ruben BS. Histology techniques for nails. In: Rubin AI, Jellinek NJ, Daniel III CR, et al, editors. Scher and Daniel's Nails: Diagnosis, Surgery, Therapy. 4th edition. Cham, Switzerland: Springer; 2018. p. 29–38.
3. Jiaravuthisan MM, Sasseville D, Vender RB, et al. Psoriasis of the nail: anatomy, pathology, clinical presentation, and a review of the literature on therapy. J Am Acad Dermatol 2007;57(1):1–27.
4. Zaias N. Psoriasis of the nail. A clinical-pathologic study. Arch Dermatol 1969;99(5):567–79.
5. Holzberg M, Ruben BS, Baran R. Psoriasis restricted to the nail in a 7-year-old child. Should biologics be an appropriate treatment modality when considering quality of life? J Eur Acad Dermatol Venereol 2014; 28(5):668–70.
6. Werner B, Fonseca GP, Seidel G. Microscopic nail clipping findings in patients with psoriasis. Am J Dermatopathol 2015;37(6):429–39.
7. Goettmann S, Zaraa I, Moulonguet I. Nail lichen planus: epidemiological, clinical, pathological, therapeutic and prognosis study of 67 cases. J Eur Acad Dermatol Venereol 2012;26(10):1304–9.
8. Fanti PA, Tosti A, Cameli N, et al. Nail matrix hypergranulosis. Am J Dermatopathol 1994;16(6):607–10.
9. Tosti A, Peluso AM, Misciali C, et al. Nail lichen striatus: clinical features and long-term follow-up of five patients. J Am Acad Dermatol 1997;36(6 Pt 1): 908–13.
10. Kim M, Jung HY, Eun YS, et al. Nail lichen striatus: report of seven cases and review of the literature. Int J Dermatol 2015;54(11):1255–60.
11. Mattos Simoes Mendonca M, LaSenna C, Tosti A. Severe onychodystrophy due to allergic contact dermatitis from acrylic nails. Skin Appendage Disord 2015;1(2):91–4.

12. Tosti A, Bardazzi F, Piraccini BM, et al. Idiopathic tra-chyonychia (twenty-nail dystrophy): a pathological study of 23 patients. Br J Dermatol 1994;131(6): 866–72.

13. Starace M, Alessandrini A, Bruni F, et al. Trachyony-chia: a retrospective study of 122 patients in a period of 30 years. J Eur Acad Dermatol Venereol 2020. https://doi.org/10.1111/jdv.16186.

14. Lawry MA, Haneke E, Strobeck K, et al. Methods for diagnosing onychomycosis: a comparative study and review of the literature. Arch Dermatol 2000; 136(9):1112–6.

15. Hsiao Y-P, Lin H-S, Wu T-W, et al. A comparative study of KOH test, PAS staining and fungal culture in diagnosis of onychomycosis in Taiwan. J Dermatol Sci 2007;45(2):138–40.

16. Gupta AK, Ricci M-J. Diagnosing onychomycosis. Dermatol Clin 2006;24(3):365–9.

17. Burkhart CN, Burkhart CG, Gupta AK. Dermatophy-toma: recalcitrance to treatment because of exis-tence of fungal biofilm. J Am Acad Dermatol 2002; 47(4):629–31.

18. Baran R, Kint A. Onychomatrixoma. Filamentous tufted tumour in the matrix of a funnel-shaped nail: a new entity (report of three cases). Br J Dermatol 1992;126(5):510–5.

19. Perrin C, Baran R, Pisani A, et al. The onychomatri-coma: additional histologic criteria and immunohis-tochemical study. Am J Dermatopathol 2002;24(3): 199–203.

20. Perrin C, Baran R, Balaguer T, et al. Onychomatri-coma: new clinical and histological features. A re-view of 19 tumors. Am J Dermatopathol 2010; 32(1):1–8.

21. Di Chiacchio N, Tavares GT, Tosti A, et al. Onycho-matricoma: epidemiological and clinical findings in a large series of 30 cases. Br J Dermatol 2015; 173(5):1305–7.

22. Reserva JL, Ruben BS, Venna SS. Asymptomatic longitudinal pachyxanthonychia of the fingernail. Skin Appendage Disord 2017;3(1):32–5.

23. Fernandez-Flores' A, Barja-Lopez J-M. Pleomorphic onychomatricoma. J Cutan Pathol 2014;41(7): 555–60.

24. Miteva M, de Farias DC, Zaiac M, et al. Nail clipping diagnosis of onychomatricoma. Arch Dermatol 2011;147(9):1117–8.

25. Tallon B, Strydom F, Emanuel PO. Nail plate clues to a remote diagnosis. J Cutan Pathol 2013;40(1):2–3.

26. Tosti A, Schneider SL, Ramirez-Quizon MN, et al. Clinical, dermoscopic, and pathologic features of onychopapilloma: a review of 47 cases. J Am Acad Dermatol 2016;74(3):521–6.

27. Miteva M, Fanti PA, Romanelli P, et al. Onychopapil-loma presenting as longitudinal melanonychia. J Am Acad Dermatol 2012;66(6):e242–3.

28. Delvaux C, Richert B, Lecerf P, et al. Onychopapillo-mas: a 68-case series to determine best surgical procedure and histologic sectioning. J Eur Acad Dermatol Venereol 2018;32(11):2025–30.

29. Perrin C, Cannata GE, Bossard C, et al. Onychocytic matricoma presenting as pachymelanonychia longi-tudinal. A new entity (report of five cases). Am J Der-matopathol 2012;34(1):54–9.

30. Bon-Mardion M, Poulalhon N, Balme B, et al. Ungual seborrheic keratosis. J Eur Acad Dermatol Venereol 2010;24(9):1102–4.

31. Baran R, Moulonguet I, Goettmann-Bonvallot S, et al. Longitudinal subungual acanthoma: one denomina-tion for various clinical presentations. J Eur Acad Der-matol Venereol 2018;32(9):1608–13.

32. Fanti PA, Tosti A. Subungual epidermoid inclusions: report of 8 cases. Dermatologica 1989;178(4): 209–12.

33. Bukhari IA, Al-Mugharbel R. Subungual epidermoid inclusions. Saudi Med J 2004;25(4):522–3.

34. Telang GH, Jellinek N. Multiple calcified subungual epidermoid inclusions. J Am Acad Dermatol 2007; 56(2):336–9.

35. Ruben BS, LeBoit PE. Subungual epidermoid inclu-sions: an underappreciated diagnostic pitfall in inter-pretation of nail unit biopsies. J Cutan Pathol 2008; 35(1):97.

36. Baran R, Simon C. Longitudinal melanonychia: a symptom of Bowen's disease. J Am Acad Dermatol 1988;18(6):1359–60.

37. Stoll DM, Ackerman AB. Subungual keratoacan-thoma. Am J Dermatopathol 1980;2(3):265–71.

38. Montes CM, Maize JC, Guerry-Force ML. Inconti-nentia pigmenti with painful subungual tumors: a two-generation study. J Am Acad Dermatol 2004; 50(2 Suppl):S45–52.

39. Malvehy J, Palou J, Mascaró JM. Painful subungual tumour in incontinentia pigmenti. Response to treat-ment with etretinate. Br J Dermatol 1998;138(3):554–5.

40. Amin B, Nehal KS, Jungbluth AA, et al. Histologic distinction between subungual lentigo and mela-noma. Am J Surg Pathol 2008;32(6):835–43.

41. Ruben BS. Pigmented lesions of the nail unit. Semin Cutan Med Surg 2015;34(2):101–8.

42. Lee JH, Lim Y, Park J-H, et al. Clinicopathologic fea-tures of 28 cases of nail matrix nevi (NMNs) in Asians: comparison between children and adults. J Am Acad Dermatol 2018;78(3):479–89.

43. Cooper C, Arva NC, Lee C, et al. A clinical, histo-pathologic, and outcome study of melanonychia striata in childhood. J Am Acad Dermatol 2015; 72(5):773–9.

44. Park S-W, Jang K-T, Lee J-H, et al. Scattered atyp-ical melanocytes with hyperchromatic nuclei in the nail matrix: diagnostic clue for early subungual mel-anoma in situ. J Cutan Pathol 2016;43(1):41–52.

45. Ruben BS, McCalmont TH. The importance of attached nail plate epithelium in the diagnosis of nail apparatus melanoma. J Cutan Pathol 2010; 37(10):1028–9, 1027.

46. Theunis A, Richert B, Sass U, et al. Immunohistochemical study of 40 cases of longitudinal melanonychia. Am J Dermatopathol 2011;33(1): 27–34.

47. Baran LR, Ruben BS, Kechijian P, et al. Non-melanoma Hutchinson's sign: a reappraisal of this important, remarkable melanoma simulant. J Eur Acad Dermatol Venereol 2018;32(3):495–501.

48. Chu A, André J, Rich P, et al. Immunohistochemical characterization of benign activation of junctional melanocytes and melanoma in situ of the nail unit. J Cutan Pathol 2019;46(7):479–83.

49. Romano RC, Shon W, Sukov WR. Malignant melanoma of the nail apparatus: a fluorescence in situ hybridization analysis of 7 cases. Int J Surg Pathol 2016;24(6):512–8.

50. Lee M, Yoon J, Chung Y-J, et al. Whole-exome sequencing reveals differences between nail apparatus melanoma and acral melanoma. J Am Acad Dermatol 2018;79(3):559–61.e1.

Concepts, Role, and Advances on Nail Imaging

Ximena Wortsman, MD

KEYWORDS

- Nail imaging Ultrasound nail • Nail ultrasound • Dermatologic ultrasound • Ultrasound dermatology
- Nail • Ultrasound

KEY POINTS

- There are several imaging techniques for studying the nail, and all of them require proper devices and trained operators.
- Currently, among imaging techniques, the better axial spatial resolution and the more extensive range of applications are provided by ultrasound, which currently is the first-choice imaging technique for evaluating nail conditions.
- A correlation of state-of-the-art clinical and imaging figures supports the review of this topic.

INTRODUCTION

Imaging of the nail has evolved from old radiographs to the generation of super–high-resolution ultrasound images that allow observing, with high-definition submillimeter alterations, of the nail unit and periungual tissues.[1]

The most common imaging techniques are radiographs, ultrasound, computed tomography (CT), and magnetic resonance imaging (MRI).[2] The capabilities of each imaging technique are dynamic and can vary significantly over time due to the constant advances in the imaging field. Nowadays, in the superficial structures field, the highest-resolution images are provided by ultrasound because its axial resolution can vary from 100 μm at 15 MHz to 30 μm at 70 MHz.[3,4] This capability implies that ultrasound can distinguish submillimeter changes that can be as small as 0.05 mm.[4]

Currently, MRI, using commercially available devices, presents a lower axial resolution compared to ultrasound that goes up to 500 μm, using 1.5T devices and up to 100 μm in the new 7T machines.[5] The latter fact means that on MRI, the lesions of the nail that measure less than 3 mm may be challenging to discriminate.[6]

In addition, MRI commonly requires the intravenous injection of contrast media (gadolinium) that

potentially can be nephrotoxic.[7] In contrast, ultrasound can detect submillimeter structures and characterize the type and velocity of the blood flow noninvasively through the color Doppler application.[1,8] Moreover, ultrasound is considered safe and commonly is performed on pregnant women and infants.

Nevertheless, MRI is useful for studying the alterations of the medulla of the bone, which are not possible to detect on ultrasound because the calcium of the bony cortex tends to stop the passage of the sound waves.[2]

CT rarely is used for studying nail conditions; however, it may be helpful in the detection of bony changes in tumoral or traumatic conditions of the fingers and toes.[9]

To date, ultrasonography can help diagnosis in a wide range of ungual conditions, such as benign and malignant tumors, inflammatory diseases, and location abnormalities.[1,2,8–10]

MRI mostly is used for studying some tumoral or pseudotumoral conditions that involve the medulla of the bone.[2,9,11]

Imaging should provide the lesional origin (ungual or periungual), size in all axes (millimeters), exact location, degree of vascularity, and involvement of adjacent tissues.[1,8,12] These anatomic

Funding: None.

Institute for Diagnostic Imaging and Research of the Skin and Soft Tissues, Departments of Dermatology, Universidad de Chile and Pontificia Universidad Católica de Chile, Lo Fontecilla 201, of 734, Las Condes, Santiago 7591018, Chile

E-mail address: xworts@yahoo.com

Dermatol Clin 39 (2021) 337–350

https://doi.org/10.1016/j.det.2020.12.010

data can help select the best site and the extent of the incision and decrease the potential cosmetic sequel of a nail biopsy.

TECHNICAL CONSIDERATIONS

Any imaging technique needs both a proper device and a trained operator, which may influence the decision of the type of examination in an institution.[13] On ultrasound, there is a growing number of publications on nail pathologies, including guidelines and international training courses.[14,15] MRI usually is part of the training of residency programs in radiology; however, the superficial structures pathologies can be a vast world that needs additional training and constant exposure.

For studying the nail, ultrasound requires multichannel devices that work with variable frequency, that are linear or compact linear, and that have probes with frequencies greater than or equal to 15 and currently can go up to 70 MHz[1,4]; these 70-MHz probes offer a much higher resolution, but their penetration into the tissues is lower.[4] Nevertheless, most of the ultrasound machines have 2 or 3 probes that work at different frequencies, which helps keep a high-definition view through all the layers.

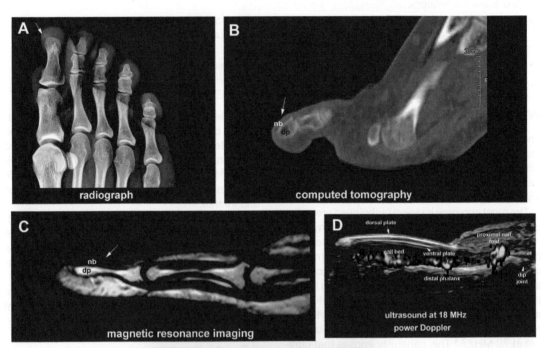

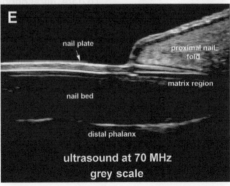

Fig. 1. Different imaging techniques for studying the nail. A, radiograph; B, computed tomography; C, magnetic resonance; D, ultrasound at 18 MHz and E, ultrasound at 70 MHz. Notice the difference in resolution between all of them. The arrows (A–C) point out the nail region. (D) Presents a power Doppler image of the nail (application of Doppler to detect slow flow) that shows the normal vascularity located in the deeper two-thirds of the nail bed. (E) At 70 MHz (gray scale), there is a higher definition of the nail unit. dip, distal interphalangeal joint; dp, distal phalanx; et, extensor tendon, nb, nail bed; np, nail plate.

The limitations of ultrasound are the detection of pigments, such as melanin and lesions, that measure less than 0.1 mm at 18 MHz and less than 0.05 mm at 70 MHz.[3,4] The limitations of MRI and CT are the detection of lesions that measure less than 3 mm to 5 mm.[6,11] MRI has issues for detecting small calcifications in the soft tissues.[16] CT does not detect pigments and MRI can track some types, such as hemosiderin depending on the amount.[9]

CT is a radiating imaging technique[13] and commonly requires intravenous injection of contrast media with a potential nephrotoxic agent. Despite complications due to radiation and nephroxicity in CT are rare its request should consider the benefits versus the potential harms.[17]

ULTRASOUND OF THE NORMAL ANATOMY OF THE NAIL

At 15 MHz to 24 MHz, the nail plate shows as a hyperechoic bilaminar band with dorsal and ventral plates with an anechoic interplate space in-between the plates.[1,2,8,10,18,19] At 70 MHz, this interplate space turns to slightly hyperechoic.[1] The nail bed appears as a hypoechoic band beneath the nail plate that turns to slightly hyperechoic at the matrix region.[1,8,18,19]

The periungual tissues show the same appearance of the normal skin (a laminar hyperechoic epidermis and a hyperechoic dermal band, less bright than the epidermis). Arterial and venous low-velocity vessels usually are detected in the deeper two-thirds of the nail bed. The bony margin of the distal phalanx appears as a hyperechoic line. In the vicinity, there is the hyperechoic band of the extensor tendon and the anechoic space of the distal interphalangeal joint (DIP). The bony margin of the distal phalanx shows as a hyperechoic line.[1,8,18,19]

On MRI, using proton density and T1-weighted images, the normal nail plate appears as a single very hypointense band and the nail bed as a hypointense space[20] (Fig. 1).

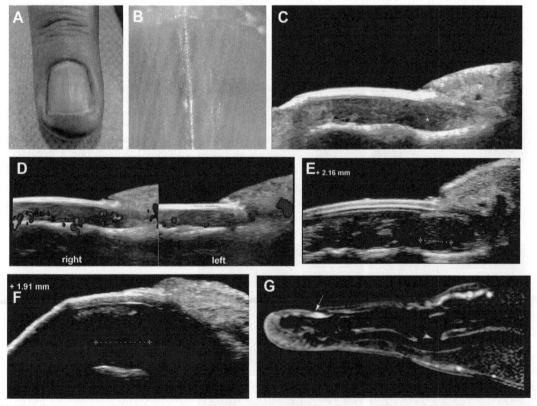

Fig. 2. Glomus tumor. (*A*) Clinical image. (*B*) Dermoscopy view. (*C*) Ultrasound (gray scale at 18 MHz) demonstrates an oval-shaped, well-defined hypoechoic structure (*asterisk*) located in the radial aspect of the proximal part of the nail bed of the right ring finger with scalloping of the underlying bony margin. (*D*) Color Doppler ultrasound (side-by-side, comparative views at 18 MHz right, showing the tumor and left presenting the normal side) shows slight hypervascularity of the proximal part of the nail bed in the right ring finger. Ultrasound at 70-MHz: (*E*) longitudinal and (*F*) transverse views present a 2.16-mm × 1.91-mm hypoechoic nodule with a higher definition (between markers). (*G*) MRI (STIR, short-tau inversion recovery sequence) demonstrates a hypertense area in the proximal part of the nail bed that corresponds to the location of the tumor (arrow).

COMMON APPLICATIONS OF ULTRASOUND IMAGING OF THE NAIL
Benign Tumors and Pseudotumors

For academic purposes, the conditions are separated according to their nature (solid and cystic).

Solid

Glomus tumors Glomus tumors are derived from the neuromyoarterial plexus, and their most common location is the nail bed.[1,2,10,11,13,21–26] They may be found, however, in the periungual tissues.[27] On ultrasound, they frequently appear as a well-defined oval-shaped nodule in the nail bed that produces scalloping of the bony margin of the distal phalanx.[1,8,18,19,21–25] On color Doppler, they commonly are hypervascular with slow flow arterial vessels; however, some less frequent variants, such as glomangiomyomas. may present hypovascularity.[1] On MRI, they appear as a well-marginated, round or oval, hypointense subungual lesions in the T1-weighted images that turn into hyperintense lesions, sometimes with a hypointense rim on the T2-weighted images (**Fig. 2**).[2,9,20] Nevertheless, small glomus tumors (less than or equal to 3 mm) may not be detected

or possible to discriminate from other subungual entities on MRI.[6,11]

Ungual and periungual fibromatous tumors The heterogeneous group of ungual and periungual fibromatous benign tumors commonly show as subungual and periungual eccentric hypoechoic structures or bands. Subungual fibromas usually involve the lateral nail fold and show as ill-defined or lobulated areas that extrinsically compress the nail plate and remodel the bony margin. Periungual fibromas frequently present as well-defined bandlike structures that involve the proximal nail fold, where they extrinsically compress the origin of the nail plate and, therefore, the matrix region.[1,2,8,23] Fibrokeratomas, another variant, usually present in their distal part an irregular hyperechoic area caused by hyperkeratosis.[1] On color Doppler, fibromas commonly show a hypovascular pattern.[1,8,23] Nevertheless, some variants, such as angiofibromas, can present prominent vascularity or a central vascular pedicle (**Fig. 3**).[1,8,23]

On MRI, fibromas show hypointensity in all the sequences; however, occasionally, due to the presence of mucoid material, they may appear

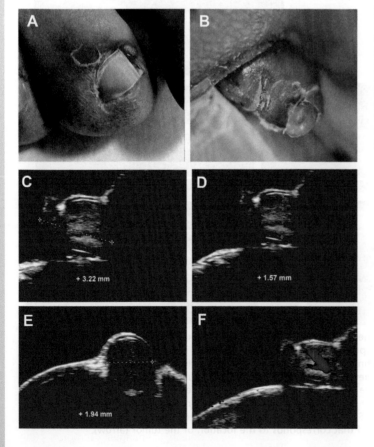

Fig. 3. Periungual angiofibroma. (*A*) Clinical photograph. (*B*) Dermoscopy view. Ultrasound images at 70 MHZ (gray scale: [*C*, *D*] longitudinal view, [*E*] transverse view, and [*F*] color Doppler) demonstrate a hypoechoic well-defined hypoechoic band measuring 3.22 mm (longitudinal) × 1.57 mm (thickness) × 1.94 mm (transverse) with a central vascular pedicle (colors [*F*] colors).

as slightly heterogeneous or hyperintense onT2-weighted images.[2,21]

Onychomatricoma Onychomatricoma is an ungual benign tumor derived from the nail matrix, and its typical ultrasound pattern is characterized by an ill-defined, eccentric, and proximal hypoechoic subungual structure with multiple hyperechoic lines that protrude into the nail plate and also may involve the proximal nail fold.[1,8,23,28] On color Doppler, it presents a variable degree of internal blood flow that can go from hypovascular to an intermediate degree of vascularity (**Fig. 4**).[1,8,23,28] On MRI, it shows on T2 as a hyperintense mass with filamentous extensions and enhancement after the injection of gadolinium.[20,21,29]

Ungual and periungual granuloma Ungual granuloma is a pseudotumor that usually is generated or associated with chronic inflammation and trauma.[1] On ultrasound, subungual granulomas show as an ill-defined thickening and hypoechoic area in the nail bed that displaces the nail plate upward.[1,8] On color Doppler, subungual vascularity is variable and can go from hypovascular to hypervascular (telangiectatic or pyogenic variant).[1,8]

The telangiectatic subungual granulomas may mimic amelanotic melanoma due to their intense hypervascularity.[30] The telangiectatic variant of granulomas, however, commonly affects the proximal nail fold and present as a network of multiple and tortuous hypervascular spaces (**Fig. 5**).[1]

On MRI, it has been described as isointense on T1-weighted images and hyperintense on T2-weighted images, and with intense enhancement after gadolinium injection.[20,21]

Subungual exostosis and osteochondromas Subungual exostosis and osteochondromas are benign bony outgrowths derived from the distal phalanx that protrude into the nail bed.

On ultrasound, exostosis show as hyperechoic bands with posterior acoustic shadowing artifact.[1,8,18,23] Osteochondromas may present as an irregular hyperechoic band; however, the cartilaginous part of this benign tumor shows a hypoechoic cap.[1,8,10,18,23] There are thickening and hypoechogenicity of the nail bed due to inflammatory and granulomatous reaction. Thickening and irregularities in the nail plate also are observed (**Fig. 6**).[1,2,8,10,18,23]

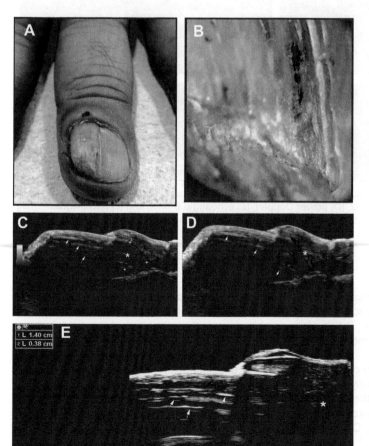

Fig. 4. Onychomatricoma. (*A*) Clinical image. (*B*) Dermoscopy view. Longitudinal ultrasound views ([*C*] gray scale and [*D*] color Doppler ultrasound at 18 MHz; [*E*] gray scale at 70 MHz) present an ill-defined hypoechoic mass (*asterisk*) in the proximal part of the nail bed measuring 1.4 cm (longitudinal) × 0.38 cm (thickness) with hyperechoic lines (*arrows*) that protrudes into the interplate space of the nail plate. (*D*) Notice the mild hypervascularity.

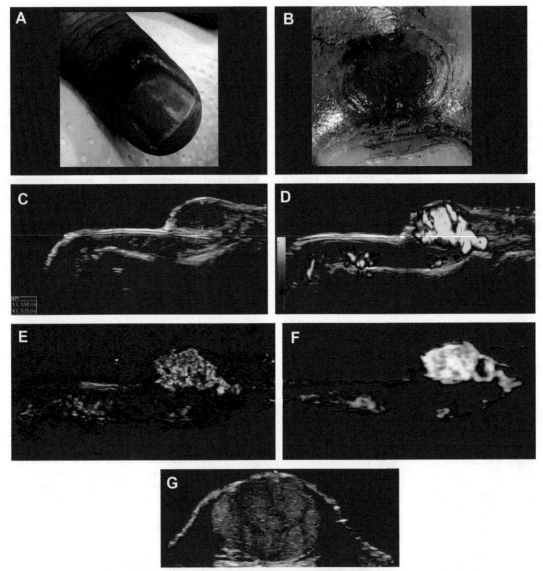

Fig. 5. Telangiectatic (pyogenic) periungual granuloma. (*A*). Clinical photograph. (*B*) Dermoscopy view.(*C–G*) Ultrasound images ([*C*] gray scale at 18 MHz, [*D*] power Doppler, [*E*] echoangio B-flow, and [*F*] microvascular imaging [*G*] gray scale at 70 MHz) presents a 5.0-mm [longitudinal] × 0.25-mm [thickness] hypervascular nodule with numerous tortuous vessels in the dermis and subcutis of the proximal nail fold.

On MRI, they present as hypointense and hyperintense areas that enhance on postcontrast T1-weighted fat-saturated sequences. The hyaline cartilage of osteochondromas is hyperintense on T2-weighted images.[2,20,21]

Radiographs would be enough to confirm subungual exostoses; however, clinically, they can mimic other ungual pathologies; therefore, it is not uncommon that subungual exostoses are imaged first by ultrasound or MRI. CT also may detect them, depending on the size.[1]

Cystic Synovial or myxoid cyst
Synovial or myxoid cysts are composed of a variable degree of proliferation of the synovium and synovial mucous fluid that extend into the proximal nail fold and rarely into the nail bed.[23]

On ultrasound, they appear as a well-defined oval-shaped structure with echoes and connected with the DIP.[1,8,10,23] Frequently, there are signs of osteoarthrosis in the DIP.[1,8,23] The nail plate commonly presents a concavity in the same axis of the periungual cyst due to the extrinsic

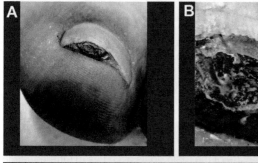
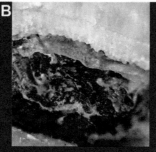
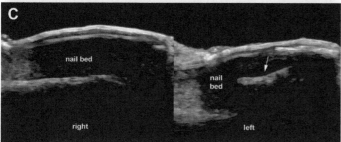
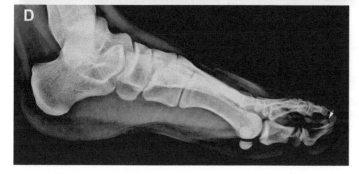

Fig. 6. Subungual exostosis. (*A*) Clinical photograph. (*B*) Dermoscopy. (*C*) Ultrasound at 18 MHz (side-by-side, comparative view; right, normal side and left side with the exostosis) shows a hyperechoic band (*arrow*) that corresponds to the exostosis located in the left big toe. Notice the difference with the normal contralateral side. (*D*) Radiograph (oblique view) shows a bony outgrowth on the surface of the left big toe (*arrow*).

compression of the nail plate.[1,8,23] On color Doppler, these cystic lesions are avascular; nevertheless, the proximal nail fold can show hypervascularity depending on the level of inflammation (**Fig. 7**).[1,23]

Ultrasound helps to locate the connection between the cyst and the DIP; therefore, recurrences may be avoided.[1,8,23]

On MRI, these cysts present as hyperintense on T2weighted images and show early peripheral enhancement in fat-saturated T1-weighted images.[2,20,21]

Malignant Tumors of the Nail

Squamous cell carcinoma

On ultrasound, squamous cell carcinoma shows as an ill-defined and eccentric hypoechoic or heterogeneous structure that commonly erodes the nail plate and the bony margin of the distal phalanx and can extend into the periungual folds. On color

Doppler, it commonly is hypervascular with irregular vessels (**Fig. 8**).[1,8,18]

On MRI, these tumors are hypointense on T1-weighted images, intermediate to hyperintense signal on T2-weighted images, and enhance after gadolinium in fat-saturated T1-weighted images.[31]

Subungual melanoma

Even though the detection of pigments, such as melanin, is one of the limitations of ultrasound,[3] it is possible in some cases to detect a masslike structure. Depending on the stage of invasion, subungual melanomas can show as an asymmetric area of hypervascularity in the nail bed without a perceptible mass or as an ill-defined hypoechoic and hypervascular subungual mass that can erode the nail plate and the bony margin (**Fig. 9**).[1,2,8]

On MRI, subungual melanomas' signal intensity depends on their amount of melanin; therefore, melanotic tumors show as hyperintense on T1-weighted images and hypointense on T2-weighted

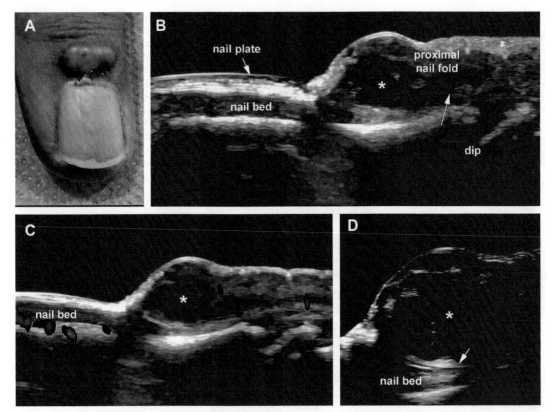

Fig. 7. Myxoid cyst connected to the DIP. (*A*). Clinical image. Ultrasound images ([*B*] gray scale and [*C*] color Doppler at 18 MHz; [*D*] gray scale at 70 MHz) demonstrate oval-shaped, slightly lobulated, anechoic cystic structure (*asterisk*) in the dermis and subcutis of the proximal nail fold connected to the dorsum of the DIP through a thin and tortuous tract ([*B*] *arrow pointing up*). (*D*) Notice the echoes inside the cyst that imply a mucous content and the extrinsic compression of the proximal nail plate ([*D*] *arrow*). dip, distal interphalangeal joint.

images, amelanotic or poorly melanotic as hypointense on T1-weighted images, and intermediate to hyperintense on T2-weighted images.[2,21]

The detection of melanoma and melanoma metastases on MRI and PET CT also depends on the size of the tumor; therefore, tumors measuring less than 3 mm on MRI or metastases measuring less than 5 mm in PET CT may present false-negative results.[32,33]

PET-CT staging of melanomas can show false-positive results under inflammation, among other causes.[32,33]

Growth and Location Alterations

In growth and location alteration abnormalities, ultrasound is the only reported technique that has described patterns of alterations.

Onychocryptosis

On ultrasound, it is possible to detect the location and size of the fragment of the nail plate that is abnormally located in the periungual region.[1,8,18]

The nail plate fragment shows as a bilaminar hyperechoic band in the lateral nail fold. The

dermis of the nail fold presents thickening and decreased echogenicity due to the inflammation. On color Doppler, there is a variable degree of hypervascularity in the periphery of the fragment (**Fig. 10**).[1,8,18]

Onychomadesis and retronychia

Onychomadesis implies a fragmentation of the nail plate, which frequently is associated with inflammation of the nail bed. On ultrasound, the nail bed is thick and diffusely hypoechoic, which commonly includes the matrix region. The fragmentation of the nail plate usually starts in the ventral plate, and, in later stages, there are fragmentation, irregularities, and thickening of both plates.[1,8,12,18]

Retronychia means a posterior embedding of the nail plate that can be alone or concomitant with onychomadesis. On ultrasound, there are 3 diagnostic ultrasound criteria for unilateral retronychia: the decrease of the distance between the origin of the plate and the base of the distal phalanx in comparison with the normal contralateral side, a hypoechoic halo surrounding the origin of the nail plate,

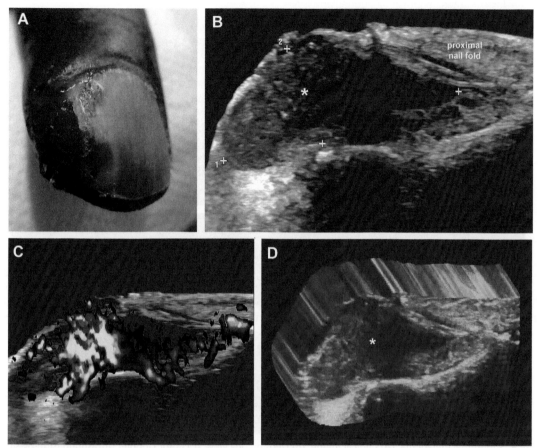

Fig. 8. Squamous cell carcinoma. (*A*) Clinical image. Ultrasound images ([*B*] gray scale; [*C*] power Doppler; and [*D*] 3-dimensional reconstruction of gray scale) show an ill-defined hypoechoic subungual mass (between markers [*asterisk*]) that extends into the radial periungual region with prominent and chaotic vascularity. There are erosions of the nail plate and bony margin.

and the thickening of the proximal nail fold in the affected side.[1,8,12,18,34] For diagnosing retronychia, at least 2 of these criteria are needed; however, the halo sign should be constant (**Fig. 11**).[1,8,12,18,34] There also are ultrasonographic criteria for diagnosing bilateral retronychia.[34]

Inflammatory Conditions of the Nail

Psoriasis

The use of ultrasound and MRI has increased in psoriasis, and there are ultrasonographic patterns of involvement of the nail bed and nail plate as well as a scoring system for evaluating psoriatic arthropathy on MRI called the PsA MRI Score.[10,35–51]

On ultrasound, psoriatic onychopathy shows thickening of the nail bed, loss of definition of the ventral plate; hyperechoic deposits in the distal part of the ventral plate; and the presence of thick, irregular, and wavy nail plates.[1,8] On color Doppler, there is a variable degree of vascularity, according to the activity of the disease.[1,8] Importantly,

ultrasound can detect the presence of synovitis, enthesitis, and erosions, which allows diagnosing early psoriatic arthropathy (**Fig. 12**).[41,49,50]

The ultrasound examination in psoriasis ideally should include all nails, bilaterally[1]; therefore, more severe cases can be detected earlier.[52] Ultrasound also can monitor biologic drugs in psoriatic onychopathy.[53]

On MRI, the reports have been more focused on the detection of psoriatic arthropathy. Thus, on MRI, thickening and irregularities of the nail plate and hyperintensity of the synovial joints and bone marrow may support the diagnosis.[21]

Fluid collections

On ultrasound, it is possible to detect anechoic or hypoechoic laminar subungual collections, such as subungual hematomas or abscesses and hidden fractures of the distal phalanx.[1,8,54] On color Doppler, the vascularity of the nail bed and periungual tissues can be variable, according to the inflammation (**Fig. 13**).[1,8,54]

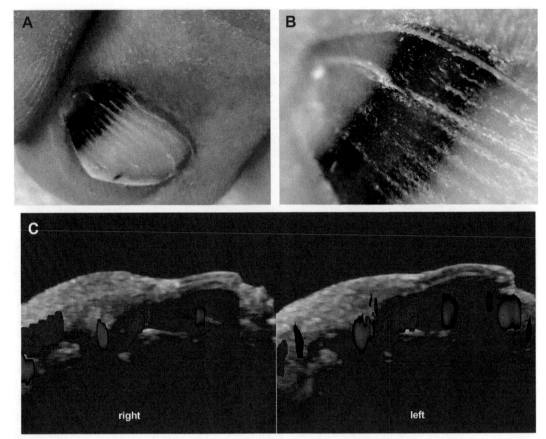

Fig. 9. Subungual melanoma. (*A*) Clinical image. (*B*) Dermoscopy view. (*C*) Color Doppler ultrasound (side-by-side views; right, normal side and left, abnormal side) demonstrate hypervascularity of the nail bed in the left third toe in comparison with the right side.

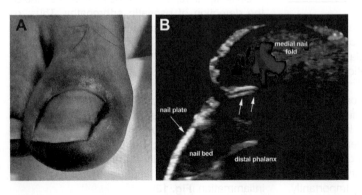

Fig. 10. Onychocriptosis. (*A*) Clinical image. (*B*) Color Doppler ultrasound (transverse view) shows a fragment of the nail plate (*arrows*) embedded in the medial periungual region. Notice the thickening, hypoechogenicity, and hypervascularity of the dermis and subcutis in the periungual area.

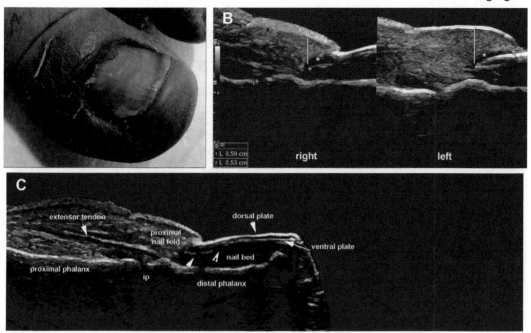

Fig. 11. Retronychia. (*A*) Clinical photograph. Ultrasound images ([*B*] Side-by-side comparative views, right side without retronychia and left side with retronychia and [*C*] gray scale panoramic view with color filter) demonstrate posterior embedding of the nail plate with decreased distance between the origin of the nail plate and the base of the distal phalanx (5.9 mm on the right and 5.3 mm on the left) and thickening of the dermis of the proximal nail fold (*vertical white lines*) in the left big toe and a hypoechoic halo (*asterisk*) in both big toes. There also is a fragmentation of the ventral plate of the left big toe due to concomitant onychomadesis (*arrowheads* [*C*]). ip, interphalangeal joint.

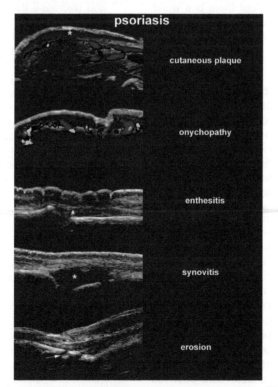

Fig. 12. Ultrasound imaging in psoriasis. Ultrasound shows the involvement of the skin, nail, tendinous insertion, joint, and bone. Color Doppler ultrasound presents an active cutaneous plaque and onychopathy (hypervascularity in the dermis, subcutis, and subungual regions). Gray scale ultrasound demonstrates decreased echogenicity and mild thickening of the insertion of the central band of the extensor tendon of the finger (*asterisk*), synovial distension with fluid in the joint, and a focal erosion of the cortex (*arrow*).

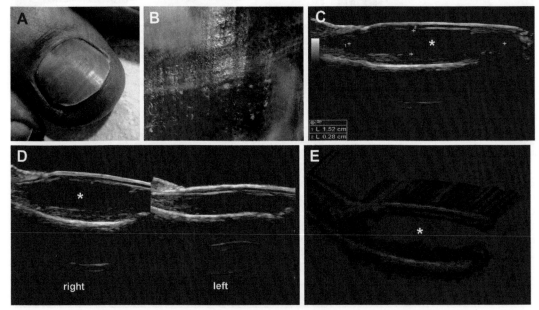

Fig. 13. Subungual hematoma. (*A*) Clinical photograph. (*B*) Dermoscopy view. Ultrasound images (gray scale, longitudinal views: [*C*] right big toe; [*D*] side-by-side comparative views, right side with the hematoma and left, normal side; and [*E*] 3-dimensional reconstruction with color filter) show anechoic subungual fluid collection (*asterisk*).

In summary, imaging can be a powerful tool to support the early diagnosis, extent, and monitoring of common conditions of the nail. This review discusses frequent pathologies, but there is a wider range of nail conditions that may be evaluated and benefited from imaging examinations.[1,2,8,10,18]

SUMMARY

In summary, imaging can be a powerful tool to support the early diagnosis, extent, and monitoring of common conditions of the nail. The choice of technique depends on the availability of the proper devices and trained operators. Nevertheless, currently, ultrasound is the first-choice imaging technique due to better axial resolution and capability to explore noninvasively and safely a more extensive range of ungual pathologies.

CLINICS CARE POINTS

Pearls
- The main applications of imaging of the nail include tumors (benign and malignant), pseudotumors (granulomas, cysts), inflammatory conditions (psoriasis, fluid collections), growth and location alterations (onychocryptosis, onychomadesis, and retronychia).
- Imaging can support critical data such as origin (ungual or periungual), size in all axes, location, degree of vascularity, and adjacent

tissues' involvement (bone, tendons, or joint). This can help manage better the pathologies, select the best site and the incision's extent, and decrease the potential cosmetic sequel of a nail biopsy.
- The selection of the imaging modality should consider the availability of a device and a trained operator. However, currently, ultrasound presents a better axial resolution in comparison with MRI and CT.

Pitfalls
- Among the limitations of ultrasound is the detection of pigments such as melanin.
- MRI and CT can present issues for discriminating lesions that measure less than 3-5 mm.

DISCLOSURE

None.

REFERENCES

1. Wortsman X. Ultrasound of nail conditions. In: Wortsman X, editor. Atlas of dermatologic ultrasound. New York: First; 2018. p. 215–77. https://doi.org/10.1007/978-3-319-89614-4-8.
2. Baek HJ, Lee SJ, Cho KH, et al. Subungual tumors: Clinicopathologic correlation with US and MR imaging findings. Radiographics 2010;30(6):1621–36.
3. Wortsman X, Wortsman J. Clinical usefulness of variable-frequency ultrasound in localized lesions of the skin. J Am Acad Dermatol 2010;62(2):247–56.

4. Wortsman X, Carreño L, Ferreira-Wortsman C, et al. Ultrasound Characteristics of the Hair Follicles and Tracts, Sebaceous Glands, Montgomery Glands, Apocrine Glands, and Arrector Pili Muscles. J Ultrasound Med 2019;38(8):1995–2004.

5. Edlow BL, Mareyam A, Horn A, et al. 7 Tesla MRI of the ex vivo human brain at 100 micron resolution. Sci Data 2019;6(1):244.

6. Al-Qattan MM, Al-Namla A, Al-Thunayan A, et al. Magnetic resonance imaging in the diagnosis of glomus tumours of the hand. J Hand Surg Am 2005;30(5):535–40.

7. Mathur M, Jones JR, Weinreb JC. Gadolinium deposition and nephrogenic systemic fibrosis: A radiologist's primer. Radiographics 2020;40(1): 153–62.

8. Wortsman X. In: Wortsman X, Jemec GB, editors. Sonography of the nail. New York, NY: Springer NY; 2013.

9. Drapé JL. Imaging of tumors of the nail unit. Clin Podiatr Med Surg 2004;21(4):493–511.

10. Aluja Jaramillo F, Quiasúa Mejía DC, Martínez Ordúz HM, et al. Nail unit ultrasound: a complete guide of the nail diseases. J Ultrasound 2017; 20(3):181–92.

11. Trehan SK, Athanasian EA, Dicarlo EF, et al. Characteristics of glomus tumors in the hand not diagnosed on magnetic resonance imaging. J Hand Surg Am 2015;40(3):542–5.

12. Wortsman X, Wortsman J, Guerrero R, et al. Anatomical changes in retronychia and onychomadesis detected using ultrasound. Dermatol Surg 2010; 36(10):1615–20.

13. Wortsman X. Common applications of dermatologic sonography. J Ultrasound Med 2012;31(1):97–111.

14. Wortsman X, Alfageme F, Roustan G, et al. Guidelines for performing dermatologic ultrasound examinations by the dermus group. J Ultrasound Med 2016;35(3):577–80.

15. Wortsman X, Alfageme F, Roustan G, et al. Proposal for an assessment training program in dermatologic ultrasound by the DERMUS Group. J Ultrasound Med 2016;35(11):2305–9.

16. Wu Z, Mittal S, Kish K, et al. Identification of calcification with magnetic resonance imaging. J Magn Reson Imaging 2010;29(1):177–82.

17. Ozkok S, Ozkok A. Contrast-induced acute kidney injury: A review of practical points. World J Nephrol 2017;6(3):86.

18. Wortsman X, Jemec GB, Villani A. Ultrasound and other imaging methods. In: Baran R, de Berker D, Holzberg M, et al, editors. Diseases of the nails and their management. 5th edition. Wiley Blackwell; 2018. p. 140–71. https://doi.org/10.1002/9781119323396.ch5.

19. Wortsman X, Jemec GBE. Ultrasound Imaging of Nails. Dermatol Clin 2006;24(3):323–8.

20. Drape J. Magnetic Resonance Imaging. In: Baran R, de Berker D, Holzberg M, et al, editors. Diseases of the nails and their management. 5th edition. Wiley Blackwell; 2018. p. 175–99. https://doi.org/10.1002/9781119323396.ch6.

21. Mundada P, Becker M, Lenoir V, et al. High resolution MRI of nail tumors and tumor-like conditions. Eur J Radiol 2019;112:93–105.

22. Wortsman X, Jemec GBE. Role of high-variable frequency ultrasound in preoperative diagnosis of glomus tumors a pilot study. Am J Clin Dermatol 2009;10:23–7.

23. Wortsman X, Wortsman J, Soto R, et al. Benign tumors and pseudotumors of the Nail: A novel application of sonography. J Ultrasound Med 2010;29(5):803–16.

24. Chiang YP, Hsu CY, Lien WC, et al. Ultrasonographic appearance of subungual glomus tumors. J Clin Ultrasound 2014;42(6):336–40.

25. Kromann CB, Wortsman X, Jemec GBE. High-frequency ultrasound of the nail. In: Humbert P, Fanian F, Maibach HI, et al, editors. Agache's measuring the skin: non-invasive investigations, physiology, normal constants. 2nd edition. Cham, Switzerland: Springer International Publishing; 2017. p. 891–6. https://doi.org/10.1007/978-3-319-32383-1_123.

26. Rodriguez-Takeuchi SY, Villota V, Renjifo M. Anatomy and pathology of the nail and subungual space: Imaging evaluation of benign lesions. Clin Imaging 2018;52:356–64.

27. Catalano O, Roldan FA, Solivetti FM, et al. Color doppler sonography of extradigital glomus tumors. J Ultrasound Med 2017;36(1):231–8.

28. Soto R, Wortsman X, Corredoira Y. Onychomatricoma: clinical and sonographic findings. Arch Dermatol 2009. https://doi.org/10.1001/archdermatol.2009.312.

29. Cinotti E, Veronesi G, Labeille B, et al. Imaging technique for the diagnosis of onychomatricoma. J Eur Acad Dermatol Venereol 2018;32(11):1874–8.

30. Silva-Feistner M, Ortiz E, Alvarez-Véliz S, et al. Amelanotic subungual melanoma mimicking telangiectatic granuloma: clinical, histologic, and radiologic correlations. Actas Dermosifiliogr 2017;108(8):785–7.

31. Quintana-Codina M, Creus-Vila L, Iglesias-Plaza A, et al. Sonographic appearance of subungual squamous cell carcinoma in the hand. J Clin Ultrasound 2018;46(3):212–4.

32. Ladd ME, Bachert P, Meyerspeer M, et al. Pros and cons of ultra-high-field MRI/MRS for human application. Prog Nucl Magn Reson Spectrosc 2018;109: 1–50.

33. Nijhuis AAG, Dieng M, Khanna N, et al. False-positive results and incidental findings with annual CT or PET/CT surveillance in asymptomatic patients

with resected stage III melanoma. Ann Surg Oncol 2019. https://doi.org/10.1245/s10434-019-07311-0.

34. Fernández J, Reyes-Baraona F, Wortsman X. Ultrasonographic criteria for diagnosing unilateral and bilateral retronychia. J Ultrasound Med 2018;37(5):1201–9.

35. Bakewell C, Aydin SZ, Ranganath VK, et al. Imaging techniques: options for the diagnosis and monitoring of treatment of enthesitis in psoriatic arthritis. J Rheumatol 2019. https://doi.org/10.3899/jrheum.190512. jrheum.190512.

36. Idolazzi L, Zabotti A, Fassio A, et al. The ultrasonographic study of the nail reveals differences in patients affected by inflammatory and degenerative conditions. Clin Rheumatol 2019;38(3):913–20.

37. Mendonça JA, Aydin SZ, D'Agostino MA. The use of ultrasonography in the diagnosis of nail disease among patients with psoriasis and psoriatic arthritis: a systematic review. Adv Rheumatol 2019;59(1):41.

38. Mondal S, Dutta S, Lahiri D, et al. Assessment of nail unit structures by ultrasound in patients with psoriatic arthritis and their correlations with disease activity indices: a case–control study. Rheumatol Int 2018;38(11):2087–93.

39. Moreno M, Lisbona MP, Gallardo F, et al. Ultrasound assessment of psoriatic onychopathy: A cross-sectional study comparing psoriatic onychopathy with onychomycosis. Acta Derm Venereol 2019;99(2):164–9.

40. Moya Alvarado P, Roé Crespo E, Muñoz-Garza FZ, et al. Subclinical enthesopathy of extensor digitorum tendon is highly prevalent and associated with clinical and ultrasound alterations of the adjacent fingernails in patients with psoriatic disease. J Eur Acad Dermatol Venereol 2018;32(10):1728–36.

41. Naredo E, Janta I, Baniandrés-Rodríguez O, et al. To what extend is nail ultrasound discriminative between psoriasis, psoriatic arthritis and healthy subjects? Rheumatol Int 2019;39(4):697–705.

42. Wortsman X, Gutierrez M, Saavedra T, et al. The role of ultrasound in rheumatic skin and nail lesions: A multi-specialist approach. Clin Rheumatol 2011;30(6):739–48.

43. Zabotti A, Errichetti E, Zuliani F, et al. Early psoriatic arthritis versus early seronegative rheumatoid arthritis: Role of dermoscopy combined with ultrasonography for differential diagnosis. J Rheumatol 2018;45(5):648–54.

44. Chaowattanapanit S, Pattanaprichakul P, Leeyaphan C, et al. Coexistence of Fungal Infections in Psoriatic Nails and their Correlation with Severity of Nail Psoriasis. Indian Dermatol Online J 2018;9(5):314–7.

45. Chaudhari AJ, Ferrero A, Godinez F, et al. High-resolution 18F-FDG PET/CT for assessing disease activity in rheumatoid and psoriatic arthritis: Findings of a prospective pilot study. Br J Radiol 2016;89(1063).

46. Choi JW, Kim BR, Seo E, et al. Identification of nail features associated with psoriasis severity. J Dermatol 2017;44(2):147–53.

47. Coates LC, Hodgson R, Conaghan PG, et al. MRI and ultrasonography for diagnosis and monitoring of psoriatic arthritis. Best Pract Res Clin Rheumatol 2012;26(6):805–22.

48. Fassio A, Giovannini I, Idolazzi L, et al. Nail ultrasonography for psoriatic arthritis and psoriasis patients: a systematic literature review. Clin Rheumatol 2019. https://doi.org/10.1007/s10067-019-04748-2.

49. Gutierrez M, Wortsman X, Filippucci E, et al. High-frequency sonography in the evaluation of psoriasis nail and skin involvement. J Ultrasound Med 2009;28(11):1569–74.

50. Gutierrez-Manjarrez J, Gutierrez M, Bertolazzi C, et al. Ultrasound as a useful tool to integrate the clinical assessment of nail involvement in psoriatic arthritis. Reumatologia 2018;56(1):42–4.

51. Idolazzi L, Gisondi P, Fassio A, et al. Ultrasonography of the nail unit reveals quantitative and qualitative alterations in patients with psoriasis and psoriatic arthritis. Med Ultrason 2018;20(2):177–84.

52. Rigopoulos D, Baran R, Chiheb S, et al. Recommendations for the definition, evaluation, and treatment of nail psoriasis in adult patients with no or mild skin psoriasis: A dermatologist and nail expert group consensus. J Am Acad Dermatol 2019;81(1):228–40.

53. Yamaoka T, Hayashi M, Tani M, et al. Value of ultrasonography findings for nail psoriasis before and after adalimumab administration. Clin Exp Dermatol 2017;42(2):201–3.

54. Gungor F, Akyol KC, Eken C, et al. The value of point-of-care ultrasound for detecting nail bed injury in. Am J Emerg Med 2016;34(9):1850–4.

Nail Cosmetics and Adornment

Zoe Diana Draelos, MD

KEYWORDS

• Nail polish • Artificial nails • Nail shellac • Nail sculptures • Nail prostheses

KEY POINTS

- Nail adornment is a popular manner of personal expression that has endured since the Egyptians first henna stained their nails in 5000 BC.
- Nail polish is based on a nitrocellulose film created by reacting cellulose fiber, from cotton linters or wood pulp, with nitric acid, followed by dissolving in organic solvents, to form a hard, glossy film. This film is modified by a toluene-sulfonamide-formaldehyde resin.
- Toluene-sulfonamide-formaldehyde resin is a possible source of allergic contact dermatitis.
- Harder chip-resistant nail shellacs are replacing nail polish, utilizing materials used in dental bonding based on polymethyl methacrylate, also known as PMMA or plexiglass.
- Nail polymers can be used to achieve nail elongation by mixing the monomer liquid ethyl or isobutyl methacrylate with the powdered polymethyl methacrylate in the presence of benzoyl peroxide.

INTRODUCTION

Nail cosmetics are a popular manner of personal expression. They allow people to nonverbally communicate how they wish to be seen by others and how they see themselves. Long nails, short nails, blue nails, black nails, multicolored nails, sparkly nails, and artificial nails are all available in most strip malls in the United States for purchase. Young girls and mature women wear nail adornment. Both the fingernails and toenails can be adorned with artwork, jewels, stencils, or simply 1 plain color.

This article examines the current state of nail cosmetics beginning with a historic perspective and then examining some of the newer polymer technology that has made elaborate nail adornment possible.

HISTORIC PERSPECTIVE

Nail adornment began with the Egyptians in 5000 BC with the use of orange henna as a vegetable-derived semipermanent stain for the nails. The color of the nails was used to indicate social status, with paler colors reserved for lower classes and red only worn by high society. Queen Nefertiti stained her fingernails and toenails a vivid red color, while Cleopatra preferred deep rust red. Henna is derived from the *Lawsonia mermis* plant, a member of the privet family. The dried leaves are collected and mashed into a paste that is applied to the nail. The lawsone migrates from the henna paste and binds to the stratum corneum.

The first true nail polish was developed by the Chinese in 3000 BC, containing gum Arabic, egg white, gelatin, vegetable dyes, and beeswax. Each dynasty had a characteristic nail polish color. The Chou Dynasty (600 BC) royalty wore silver and gold nails, while the Ming Dynasty (1300 AD) wore red and black nails.

Nail adornment in the United States prior to 1920 used an abrasive powder to shine the nails followed by a colored stain. The first true nail polish was introduced in 1930 by Charles Revson, who had the idea that car paint technology could be applied to nails. He first marketed a clear nail polish and then added a variety of pigments to found Revlon in 1932. The modern era of nail adornment in the United States had been invented.

NAIL POLISH

Nail polish was based on creating a nitrocellulose film by reacting cellulose fiber, from cotton linters

Dermatology Consulting Services, PLLC, 2444 North Main Street, High Point, NC 27262, USA
E-mail address: zdraelos@northstate.net

Dermatol Clin 39 (2021) 351–359
https://doi.org/10.1016/j.det.2021.01.001
0733-8635/21/© 2021 Elsevier Inc. All rights reserved.

or wood pulp, with nitric acid, followed by dissolving in organic solvents. Following evaporation of the solvents, a hard, glossy film of nitrocellulose was produced, known as a lacquer. This technology was used in the automobile industry to paint cars, but was adapted to nail adornment.[1]

The basic constituents of nail polish are described.[2]

Primary Film-Former

This includes nitrocellulose, methacrylate polymers, and vinyl polymers. Nitrocellulose is the major film former in nail polish. However, it is highly explosive during the manufacturing process; thus there are few nail polish plants in the United States.

Secondary Film-Forming Resin

The secondary resins, including formaldehyde, p-toluene sulfonamide, polyamide, acrylate, alkyd, and vinyl resins, add resistance to nail polish chipping.

Plasticizers

Plasticizers, including dibutyl phthalate, dioctyl phthalate, tricresyl phosphate, and camphor, are used in nail polish to keep the product soft and pliable. Dibutyl phthalate is a controversial chemical outlawed in states such as California in September 2006, for its ability to act as an endocrine modulator. This only occurs when the chemical is ingested, which is a reason not to consume chipped nail polish.

Solvents and Diluents

These include acetates, ketones, toluene, xylene, and alcohols. Nail polish ingredients are dissolved in a solvent that dries rapidly, leaving the colored film on the nail surface. Diluents, such as toluene and isopropyl alcohol, lower the viscosity of the nail polish while also lowering cost.

Colorants

These include organic D&C pigments and inorganic pigments, chromium oxide greens, ferric ferrocyanide, titanium dioxide, iron dioxide, carmine, ultramarine, and manganese violet. Organic and inorganic colors can be used to pigment nail polish. Organic pigments can be selected from a US Food and Drug Administration-approved list of certified colors. Inorganic colors and pigments may also be used, but must conform to low heavy metal content standards.[3]

Specialty Fillers

These include guanine fish scale, titanium dioxide-coated mica flakes, bismuth oxychloride, and metal particles.

There are many different types of polish sold to create various nail appearances. For example, light reflective ingredients, such as guanine fish scale, titanium dioxide-coated mica, or bismuth oxychloride, may be added to achieve a pearl-like nail appearance. Metal particles, such as aluminum, silver, and gold, are used to create a metallic shine.

The most commonly used resin to modify the nitrocellulose lacquer is toluene-sulfonamide-formaldehyde, which is a cause of allergic contact dermatitis. The resin is found on the standard dermatology patch test tray. The North American Contact Dermatitis Group noted 4% of positive patch tests are due to toluenesulfonamide/formaldehyde resin.[4] Even though the allergic reaction is most commonly caused by wet nail enamel, Tosti and colleagues noted 11 out of 59 patients reacted to both the wet and dry nail polish.[5] Nail polish can be tested as is, but should be allowed to thoroughly dry as the solvent can cause irritant contact dermatitis if not allowed to evaporate. The toluenesulfonamide/formaldehyde resin can be also tested alone in 10% petrolatum.[6] Hypoallergenic nail polish has been developed for toluene-sulfonamide-formaldehyde allergic individuals. A polyester resin or cellulose acetate butyrate may be used to avoid allergic contact dermatitis; however, sensitivity is still possible. Hypoallergenic nail polish has not captured the consumer market because of reduced wear and increased polish peeling.[7]

NAIL POLISH VARIANTS

There is tremendous variety in the types of nail polish currently available for sale. Clearly imagination rules when it comes to nail appearance. The various currently fashionable nail polishes are discussed next.

Nail Polish Finishes

The finish of a nail polish determines the visual optical characteristics of the film. **Box 1** presents these different finishes for consideration. Each finish is created by adding specialty ingredients to create the surface appearance, and many of the additives are proprietary to certain nail polish brands.

Photochromic Nail Polish

Photochromic nail polish uses the same chemistry as the sunglasses that automatically darken when placed in sunlight. The nail polish contains a UV-sensitive compound that changes conformation

---

Box 1
Nail polish finishes

- Shimmer
- Microshimmer
- Microglitter
- Frost
- Luster
- Crème
- Translucent
- Prismatic microglitter or microshimmer
- Iridescent
- Opalescent
- Matte
- Duo-chrome
- Jelly

---

from the leuco form to the colored form when outdoors. The nail polish is a milky white and becomes pink when exposed to sunlight as a result of the photochromic property.

Thermochromic Nail Polish

Thermochromic nail polish undergoes a chemical change like photochromic nail polish; however, the change is induced by temperature. The nail polish is a lighter color when the fingers are cold and a darker color when the fingers are warm. These types of nail polish are said to express mood.

Caviar Nail Polish

Caviar nail polish is a special effect that is produced on the nail surface. Nail caviar is made of small spherical beads that are pushed into the wet nail polish and then become part of the surface texture. The beads are said to look like caviar, hence the name. The small beads are physically removed from the nail film over time and must be replaced. The effect is temporary until the nail polish is removed.

Magnetic Nail Polish

Magnetic nail polish contains magnetic particles that orient themselves along magnetic lines when the wet nail polish is exposed to a surface magnet. Nickel, cobalt, iron, gadolinium, terbium, erbium, and/or iron oxide can be used as the magnetic particle in the polish. The particles are oblong and asymmetric, creating interesting lines and

patterns on the nail surface. This type of nail polish might be a problem for nickel-allergic patients.

Crackle Nail Polish

A crackle appearance to the nails was actually discovered by accident and the commercialized. The crackle effect is achieved by applying a regular nail polish first, followed by the crackle polish and then a clear coat to keep the crackle texture from peeling. The crackle polish is overt diluted nail polish created by pouring ethyl alcohol into a bottle of regular nail polish. The ethyl alcohol creates uneven drying of the polish and the crackle effect. More ethyl alcohol leads to thinner cracks, while less ethyl alcohol produces thicker cracks.

Breathable Nail Polish

Breathable nail polish was created to meet the needs of Muslim women to cannot wear nail polish because of wudu-washing required in preparation for prayer. Wudu-washing mandates that all body surfaces, including the nails, must be washed. Conventional nail polish is not water permeable, but breathable nail polish meets wudu requirements. The nail film that is both water and oxygen permeable uses resin technology adapted from the extended wear contact lens industry to achieve this effect.

Nail Stickers and Strips

After the application of nail polish, further adornment can be achieved through the embellishment of the nail with stickers and color strips. Traditional nail polish is applied first, followed by the stickers that are pressed onto the dry nail polish. Color strips can also be cut and laid across the nail. A clear top coat of nail polish, discussed next, is then placed to seal the embellishment in place. The nail stickers and strips may contain a metracylate-based glue, problematic in methacrylate-allergic individuals.

NAIL POLISH APPLICATION TECHNIQUE

Three layers of nail polish are required to achieve a chip-free long-wearing nail effect. The 3 coats are a base coat, pigmented nail enamel, and top coat. The base coat is much like the primer used when painting a wall. The base coat ensures good adhesion to the nail plate and prevents polish chipping, but also can fill in ridges in the nails that appear with advancing age. It contains no pigment, less primary film-former, and more secondary film-former resin; it is of a lower viscosity, as a thinner film is desirable. The second layer is the actual pigmented nail enamel. The top coat, or third layer, provides gloss and resistance to chipping while speeding drying of the films. It contains increased amounts of primary film former, more plasticizer, and fewer secondary film-forming resins. Some top coats may contain sunscreens but do not contain pigment.

NAIL POLISH REMOVAL

Nail polish removers strip nail polish from the nail plate, and may dehydrate and damage the nail in the process. They may contain solvents such as acetone, alcohol, ethyl acetate, or butyl acetate. Conditioning nail enamel removers are available containing fatty materials such as cetyl alcohol, cetyl palmitate, lanolin, castor oil, or other synthetic oils. It is thought that these oily substances act as occlusive nail moisturizers retarding water evaporation, but cannot overcome the dehydrating effect of the solvent.

Nail enamel remover is applied to a tissue or cotton ball and wiped across the nail plate to remove old or unwanted nail polish. Several applications and rubbing may be required to remove the polish, if several coats have been applied. Under some circumstances, the nail with polish may actually be soaking in a cup of nail polish remover, or the nail polish remover can be applied on a cotton ball that is left on the nail and covered by aluminum foil. Nail polish remover can irritate and dry the nail plate and paronychial tissues.[8] It also can contribute to nail dryness, resulting in brittleness. These problems can be minimized by using the product sparingly and infrequently.

NAIL SHELLAC

Nail polishes are being replaced with harder chip-resistant films known as nail shellacs or SNS nails or nail gels. The material used is similar to the materials used in dental bonding based on polymethyl methacrylate, also known as PMMA or plexiglass. Some of these materials require photocuring, while the newer more popular materials are not UVC cured. The polymerization process occurs on the nail plate when methacrylate monomer is exposed to benzoyl peroxide as the initiator. Homolytic bond cleavage occurs when the benzoyl peroxide forms 2 oxygen radicals that decompose to release carbon dioxide adding one methacrylate double bond. The process repeats until 2 carbon-centered radicals combine. Thus, plexiglass formation through polymerization occurs on the nail plate to create the robust film.

These films must be applied in a professional nail salon, but the application is rapid, requiring 20 to 30 minutes in the hands of an experienced nail technician. The steps required to complete the application are discussed and presented in a figure atlas. The old nail polish must first be removed down to the bare nail plate. A drill is used to loosen the old polymer, which should not be inhaled, or particulate pneumonitis can occur (**Fig. 1**). Once the old polymer has been loosened, it must be completely removed from the nail plate by soaking the nails in acetone-based nail polish remover. Increased exposure to the remover is achieved by placing a soaked cotton ball in aluminum foil over the fingertips (**Fig. 2**). It may take around 20 minutes to loosen the old polymer (**Fig. 3**). Once the polymer is loosened, the drill is used again to grind away the loosened film. This procedure must be done carefully or the nail natural plate can also be damaged, roughened, and removed (**Fig. 4**). The natural nail is intentionally roughened to increase the surface area for adhesion of the new polymer film that will be placed (**Fig. 5**).

Once the nail plate has been prepared, the new film can be created. The benzoyl peroxide catalyst is painted on the nail plate (**Fig. 6**), followed by dipping the nail into clear powdered methacrylate monomers (**Fig. 7**). This begins the polymerization process, and the clear first polymer layer is allowed to dry. Another layer of colored methacrylate, in this case red glitter, is polymerized on the nail plate to provide the nail color film (**Fig. 8**).

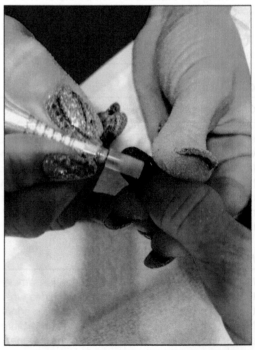

Fig. 1. Grinding removal of old polymer. (*Courtesy of* Z, Draelos, MD, High Point, North Carolina.)

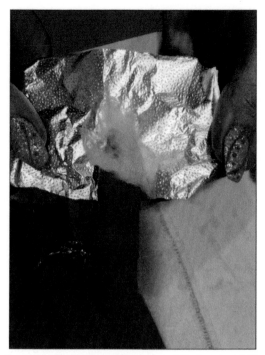

Fig. 2. Acetone soak. (*Courtesy of* Z, Draelos, MD, High Point, North Carolina.)

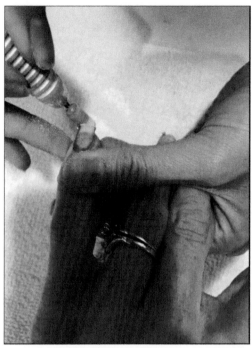

Fig. 4. Loosened material removal with grinding. (*Courtesy of* Z, Draelos, MD, High Point, North Carolina.)

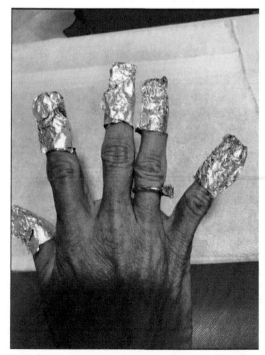

Fig. 3. Nail wrapped in foil with acetone soak. (*Courtesy of* Z, Draelos, MD, High Point, North Carolina.)

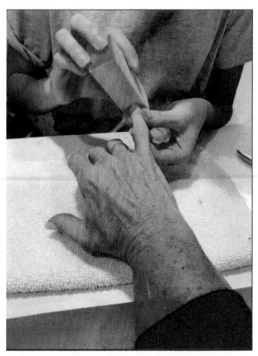

Fig. 5. Nail surface buffed and roughened. (*Courtesy of* Z, Draelos, MD, High Point, North Carolina.)

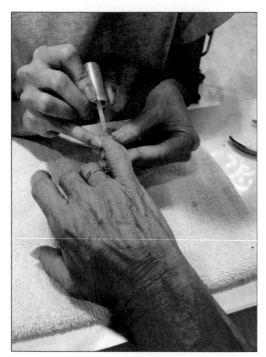

Fig. 6. Benzoyl peroxide catalyst. (*Courtesy of* Z, Draelos, MD, High Point, North Carolina.)

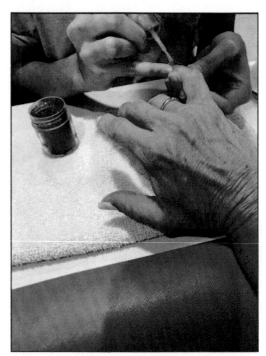

Fig. 8. Colored methacrylate monomer. (*Courtesy of* Z, Draelos, MD, High Point, North Carolina.)

Finally, the nail is dipped again into a clear methacrylate monomer to create the final shiny top coat (**Fig. 9**). The nail is then buffed with a polishing drill to smooth the polymer surface and remove any extra polymer to create the final nail appearance (**Fig. 10**). Variants of gel nails are dominating the professional nail market.

ARTIFICIAL NAILS
Preformed Artificial Nails

Long nails have been considered a sign of beauty and upward mobility throughout human history. Perhaps long nails are a sign that the individual does not perform manual labor, as long nails can prohibit use of the hands, but will also break with hand use. This human need for strong long nails has led to the development of preformed artificial nail prostheses that can be purchased at most drug stores and mass merchandizers in the United States. These nails are available in a variety of styles: precolored, uncolored, precut, and uncut. The nails also come in a variety of sizes and shapes to match the patient's natural nail plate.[9] In addition, several different types are available for purchase: press-on and unglued.

The press-on nails are the most popular, because no additional glue is applied. The nails are removed from the packaging already coated on the inner surface with a methacrylate-based adhesive and simply pressed on the natural nail

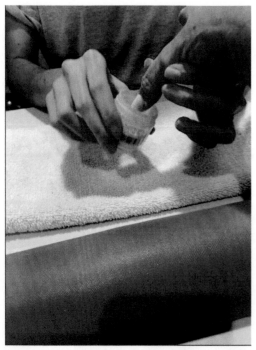

Fig. 7. Clear methacrylate monomer. (*Courtesy of* Z, Draelos, MD, High Point, North Carolina.)

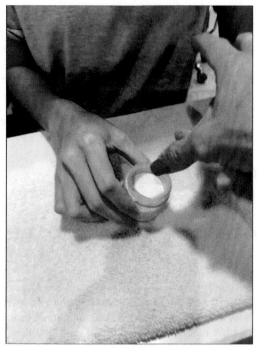

Fig. 9. Clear methacrylate monomer. (*Courtesy of Z, Draelos, MD, High Point, North Carolina.*)

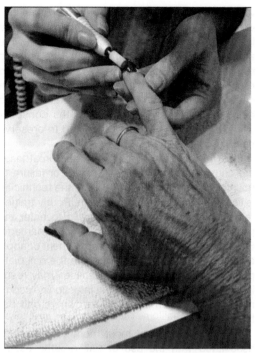

Fig. 10. Polishing polymer coated nail. (*Courtesy of Z, Draelos, MD, High Point, North Carolina.*)

plate firmly for the prosthesis to adhere. The artificial nail can be cut or trimmed to any length or shape desired. The prostheses are easily removed with trauma and designed to be worn short term, usually less than 1 week. Traumatic removal of artificial nails may result in nail peeling, known as onychoschizia, and nail plate pitting.[10] These nails may be problematic in methacrylate-allergic individuals.

Custom Artificial Nails

Preformed nails do not always match the nail contour of the individual and are designed to be temporary. This need has resulted in another professional nail procedure where custom-made nail elongation is achieved using a similar polymer technology discussed under nail shellacs. Sometimes this technique is known as nail sculptures, since a custom-designed nail elongation is sculpted to fit the fingertip of the client.

This technique uses liquid ethyl or isobutyl methacrylate as the monomer that is mixed with the powdered polymethyl methacrylate polymer. The product is allowed to polymerize in the presence of a benzoyl peroxide accelerator, and a formable acrylic is made that hardens in 7 to 9 minutes.[11] Usually, hydroquinone, monomethyl ether of hydroquinone, or pyrogallol is added to slow down polymerization.[12] A template form is placed inside the natural nail plate, and the new nail elongation

is built over the natural nail plate extending onto the form. The acrylic is mixed and applied with a paint brush to cover the entire natural nail plate and extended onto the template to the desired nail length. A clear acrylic is used over the natural nail plate attached to the nail bed so that the natural pink color shows through. A white acrylic is used from the nail plate's free edge distally. This creates a natural-appearing nail, or nail polish can be used to cover the entire nail sculpture.

The nail sculpture is a durable plexiglass plate that many wearers use as a tool, due to its hardness. The artificial nail can be used as a screwdriver or scrapper, but damage to the natural nail plate occurs. The bond between the nail sculpture and the natural nail is stronger than the bond between the natural nail plate and the nail bed. This means onycholysis is a common occurrence. With wearing, the nail sculpture will grow out with the natural nail plate, requiring new polymer to be placed at the proximal new nail growth. In addition, the edges of the nail sculpture will loosen and need to be trimmed and repaired. Nail sculptures require professional attention every 3 weeks. Failure to maintain the nail prosthesis will result in onycholysis or damage to the natural nail plate.

Nail Prostheses Dermatologic Problems

Nail prostheses are damaging to the natural nail plate, even in the conscientious patient. After 2 to 4 months of wear, the natural nail plate becomes yellowed, dry, and thin because of a lack of oxygen exchange across the nail plate and the repeated trauma from the drilling required to remove the nail prostheses and roughen the nail plate prior to prostheses application. For this reason, sculptured nails should not be worn for more than 3 months consecutively, allowing a 1 month rest period to preserve nail health.

Most problems that arise with nail prostheses are caused by poor technician skills or failure to maintain the nails properly. Be sure the technician is licensed, and the facility is clean. Poorly trained technicians may allow liquid acrylic to enter the proximal nail fold, resulting in nail matrix damage. Furthermore, failure to sterilize equipment or apply antifungal, antibacterial solutions to the nail plate prior to application of the prostheses may result in fungal, viral, and/or bacterial infections. A common infection seen in nail salon owners and patrons is flat warts.

Onycholysis is the most common problem associated with the use of nail prostheses, as the bond between the sculpture and the natural nail plate is stronger than the adhesion between the natural nail and nail bed. Additionally, sensitivity to the acrylic can cause onycholysis,[13,14] or even loss of the natural fingernails.[15] Interference with the nail vapor exchange and nail trauma during the prostheses application and removal process leave the natural nail plate thinned and yellowed.

Allergic contact dermatitis may occur as isobutyl, ethyl, and tetrahydrofurfuryl methacrylate are strong sensitizers[16,17]; however, the polymerized, cured acrylic is not sensitizing, only the liquid monomer.[18] If allergic contact dermatitis is suspected, patch testing can be conducted with 10% methacrylate monomer in olive oil.[19]

SUMMARY

Nail adornment is a popular human activity that has endured through the ages. Nail polish, originally adapted from automobile paint, has expanded to include tremendous variety in colors, finishes, special effects, and durability. The desire to have long fingernails has resulted in the adaptation of dental restoration techniques to nail prostheses. Fashion and imagination are the driving factors behind innovation in nail cosmetics.

CLINICS CARE POINTS

- Nail polish is a source of allergic contact dermatitis and should be considered when evaluating contact dermatitis of the face.
- Nail prostheses decrease oxygen transfer across the nail plate and may cause nail dystrophy.
- Onycholysis is a common side effect of nail prostheses.

DISCLOSURE

The author has nothing to disclose.

REFERENCES

1. Wimmer EP, Scholssman ML. The history of nail polish. Cosmet Toilet 1992;107:115–20.
2. Wing HJ. Nail preparations. In: deNavarre MG, editor. The chemistry and manufacture of cosemtics. Wheaton (IL): Allured Publishing Corporation; 1988. p. 983–1005.
3. Schlossman ML. Nail polish colorants. Cosmet Toil 1980;95:31.
4. Adams RM, Maibach HI. A five-year study of cosmetic reactions. J Am Acad Dermatol 1985;13:1062–9.
5. Tosti A, Buerra L, Vincenzi C, et al. Contact sensitization caused by toluene sulfonamide-formaldehyde resin in women who use nail cosmetics. Am J Contact Dermatitis 1993;4:150.
6. deGroot AC, Weyland JW, Nater JP. Unwanted effects of cosmetics and drugs used in dermatology. 3rd edition. New York: Elsevier; 1994.
7. Schlossman ML. Nail-enamel resins. Cosmet Technology 1979;1:53.
8. Wallis MS, Bowen WR, Guin JD. Pathogenesis of onychoschizia (lamellar dystrophy). J Am Acad Derm 1991;24:44–8.
9. Brauer EW. Selected prostheses primarily of cosmetic interest. Cutis 1970;6:521–4.
10. Lazar P. Reactions to nail hardeners. Arch Dermatol 1966;94:446–8.
11. Barnett JM, Scher RK, Taylor SC. Nail cosmetics. Dermatol Clin 1991;9:9–17.
12. Viola LJ. Fingernail elongators and accessory nail preparations. In: Cosmetics, science and technology. 2nd edition. New York: Wiley-Interscience; 1972. p. p. 543–552.
13. Goodwin P. Onycholysis due to acrylic nail applications. J Exp Dermatol 1976;1:191–2.
14. Lane CW, Kost LB. Sensitivity to artificial nails. Arch Dermatol 1956;74:671–2.
15. Fisher AA. Permanent loss of fingernails from sensitization and reaction to acrylic in a preparation designed to make artificial nails. J Dermatol Surg Oncol 1980;6:70–1.

16. Marks JG, Bishop ME, Willis WF. Allergic contact dermatitis to sculptured nails. Arch Dermatol 1979; 115:100.

17. Fisher AA. Cross reactions between methyl methacrylate monomer and acrylic monomers presently used in acrylic nail preparations. Contact Dermatitis 1980;6:345-347,

18. Fisher AA, Franks A, Glick H. Allergic sensitization of the skin and nails to acrylic plastic nails. J Allergy 1957;28:84.

19. Baran R, Dawber RPR. The nail and cosmetics. In: The nails in disease. 4th edition. Chicago: Yearbook Publishers; 1986. p. 129.

Moving?

Make sure your subscription moves with you!

To notify us of your new address, find your **Clinics Account Number** (located on your mailing label above your name), and contact customer service at:

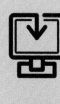

Email: journalscustomerservice-usa@elsevier.com

800-654-2452 (subscribers in the U.S. & Canada)
314-447-8871 (subscribers outside of the U.S. & Canada)

Fax number: 314-447-8029

Elsevier Health Sciences Division
Subscription Customer Service
3251 Riverport Lane
Maryland Heights, MO 63043

*To ensure uninterrupted delivery of your subscription, please notify us at least 4 weeks in advance of move.

ELSEVIER

Moving?

Make sure your subscription moves with you!

To notify us of your new address, find your Clinics Account Number (located on your mailing label above your name), and contact customer service at:

Email: journalscustomerservice-usa@elsevier.com

800-654-2452 (subscribers in the U.S. & Canada)
314-447-8871 (subscribers outside of the U.S. & Canada)

Fax number: 314-447-8029

Elsevier Health Sciences Division
Subscription Customer Service
3251 Riverport Lane
Maryland Heights, MO 63043

Printed and bound by CPI Group (UK) Ltd, Croydon, CR0 4YY

03/10/2024

01040372-0002